*The Corporation
In American Politics*

The Corporation
in American Politics

EDWIN M. EPSTEIN
University of California, Berkeley

PRENTICE-HALL, INC. *Englewood Cliffs, New Jersey*

P–13–173153–X
C–13–173161–0

Library of Congress Catalog Card No.: 74–75632

Current Printing (Last Digit):
10 9 8 7 6 5 4 3 2 1

Printed in the United States of America

PRENTICE-HALL INTERNATIONAL, INC., *London*
PRENTICE-HALL OF AUSTRALIA, PTY. LTD., *Sydney*
PRENTICE-HALL OF CANADA, LTD., *Toronto*
PRENTICE-HALL OF INDIA PRIVATE LTD., *New Delhi*
PRENTICE-HALL OF JAPAN, INC., *Tokyo*

To My Wife, Soni,
Who Has Helped in So Many Ways

Preface

This project originated in early 1966 when I was invited to be a member of a panel discussing "The Business Corporation and the Political Process" as part of the Executive Program sponsored by the Schools of Business Administration of the University of California, Berkeley. My specific task was to discuss the theoretical and practical implications of corporate involvement in the political process with a group consisting primarily of middle-management-level corporate and government executives. From the dialogue that followed my presentation, it was apparent that many of the members of the generally sophisticated audience were uninformed or misinformed concerning both the general nature of the political process and the particular role of business corporations in American politics. Similarly, college students frequently demonstrate unawareness and naïveté regarding corporate political involvement, since the subject is commonly given short shrift in courses on American Government, Interest Groups in American Politics, or The Political and Social Environment of Business. This lack of academic attention is primarily a consequence of the large number of issues customarily dealt with in such courses and of the paucity of materials that specifically treat the question of the corporation in politics. Hopefully, this volume will remedy, at least in part, the latter shortcoming. My research and thinking about the subject of business and politics has convinced me of the possible usefulness of a book dealing exclusively with the topic of corporate political activity that would provide a source of reference for scholars, students, and members of the general public who are interested in this subject.

This book also constitutes an effort to clarify and to re-evaluate my thinking about the involvement of corporations in the political process. The approach in this volume is analytical and descriptive rather than empirical. I have focused attention equally upon issues of political theory and public policy and upon the actual political behavior of business firms. Although I am fully aware of the importance and extensiveness of corporate political activities in the international sphere, I have emphasized the domestic scene, except in a few isolated instances. The subject of the corporation in foreign affairs is deserving of separate treatment by experts in international politics. Accordingly, this book is national rather than comparative in nature and deals with American business corporations in the context of the political process within the United States.

Because, in certain ways, this work is a seminal effort in its particular field, some of the hypotheses in which I have indulged have not been tested by myself or others; indeed, a number of them can not be tested, given our present state of knowledge. During the next several years, I hope to test a number of these hypotheses through empirical field research on some of the questions posed in the Appendix. Hopefully, thereby, our information regarding the political role of the corporation will be increased and our efforts to formulate a theory concerning corporations as political participants enhanced.

It is also necessary for me to point out that in a certain sense, this book is patently normative in character. On the basis of my analysis of corporate political activity, I have formulated a political theory of the firm that recognizes corporations as legitimate participants in the American political process. In light of this theory, I shall urge the necessity both of reevaluating our traditional concepts of corporate political activities and of removing—or, at very least, modifying—the present prohibitions against certain forms of corporate participation.

A personal note is necessary at this juncture. I have arrived at my present view of the legitimacy of corporate political activity only after long and, hopefully, careful analysis of the relevant issues. In truth, in some respects my conclusions are contrary to the views that I held when I began this project. In the past, corporations and their leaders have not infrequently utilized their political resources in support of policies and persons with whom I have felt little sympathy as a matter of personal political philosophy. I view it, however, as the obligation of the social scientist to formulate his conclusions on the basis of his analysis of the relevant information. He should arrive at his position as objectively as possible, full-well recognizing, but, as far as possible, disregarding his own biases. I have sought to adopt such a posture in writing this book.

It is my hope that *The Corporation in American Politics* accomplishes the several objectives set forth above. In any event, it constitutes an effort to search for the answers to the "important and ever urgent questions" to which Robert A. Dahl referred a few years ago when he urged political scientists to concern themselves with the interface of business and politics.*

As is usually the case with all such writing efforts, the author is in the debt of a number of individuals. I hereby express my appreciation to the directors and personnel of the Institute of Governmental Studies and the Institute of Business and Economic Research, both of the University of California, Berkeley, which supported this research financially and in terms of organizational assistance. I also acknowledge gratefully the contributions of John A. Edie,   Earl A. Molander,   Kenneth D.

*Robert A. Dahl, "Business and Politics: A Critical Appraisal of Political Science," in Robert A. Dahl, Mason Haire, and Paul F. Lazarsfeld, *Social Science Research on Business: Product and Potential* (New York: Columbia University Press, 1959), pp. 3, 44.

Walters, and especially Terry H. Coyne, who assisted in the researching of materials. To my professorial colleagues Richard M. Abrams, Michael P. Rogin, Dow Votaw, and Aaron Wildavsky, all of the University of California, Berkeley; L. Vaughn Blankenship, the State University of New York at Buffalo; Ivar Berg and Clarence C. Walton, both of Columbia University; R. Joseph Monsen, the University of Washington; and Joseph C. Palamountain, Jr., Skidmore College, my thanks for reviewing and criticizing various drafts of the manuscript. I have benefited from your comments. None of the above named persons is, however, responsible for the shortcomings of this book. Thoughtful and competent assistance was given in the typing of the final draft of this manuscript by Mrs. Florence Myer. The excellent editorial advice of Miss Ellen Seacat and the assistance of Miss Pamela Fischer, Mr. James F. Beggs, and Mr. Charles Briqueleur of Prentice-Hall are sincerely appreciated.

Lastly and most importantly, I thank my family—my wife, Soni, and our children, Mimi and Danny—for their forbearance and encouragement during the "long, hot summer" (extending nearly three years) of the writing of this book. It was they who suffered the attention not paid and the aggravations shared until this project was completed.

EDWIN M. EPSTEIN

Berkeley, California
February, 1969

Contents

The Corporation
In American Politics

Chapter One

Introduction

Neither American constitutional law nor political theory can account for the corporate presence in the political arena. Indeed, early in United States history, Chief Justice John Marshall stated emphatically:

This being [the corporation] does not share in the civil government of the country, unless that be the purpose for which it was created. Its immortality no more confers on it political power, or a political character, than immortality would confer such power or character on a natural person.[1]

So too, political philosophers generally have been hostile to according "political personality" to corporations or to other social groups.

However, political activity by business corporations is a basic fact of the American political scene and has been so from the beginning of the nineteenth century. There is little likelihood, moreover, that this involvement will diminish in the foreseeable future, since the increasingly "mixed" character of American society has thrust public and private institutions (particularly business firms) into a state of permanent interdependence. John Kenneth Galbraith may be premature in perceiving the emergence of the New Industrial State, marked by a symbiotic relationship between the "industrial system" and the state;[2] but the previously sacrosanct line between publicness and privateness has unquestionably been blurred in recent years and probably will become less and less distinct.

Despite the long history of successful political involvement of corporations, scholars have devoted relatively little attention to the subject of the business firm as a political participant. A few years ago, political scientist Robert A. Dahl remonstrated with his professional colleagues:

> For all the talk and all the public curiosity about the relations between business and politics, there is a remarkable dearth of studies on the subject. What *is* written is more likely to come from the pen of a sociologist, an historian, a lawyer, or an economist than from a political scientist.[3]

Published studies have dealt primarily with a limited number of topics—government regulation of economic activity, the influence of business leaders on specific legislation or on public issues, the politics of administrative regulation, the lobbying process, corporate managers as an elite group in the community power structure, corporate political ideology, and the corporation as a general repository of political (and social and economic) power. In the available literature, examinations of corporate political activities are usually subsumed in general discussions about trade or industry associations and their political endeavors. A few recent works have focused some attention on political participation by corporations, but such contributions are rare.

Existing studies do not emphasize corporate political behavior as an organizational activity. Few social scientists have examined business political endeavors from the perspective of the firm—that is, few have studied the entire range of an organization's political inputs in order to analyze the motivations, methods, and over-all significance of political involvement. Historically, scholarly interest in such involvement has been systemic, viewing corporate activities in the context of the over-all political process, in which business firms are considered as merely one type of participant in a diverse universe of interest groups. However, certain characteristics of the corporation distinguish it from other political actors and give rise to a number of questions that are peculiar to the corporate area. It is rather surprising, therefore, that students of the political process have not concentrated more frequently on business firms.

Four major factors have contributed to this lack of interest in and of attention to the corporations. (1) Scholars have been preoccupied with the behavior of other, more traditional, political participants, such as the electorate; public officials in various branches and on different levels of government; social, economic, military, and professional elites; ethnic and racial groups; and the multitude of formal and ad hoc interest groups. (2) Collection of information about corporate political activities is difficult because of both the great reluctance of most firms to disclose their actions and the diffused quality of corporate efforts, which take place on many fronts and on the part of many persons. (3) The distinction between organizational political activity and the activities of corporate executives who are acting as individual citizens cannot easily be assessed. (4) Scholars until fairly recently have failed to view business firms (as distinguished from their managers) as entities which possess noneconomic dimensions that give them specific organizational political interests and goals and necessitate political involvement as a *corporate* activity.

The above comments should be construed, not as an indictment of nonfeasance against the scholarly community (particularly political scientists), but rather as an underlining of the purposes of this book. In these pages, I have undertaken several tasks:

1. The examination, from the *internal* perspective of the large business organization, of the nature, techniques, and rationale underlying corporate political involvement.

2. The evaluation of the legitimacy of such involvement, in terms of both the over-all political process and the unique character of the corporation, and assessment of common arguments in favor of and in opposition to corporate political activity.

3. The development of a framework of analysis within which corporate political involvement can be evaluated and, as possible, the impact of this involvement on the political process can be examined.

4. The presentation, for those who are interested in both American politics and business organizations, of a compact but systematic overview of corporate political activities, which, hopefully, may stimulate interest in further study of the many problems in this area.

5. The establishment of a perspective on the theory and practice of corporate political action, which will reveal the significance of such action for both the American social order and the corporate system.

6. The development of recommendations for substantial change in both the philosophy and the content of legal regulation of corporate political activities.

7. The delineation of certain areas, now largely neglected, in which research relating to corporate political activity could contribute to better understanding of the implications of this involvement for the American political system.

We now turn our attention to these matters.

NOTES

[1]*Dartmouth College* v. *Woodward*, 4 Wheaton 518, 636 (1819).

[2]John Kenneth Galbraith, *The New Industrial State* (Boston: Houghton Mifflin Company, 1967), especially pp. 296–324, 379–412.

[3]Robert A. Dahl, "Business and Politics: A Critical Appraisal of Political Science," in Robert A. Dahl, Mason Haire, and Paul F. Lazarsfeld, *Social Science Research on Business: Product and Potential.* (New York: Columbia University Press, 1959), p. 3.

Chapter Two

Corporations and Politics: An Overview of the Issues

The "business-in-politics" movement, which persists after flourishing briefly during the 1950's and early 1960's, reactivated an ever-recurring issue in American politics: Should business corporations engage in political activities? While answers to this question have ranged from resounding Yes's to equally emphatic No's, the No's have prevailed for both managers and scholars. For purposes of analysis, the broad question of the propriety of corporate political involvement should be divided to highlight the two major issues involved: (1) whether it is necessary and desirable for business firms, as a matter of corporate policy, to engage in politics; and (2) whether, given the fact of corporate political involvement, this involvement is legitimate (that is, rightful). A number of subsidiary issues must be considered. Relevant subissues of the first question include the manner of corporate political participation, the costs and benefits corollary to such participation, the objectives of the company, the existence of policy alternatives for business firms, the probable consequences to the firm of nonparticipation, and the rationale underlying corporate activities. The second question (of legitimacy) demands consideration of the following points: the *internal* legitimacy of the corporation as a political participant, as determined by its organizational purpose, constituency, sources of managerial authority, and patterns of governance, and its *external* legitimacy, as evaluated in terms of theories of democracy, the implications of corporate political activity for other social interests, and the impact of this activity upon the maintenance of an "open" political order in the American polity.

These issues will be treated at length in subsequent chapters; however, a few general remarks are appropriate at this point.

THE INEVITABILITY OF CORPORATE
POLITICAL ACTIVITY

American business corporations have been, *are*, and, in the foreseeable future, will undoubtedly continue to be involved in the political process. This involvement results from the corporate presence in a pluralistic democracy in which diverse social interests seek to enhance their economic positions vis-à-vis each other. Moreover, the extent of corporate political activity will probably increase. A partial explanation for this likely development is that

> no other institution in society exercises more influence on the economy than government does. . . . Indeed, in the middle of the twentieth century, there is no democracy, large or small, in which the state does not undertake major responsibilities of an economic character. . . . It follows, when most citizens are keenly aware that their livelihood depends heavily on the state, that much of the controversy which creates the substance of politics consists either in justifying the programs of the government or in finding a reasoned case to oppose them.[1]

If two additions are made to this statement, the necessity of corporate political involvement becomes apparent. First, the dependence upon government experienced by individual citizens in earning their livelihoods is duplicated or, more likely, exceeded by the dependence of business organizations upon the state. For a significant number of companies, government contracts, subsidies, or franchises are the lifelines to survival; and for all business firms, legislative and administrative guidelines by local, state, and federal governments structure the environment within which they operate. Thus, even the most economically insignificant enterprise is vitally affected by governmental policy.

Second, "the controversy which creates the substance of politics" in this country includes more than merely the justifying and the opposing of governmental programs. It involves the determination of relationships of power and influence among diverse social interests (including business corporations) and the many organs of government. The achievement of interest-group goals is the prize at stake.

An ironic aspect of the expanding importance of governmental involvement in the operations of the economy is that, as an unintended consequence, it has resulted in the necessity of increased corporate political involvement. However, the growth in importance of the business corporation in terms of both size and social significance has made inevitable the growth of government, since

> wherever technology advances, wherever private business extends its range, wherever the cultural life becomes more complex, new tasks are imposed on government. This happens apart from, or in spite of, the particular philosophies that governments cherish. . . . In the longer run the tasks undertaken by government are dictated by changing conditions, and governments on the whole are more responsive than creative in fulfilling them.[2]

Corporations have been prime catalysts for the technological advances that have resulted in new forms of economic activity. These activities, together with the spread of industrialization and urbanization, have shaped the complex character of contemporary American life and have necessitated governmental expansion. Short of some totally unforeseeable change in the basic nature of our society, all these conditions will be with us in the future. Economic development and governmental growth appear to be inseparable companions.

CORPORATE POLITICS:
AN ECONOMIC ABERRATION?

The preceding thesis (the inevitability of corporate political involvement) comports with neither the historical role of business enterprise nor the classical model of capitalism formulated by economic theorists. Historically (and even today, except for highly industrialized nations), "business" activity has been primarily commercial and financial and has been carried on by individuals or small-scale enterprises. During the preindustrial stages of economic development, except in a few instances (notably the Italian city-states and the Hanseatic woolen centers), social status and political power have been associated, not with business activity, but rather with the control of the landed resources of the society. In this situation, the society has considered business activity of marginal importance; consequently, the businessman has led a precarious existence in terms of security and autonomy. A number of the preindustrial countries of the Middle East, Southeast Asia, Africa, and Latin America are still in this stage.[3]

In western Europe and the United States, the spread of industrial capitalism and the political ascendancy of business interests have burgeoned in the past one hundred fifty years, with the greatest development occurring during the past century. The dominance of manufacturing was established in Great Britain during the middle third of the nineteenth century, but not in the United States until after the Civil War. By 1900, however, virtually the entire Western world was committed to industrialism as an economic way of life. It is hardly coincidental that during this period industrial activity became increasingly concentrated in large-scale organizations, which evolved into institutions of critical social importance. Businessmen and business firms were transformed from bit players on the stage of politics to star performers.

Economic theory has offered little to explain political activity by economic organizations. In the classical model of the market economy, firms are concerned solely with producing and distributing the goods required by the society at the lowest possible level of cost so that the margin of profit of those supplying capital is maximized. Since the market operates independently of other social institutions and is controlled by the operation of "immutable" laws which determine the best allocation of scarce resources, noneconomic factors are irrelevant to the operations of each economic unit. Under the Smithian concept of an "invisible hand" that guides the economic destinies of society, there is no reason to attribute any importance to political influences. When Adam Smith was writing in the 1770's, enterprises were small and new markets were developing rapidly; therefore, this perspective was, to a degree, accurate. However, the state of perfect market competition existing without any external influences, which was assumed by Smith and his disciples, was hardly validated by the situation at the end of the nineteenth century.

Nevertheless, with few exceptions, philosophers of the "Dismal Science" theorized about an economy that functioned without intrusion of noneconomic variables. Indeed, except for Karl Marx, economists have given explicit recognition to the importance of governmental influence on the environment of economic activity only since the publication, in 1936, of John Maynard Keynes's *General Theory of Employment, Interest and Money*.[4] Marx, it will be recalled, considered government, together with all other social institutions, as the superstructure imposed by the class controlling the means of production in order to strengthen its position.[5] Although post-Keynesian economists have been aware of the vital economic role of government, they have not shown greatly increased appreciation of the importance of the political process in determining governmental policy. For example, econometricians seldom include political variables among the inputs for their models of the economy—undoubtedly because of the difficulty in measuring these variables. The reasons notwithstanding, the failure of the models to encompass political factors renders them suspect in terms of reliability. Unlike other social scientists, economists have not generally recognized that the economy is merely one among many social subsystems of a society that exists in intimate association with the other subsystems.[6] The economy is like a fragment in a mosaic and must be viewed in relation to the other fragments (consisting of a wide variety of human interactions) in order to obtain a comprehensive picture of a society.

The net effect of the two elements discussed in this section (the historical newness of industrial capitalism and the failure of economic theory to take account of political variables) has been to reinforce a narrow perspective of the political process—a perspective that does not explain the presence of a most important participant, the business corporation.

THE NATURE OF POLITICS AND THE POLITICAL PROCESS

Analysis of corporate political activity has not been adequately developed as yet, in part because of inherent ambiguities in the terms *politics, political process,* and *corporate involvement.* As a prelude to rigorous analysis, these concepts must also be clarified in order to provide the appropriate analytical framework. The nature of politics and of the political process will be considered in this section, while the question of what constitutes corporate involvement will be treated in the following section.

Particularly in the managerial literature, there has been an unfortunate tendency on the part of some commentators on the subject of business and politics to restrict their concepts of "political" to partisan electoral involvement. This narrow view, which is not supported in political theory, excludes from the realm of politics a number of activities that are of great significance to the governmental process.

Politics is the process that has been designated variously

as a relationship of "governance," "power," "influence and the influential," and "control" between and among individuals and groups in society.[7] More pragmatically, Harold D. Lasswell has defined politics as "the study of who gets what, when, and how."[8] As treated here, the political process focuses upon the operations of government and the relation of the state to the many constituencies present within it. The essential ingredient of politics is the attempt by social interests (individual and collective) to achieve access to and impact upon the diverse foci of governmental decision making. Politics, therefore, encompasses *all* activities engaged in by social interests with the intention or the consequence (or both) of guiding, affecting, or influencing governmental action. It is both a source of conflict and a mode of activity that seeks to resolve social conflicts and to promote readjustment.

This interpretation of the political process is narrow in the sense that it tends to focus attention "on *structures* that deal with politics on a full-time basis and that are explicitly labeled as pertaining to the political or governmental subsystem of the society [emphasis added]."[9] It is broad, however, in that it "focuses on political *functions* and treats politics as a process" or as "a variety of activities that may constitute only a part-time consideration for a given actor and that may even be far from the actor's main concern in operating in its own arena."[10] In terms of the primarily theoretical distinction between a broad and a narrow view of politics, the perspective presented in these pages is mixed—that is, the term *politics* includes not only the relationship of corporations to the specific structures of governmental decision making, but also the process or dynamics by which business firms seek to maximize their interests with regard to other social interests.

In the analysis of political involvement, *electoral* activities should be distinguished from *governmental* activities. The failure to recognize the existence of this dichotomy goes to the heart of the ambiguity of the terms *politics* and *political process*. *Electoral* politics includes activities related directly to the selection and support (financial and otherwise) of candidates or issues to be decided upon by the public. *Governmental* politics includes political involvement, normally associated with interest groups, directed toward the formulation, implementation, and enforcement of policy by legislative, executive, administrative, or judicial bodies. Also included in this category are activities intended to influence public opinion concerning such matters as the operations of government, the behavior of opposing social interests, and the needs and goals of the political participant.

Although electoral politics have a more dramatic quality because of the pomp and circumstance connected with the election process, social groups attempt on a day-by-day basis to achieve their ends through governmental politics. Accordingly, this examination of the relation of the corporation to politics and the political process deals with more than corporate efforts in the electoral arena. Rather, all interactions by business firms with the formal or informal institutions of government and all efforts by corporations to maximize their position in society are considered to be relevant.

CORPORATE POLITICAL INVOLVEMENT:
COLLECTIVE OR INDIVIDUAL?

The fundamental issue in the question of what constitutes "corporate" political activities is whether business political involvement should be viewed strictly in terms of the behavior of individual managers or whether it should be considered as an organizational activity intended to accomplish the political objectives of the firm. Implicit in the discussion presented in the preceding pages has been the assumption that corporations engage in the broad spectrum of political activities and that this involvement is corporate activity rather than merely the independent undertakings of individual managers. It is important, however, to test this assumption, since it goes to the heart of the analysis presented in the remainder of the book.

Corporations have political interests that are important to the well-being of the organization. While these interests may and usually do coincide with the interests of leading officers and directors of the company, this need not invariably be the case. Andrew Hacker's whimsical tale of the corporation, without shareholders and employees, whose ten directors (the only humans involved with the organization) freely acknowledged that "at least eight of the ten of us, as private citizens that is, did not favor the legislation we were supporting . . . in the company's interest"[11] is apocryphal; however, it requires little imagination to think of instances of potential conflict between the manager's individual interest and the objectives of the organization. For example, while tariff barriers aid a firm in a protected domestic industry, they may also have the effect of increasing prices of other items consumed by the corporate officer. Similarly, defeat of air- or water-pollution control measures lowers the operating costs of a company but increases the health hazards faced by the corporate manager. It is even conceivable that an executive of a major defense contractor may be personally opposed to government foreign policy, although his firm is a prime beneficiary of such a policy.

As a general rule, however, the political interests of the manager are in harmony with the objectives of his organization. Once again, examples readily come to mind. The executive is seeking to further corporate purposes when he attempts to influence the passage of legislation, the appointment of an administrator of a regulatory agency, or the awarding of a research and development contract. Indeed, in these instances the manager's individual interest is a direct consequence of the corporate interest. As a private citizen, he would probably be indifferent about which of two airlines should be awarded a passenger route; however, the matter is of crucial importance to him as an airlines executive, solely as a result of his company affiliation. It is critical, therefore, to any examination of corporate political involvement to distinguish wherever possible the activities of the organization from those of a manager acting in a personal capacity. This is not to say that every political act by an individual who happens to be by profession a corporate manager is the act of the corporation. However, it is often difficult, if not impossible, to determine if a corporate official is speaking or acting *ex cathedra* or if he has put aside the cloak of office and is behaving as a private citizen. This difficulty holds particularly for a high-ranking corporate manager who is closely identified with his firm and who, in the eyes of the public, may indeed be the personification of the company. For example, when a corporate officer makes a financial contribution to a political party, is this an individual or a corporate act? Similarly, when Henry Ford II makes pronouncements of political significance, are the words and positions those of a resident of Grosse Pointe Farms, Michigan, or of the chairman of the board of the Ford Motor Company? Similar questions could have been asked about Roger Blough of U.S. Steel and David Sarnoff of R.C.A., to cite but a couple of the most obvious examples. Even if, as John Kenneth Galbraith suggests in *The New Industrial State*, the time is fast approaching when the public will no longer know the names of our leading corporate executives,[12] the problem will not be completely resolved. The relevant public—consisting of government officials and political leaders—will still be aware of the identities of corporate executives. On a somewhat lower plane, the political views of the plant manager of an important corporate employer in a local community at least by implication carry the imprimatur of his company, even if the company has not taken an official stance on the specific issue.

When corporate political involvement is viewed at a more theoretical level, corporations *never* act. Only human beings can manifest behavior, whether it be political, economic, or social. A corporation is in reality an intellectual abstraction—an organization infused with a legal existence, status, or capacity of its own for the performance of socially recognized activities in a form and in a manner specified by the state.[13] If by some divine decree the legal status of "corporation" were abolished forthwith, it is quite clear that organizations which today are designated as business corporations would continue to exist and to perform their economic tasks in a way virtually indistinguishable from their present operations.

> The entities [corporations] would be found to be not fictitious, but factual. The railroad would go right on running. The mail order house would continue to ship to its customers. The steel company would continue to transport ore and process it into

steel. The men grouped in these concerns would continue to do what they were accustomed to do.[14]

The continuance of General Motors and American Telephone and Telegraph, for example, depends not on their corporate status but on the critical functional roles that they play in American society. Furthermore, organizations that bear striking resemblances to corporations and function in much the same way do exist in socialist and communist societies, which do not legally recognize corporate status. In all industrial societies, large-scale organizations constitute the basic economic units, regardless of the name given to that kind of organization.

The foundation of any organization, however, is the coordinated efforts of men who are attempting to further their own objectives, while also furthering a collective interest.[15] All organizations (including corporations) have particular organizational goals to which individuals subordinate their own interests and desires. At the same time, however, individuals influence organizational objectives through their own contributions. Accordingly, when managers engage in certain activities in the name of, with the resources of, and for the alleged interests of the organization, we can safely assume that the participation is that of the corporate entity. This assumption is particularly valid if the formulation and execution of a given policy have involved so many individuals or the policy has been of such long standing that it is difficult to associate it with any single person or any group of persons within the organization.

In the succeeding pages, the distinction between a corporate executive's organizational and personal political identities and activities will, where possible, be maintained. Where, however, the line between the individual and corporate activity is ill-defined and tenuous, the two will be considered as one.

SUMMATION AND PRELUDE

In this chapter the reader has been introduced to a number of the critical issues that arise from corporate political participation, including the propriety of such participation in terms of organizational purpose, the internal and external legitimacy of this participation, the relations between the corporation and the state, the nature of the interaction between the corporation and other social interests, the utility of economic theory in explaining corporate political activities, the character of politics and the political process, and the distinction between the organizational and individual political participation of corporate managers. This discussion will provide the necessary background for the succeeding chapters.

In the pages that follow, we shall (1) discuss the history, form, and techniques of corporate political activities; (2) analyze the arguments in support of and in opposition to corporate involvement in the political sphere; (3) examine the nature and the extent of corporate political power; and (4) advance the thesis that corporations, just like other collective social interests, have legitimate political concerns, which are a consequence of organizational goals and which therefore make political involvement inevitable.

While points will usually be illustrated by citing examples of the activities of large national firms, particularly with regard to their relations with the federal government, the activities of smaller business firms and political involvement of corporations on the state and local levels will be considered. Like the pigs of George Orwell's *Animal Farm*, some corporations are "more equal" than others—in terms of both their political resources and their impact upon the political process. Accordingly, relevant distinctions will be made between the political roles of large national firms and those of smaller corporations.

It will be argued in conclusion that corporations should not, as a policy matter, be relegated to the underworld of politics but should be placed on a legal parity with other social interests and be recognized as legitimate political participants in the democratic process.

NOTES

[1]Leslie Lipson, *The Democratic Civilization* (Fair Lawn, N.J.: Oxford University Press, Inc., 1964), p. 194.

[2]R. M. MacIver, *The Web of Government*, rev. ed. (New York: The Free Press, 1965), p. 236. Copyright R. M. MacIver 1965.

[3]Readers who are interested in this period of social and economic history are referred to Miriam Beard, *A History of Business: From Babylon to the Monopolists* (Ann Arbor, Mich.: Ann Arbor Paperback, The University of Michigan Press, 1962), pp. 124–58; Henri Pirenne, *Economic and Social History of Medieval Europe* (New York: Harvest Books, Harcourt, Brace & World, Inc., 1937); Max Weber, *General Economic History* (New York: Collier Books, A Division of the Crowell-Collier Publishing Co., 1961); and Robert L. Heilbroner, *The Making of Economic Society* (Englewood Cliffs, N.J.: Prentice-Hall, Inc., 1962).

[4]New York: Harcourt, Brace & World, Inc., 1936.

[5]See, for example, Karl Marx, *A Contribution to the Critique of Political Economy*, trans. N. I. Stone (Chicago: Charles H. Kerr & Company, 1904), pp. 11–13; and M. M. Bober, *Karl Marx's Interpretation of History*, 2d ed., rev. (New York: W. W. Norton & Company, Inc., Publishers, 1965), pp. 3–63.

[6]See, for example, Talcott Parsons and Neil J. Smelser, *Economy and Society* (New York: The Free Press, 1956); and Wilbert E. Moore, *The Impact of Industry* (Englewood Cliffs, N.J.: Prentice-Hall, Inc., 1965).

[7]The quoted definitions can be found respectively in: V. O. Key, Jr., *Politics, Parties, and Pressure Groups*, 5th ed. (New York: Thomas Y. Crowell Co., 1964), p. 2; Max Weber, "Politics as a Vocation," in H. H. Gerth and C. Wright Mills (eds. and trans.), *From Max Weber: Essays in Sociology* (Fair Lawn, N.J.: Oxford University Press, Inc., 1958), p. 78; Harold D. Lasswell, *Politics: Who Gets What, When, How* (Gloucester, Mass.: Peter Smith, 1950), p. 3; and George E. G. Catlin, *A Study of the Principles of Politics* (London: George Allen & Unwin, Ltd., 1930), pp. 68–69.

[8]Harold D. Lasswell, *World Politics and Personal Insecurity* (New York: The Free Press, 1965), p. 3.

[9]Oran R. Young, *Systems of Political Science*, Foundations of Modern Political Science Series (Englewood Cliffs, N.J.: Prentice-Hall, Inc., 1968), p. 4.

[10]Young, *Systems of Political Science*, p. 4.

[11]Andrew Hacker, "Introduction," in Andrew Hacker (ed.), *The Corporation Take-over* (New York: Harper & Row, Publishers, 1964), pp. 3–5.

[12]John Kenneth Galbraith, *The New Industrial State* (Boston: Houghton Mifflin Company, 1967), p. 2.

[13]There are two basic theories about corporations, the "concession" theory and the "inherence" theory. Anglo-American legal theory has generally reflected the former theory which views corporateness as an attribute that can be bestowed only by the state, by means of a concession of power given to specific individuals (incorporators). A classic expression of this theory is that

> a corporation is an artificial being, invisible, intangible, and existing only in contemplation of law. Being the mere creature of law, it possesses only those properties which the charter of its creation confers upon it, either expressly, or as incidental to its very existence. (*Dartmouth College* v. *Woodward*, 4 Wheaton 518, 636 [1819].)

The inheritance theory views corporateness as the inherent right of any group of individuals to come together to form organizations through which they can act collectively, independent of any act of indulgence by the state. For additional discussion of the distinctions between these two theories, see John P. Davis, *Corporations* (New York: Capricorn Books, G. P. Putnam's Sons, 1961), esp. pp. 13–34, 209–47; and Dow Votaw, *Modern Corporations* (Englewood Cliffs, N.J.: Prentice-Hall, Inc., 1965), pp. 9–10. Analyses of the legal attributes of American business corporations can be found in Votaw, *Modern Corporations*, pp. 29–84; Henry Winthrop Ballantine, *Ballantine on Corporations*, rev. ed. (Chicago: Callaghan and Company, 1946); and Norman D. Lattin, *The Law of Corporations* (Brooklyn: Foundation Press, Inc., 1959).

[14]Adolf A. Berle, Jr., *The 20th Century Capitalist Revolution* (New York: Harvest Books, Harcourt, Brace & World, Inc., 1954), pp. 18–19.

[15]Douglas McGregor, *The Professional Manager* (New York: McGraw-Hill Book Company, 1967), p. 30. For a sampling of the literature on human behavior in organizations, see Chester I. Barnard, *The Functions of the Executive* (Cambridge, Mass.: Harvard University Press, 1938); Herbert A. Simon, *Administrative Behavior*, 2d ed. (New York: The Free Press, 1965); Philip Selznick, *Leadership in*

Administration (New York: Harper & Row, Publishers, 1957); Robert T. Golembiewski, *Men, Management, and Morality* (New York: Mc-Graw-Hill Book Company, 1965); Amitai Etzioni, *Modern Organizations*, Foundations of Modern Sociology Series (Englewood Cliffs, N.J.: Prentice-Hall, Inc., 1964); James G. March and Herbert A. Simon, *Organizations* (New York: John Wiley & Sons, Inc., 1963); Peter M. Blau and W. Richard Scott, *Formal Organizations* (San Francisco: Chandler Publishing Company, 1962); and Leonard R. Sayles and George Strauss, *Human Behavior in Organizations* (Englewood Cliffs, N.J.: Prentice-Hall, Inc., 1966).

Chapter Three

Corporate Political Involvement: A Long-Standing Fact

Some commentators have suggested that the emphasis placed by corporations upon *electoral* activities as distinguished from the more typical concentration on *governmental* activities has been a novel aspect of corporate political involvement since World War II. However, critical analysis of American political history does not substantiate this perceived novelty. Corporations have been involved in both electoral and governmental activities since the opening decades of the nineteenth century.

THE COLONIAL AND REVOLUTIONARY ERAS

Political involvement by business interests preceded both our national existence and the concentration of economic activity in the corporate form. Private business enterprise, frequently operating in the form of a joint stock company, played an important part in the settlement of the original colonies during the seventeenth century. The Virginia Company and the Plymouth Company are examples of the joint stock company organized to promote settlement. Political power belonged to those directing the company. Economic motivations were not exclusive or, in some instances, even primary in the establishment of the American colonies; however, business goals have been indigenous to our national development, as have the efforts of those with economic interests to implement such goals through political means. Two of the great issues in American historiography are (1) whether the American Revolution was a revolt by colonial business interests against the mercantile policies of Britain, and (2) whether, as Charles A. Beard has argued, the Constitution of 1787 "was an economic document drawn with superb skill by men whose property interests were immediately at stake; and as such it appealed directly and unerringly to identical interests in the country at large."[1]

THE JEFFERSONIAN-HAMILTONIAN DEBATE

During the first decade of our national existence, a key debate between the Federalists headed by Alexander Hamilton and the Democratic-Republicans led by Thomas Jefferson was whether the new nation was to encourage manufacturing or agrarian interests. As expressed in his *Report on the Subject of Manufactures*, Hamilton recommended that government should assist and protect manufacturing. This recommendation ultimately prevailed, and the foundation was thus laid for the transformation within a century of a predominantly agricultural country into an industrial nation.

In the realm of political theory, the dispute between Jefferson and Hamilton reflects two variant and potentially contradictory democratic traditions which competed for supremacy during the nineteenth and the early twentieth centuries. One tradition originated in the writings of the Puritan left during the seventeenth century and was "primarily a humane doctrine, emphasizing the worth of the individual, and assigning the rights of private property to a subordinate, instrumental position."[2] This tradition was embodied primarily in the Declaration of Independence and is associated with Jeffersonian democracy. The second tradition draws its heritage from John Locke, and while it "is not indifferent to these humane values, to be sure, . . . it elevates the property right to the same plane" as the concept of moral liberty.[3] During the nineteenth century, latter-day Hamiltonians adopted this second view as their own, and it became the dominant theory of democracy during the Gilded Age of American Capitalism after the Civil War. This theory of democracy, which served to strengthen the economic and political position of the rapidly expanding corporations of the period and was sanctified by the decisions of the United States Supreme Court, contributed to the widespread and overt character of corporate political activity during the years 1870 to 1910.

PRE-CIVIL WAR CORPORATE POLITICS

For convenience, the beginning of corporate political involvement in the United States can be set at 1820. At that time, the approximately three hundred corporations of the entire country were concentrated in strategic economic activities—road and canal building, banking, and land development. During this early era, before the enactment of general incorporation laws, the attainment of corporate status required political activity by persons seeking such status, since corporateness could be conferred only by a special act of the legislature. Because of the public nature of the activities carried on by many of the early companies and because of the general shortage of capital, governmental assistance in the form of land or cash subsidies was also required. Such assistance was particularly necessary for railroad construction throughout the nineteenth century. Moreover, the new corporations were frequently given monopoly privileges in the exercise of their activities; the result was favoritism and corruption in the granting of corporate charters. No wonder it seemed to contemporaries that "the bargaining and trucking away chartered privileges is the whole business of our law-makers."[4]   It is not surprising that existing corporations, which held monopoly positions, waged bitter opposition to the passage of the general incorporation acts that were introduced in state legislatures during the 1830's. Despite this opposition, general acts were adopted facilitating the widespread use of the corporate form which, in the post-Civil War era, became the dominant means for conducting important economic activity.

The first historically notable confrontation between the national government and an important economic interest involved the attempt by the Second Bank of The United States to renew its corporate charter. President Andrew Jackson's veto of the congressional act renewing the charter was both an attack on the Bank's monopoly position under its charter and, significantly, an attempt to implement *laissez faire* as the guiding norm of economic democracy.[5]

Developments in the Jacksonian Era are relevant to our subsequent analysis of the political role of the corporation in the United States because the history of the period indicates that, from virtually the beginning of this country, the relationship between the corporation and the state has been close, yet beset with tension.   The closeness has involved a conferring by the state upon the corporation of significant privileges in exchange for the performance of important social tasks.   The tension has resulted from the efforts of other social interests, as represented by the state, to constrain the expansion of corporate power and from the attempts by corporations to maximize their position vis-à-vis these other interests and each other.   This anomalous relationship has manifested itself in virtually every period of American history.

THE POST-CIVIL WAR ERA

In the years following the Civil War, the number of corporations expanded rapidly until by the end of the nineteenth century there were approximately 500,000 corporations in the United States.   Notwithstanding this growth in the number of incorporated businesses, the most important characteristic of the era was the consolidation of industrial activity into large national units. During the 1880's, railroads, steel, and oil became prototypal of the concentration that was to characterize a number of basic industries within a few years.

The Age of Enterprise, as this era is commonly known, introduced not only a revolution in the mode of economic activity but also a significant change in the conduct of American politics. In many parts of the country, but particularly along the Atlantic seaboard, political power shifted from agricultural and patrician interests to the new class of entrepreneurs. Democracy came to be equated with economic freedom and the rights of property; and in 1886 the Supreme Court provided constitutional protection to corporate efforts to escape state regulation by declaring that corporations were "persons," thus coming within the purview of the Fourteenth Amendment.[6] With the election of William McKinley as President ten years later, the question of whether business or agriculture was to govern the country was conclusively resolved in favor of the former.

Corporate political activity during this period was equally apparent within the governmental and electoral spheres. In governmental politics, corporate interests exerted continual efforts to purchase the support of political decision makers in municipal offices, state legislatures, and Congress. Probably the classic instances of the outright money purchase of support are the infamous struggle in the New York legislature for control of the Erie Railroad and the activities of the Southern Pacific Railroad in controlling the California legislature.[7] On the national scene, the House of Representatives was described by one of its members as "like an auction room, where more valuable considerations were disposed of under the Speaker's hammer than in any other place on earth."[8]

At stake for the corporations of the day were railroad land grants running into the hundreds of millions of acres, utility rates, construction subsidies, franchised rights of way, monetary policies, protective tariffs, and mining and timber interests. Also at issue were numerous threats to corporate autonomy in the form of hostile legislation offered by dissident social interests.

Despite bitter railroad opposition, Granger laws were passed in a number of midwestern states during the 1870's; but within a few years many of these acts were repealed. Where attempts at repeal failed, the laws were frequently contemptuously ignored or the officials enforcing them were corrupted.

In a few instances, the public clamor for regulation, particularly on the part of shippers, could not be ignored by Congress. Even in these instances, corporate interests were effective in either weakening or substantially mitigating the potential impact of such legislation. In 1887, Congress passed the Interstate Commerce Act, ending nearly two decades of failure by proponents of railroad regulation. However, the act had little effect on the operations of the carriers, since the Interstate Commerce Commission (ICC), which was established under its provisions, was merely a fact-finding agency with no coercive powers. In dealing with the Commission, moreover, the railroads followed a pattern of behavior that has characterized corporate-agency relations to the present—that of influencing the regulatory body to become sympathetic to the needs of the regulated firms and of using the agency as a buffer between the industry and the public. In addition, the courts consistently refused to uphold the Commission's cease and desist orders. The act "was a sop to the malcontents in American political society, the minimum concession by Big Business politicians to a balking electorate."[9] While the Hepburn Act of 1906 enlarged the ICC's jurisdiction, it did not measurably improve its enforcement power. The second great regulatory milestone, the Sherman Antitrust Act of 1890, had a similar history. Passed despite opposition by leading corporations, particularly the Standard Oil Company, the act was sufficiently limited and ambiguous to be easily circumvented. The primary effect of both pieces of legislation was to provide expensive nuisances for the affected corporations and to delude the public into believing that effective regulation existed.

On the state level, while a number of states passed legislation governing wages and hours, restricting the employment of women and children, and establishing factory safety standards, such measures were successfully opposed by business firms in other jurisdictions. Moreover, the corporate opponents of such legislation were assisted by the Supreme Court, which consistently held state regulatory efforts to be unconstitutional violations of "substantive due process."

Corporate electoral politics was not neglected during this era. Corporate participation generally took three forms: personal electoral candidacy by business leaders, the actual selection and financing of legislative candidates by corporate officials, and the screening and support of those candidates presented by the party. In the 1880's, since the representation of business interests by politicians often proved costly and capricious, corporate leaders themselves stepped boldly into the political arena. The Senate in 1889 was known as the "Millionaires' Club" and its roster included such business luminaries as Leland Stanford of the Southern Pacific, George Hearst of mining and newspaper fame, Chauncey DePew of the New York Central, and Henry B. Payne of Standard Oil.

While personal participation on the part of leading business figures had largely come to an end a few years later, corporations were often represented by hand-picked candidates. It could be reported that

> a United States senator . . . represented something more than a state, more even than a region. He represented principalities and powers in business. One senator, for instance, represented the Union Pacific Railway System, another the New York Central, still another the insurance interests of New York and New Jersey. . . . Coal and iron owned a coterie from the Middle and Eastern seaport states. Cotton had half a dozen senators. And so it went.[10]

Lastly, in accordance with custom, corporations kept the party wheels well greased with generous lubrications of cash and exercised the prerogative of "clearing" candidates proposed by the parties. A crowning touch to the corporate-political relationship was the "systematic assessment" plan instituted by Mark Hanna, under which a company was expected to contribute to the Republican party according to both its stake in the general prosperity of the country and its special regional interests.[11]   In 1896, the Standard Oil Company alone gave $250,000 to support the successful Presidential candidacy of William McKinley.

While the term *corporation* has been used indiscriminately in the above paragraphs, it should be clear that far and away the majority of business firms performing on the stage of American politics were the large national enterprises ("trusts") that were beginning to predominate in a number of industries.   Perhaps the outstanding characteristic of corporate politics in the Progressive Era was the conflict that pitted the large corporations against small business interests.   This contest has been described as a "struggle over organization"[12] and, in part, involved an effort by an essentially middle-class segment of American society to limit their loss of economic, social, and political power to large corporations.   While Progressives such as Louis D. Brandeis believed that the "trusts" represented a threat to the democratic process and to individual political liberty in America,[13] small businessmen feared for their economic survival.

During the 1960's, there has developed respectable scholarly opinion that challenges the commonly accepted view of the business community as a monolithic opponent of Progressivism. In the area of economic regulation, for example, business interests did much to shape what has traditionally been regarded as reform legislation, such as the establishment of a scientific tariff commission, the development of the Federal Reserve System, and the passage of the Federal Trade Commission and Clayton Acts.   While businessmen opposed virtually all social welfare measures and generally dragged their heels on questions of political reform, "questions of economic regulation aroused a very different response: at least one segment of the business community supported each major program for federal control.   In this area businessmen exercised their greatest influence on reform and laid their claim as progressives."[14]   These efforts on the part of business reformers to regulate the activities of economic interests frequently took the form of small versus large, one industry group against a competing industry, or firms operating in one part of the economy in opposition to hostile business interests functioning in another sector.

In short, according to this recent reinterpretation of the Progressive Era, business efforts in support of government economic regulation constituted a demonstration of the exercise of what John Kenneth Galbraith has termed "countervailing power" —in this instance, the effort by smaller business to utilize government to restrain corporate giantism. However, this view of Progressivism has been challenged by some business historians. After examining the widespread participation by economic interests in obtaining the passage of regulatory legislation, Gabriel Kolko contends that the period between 1906 and 1916 was an era marked by the "triumph of conservatism," in which the needs and desires of the corporate community were the major determinants of so-called Progressive legislation.

> It is business control over politics (and by "business" I mean the major economic interests) rather than political regulation of the economy that is the significant phenomenon of the Progressive Era. Such domination was direct and indirect, but significant only insofar as it provided means for achieving a great end —political capitalism. *Political capitalism* is the utilization of political outlets to attain conditions of stability, predictability and security—to attain rationalization—in the economy.[15]

Although historians continue to debate about the motivations for and consequences of business political participation in the Progressive Era, corporations indisputably helped to shape the regulatory legislation of the day in an effort to maximize their respective economic interests.

Significantly, the impact of business upon government was felt in yet another way, which was to have importance in the years to come. In the field of public administration, reformers during the early decades of this century accepted business ideology and business procedures "enthusiastically and practically without reservation."[16] Indeed, business organization, particularly the corporate form, was used as a model for the reorganization of governmental bodies in order to increase efficiency.

One issue on which business corporations as a class met legislative defeat related to the channeling of corporate funds into political campaign chests. In 1907, Congress passed the Tillman Act, which prohibited corporate contributions to the campaigns of parties and candidates in federal elections. As a matter of actual political practice, however, statutory restrictions proved inadequate to prevent corporate interests from continuing to support parties and candidates in subsequent years. In 1936, for example, the Du Ponts and the Pews of Sun Oil Company together gave $1 million to the unsuccessful Republican effort to defeat President Franklin D. Roosevelt.[17] Donations were made individually by contributors who were so closely aligned with their respective corporations, in terms of both share ownership and managerial activity, as to make company "participation" in the gift unquestionable.

CORPORATE POLITICS 1912–1946

Despite the rhetoric of the Progressive Era and of the New Deal, throughout most of this century government has been reflective of business needs and values—an indication of the success of corporate political involvement. Indeed, corporate interests actually received encouragement from the federal government in their *governmental* political endeavors. In 1912, a conference, held in Washington under the sponsorship of the Secretary of Commerce and Labor, led to the formation of the Chamber of Commerce of the United States, which soon became one of the most important business lobbying groups. A dozen years later, Secretary of Commerce Herbert Hoover encouraged trade associations to draw up codes of business practice and ethics, which were then promulgated into standards of industry fair practice. Interestingly enough, this approach was implicitly adopted by President Franklin D. Roosevelt during the early days of the New Deal with the establishment of the short-lived National Recovery Administration.

Three dimensions of corporate political involvement during the period under discussion warrant particular mention: the extensive utilization of trade associations; the importance of public relations; and the co-optation of corporate leaders into the administrative branches of government.

TRADE ASSOCIATION ACTIVITIES

The first dimension—trade association activity—has been suggested earlier in this section. The Chamber of Commerce, the National Association of Manufacturers, the Edison Electric Institute, and the American Bankers Association, to mention but a few of the more prominent business organizations, attempted to further the political interests of constituent corporations. From the beginning of the twentieth century, interest-group activity expanded greatly as a consequence of the increasing specialization in the production and distribution of goods and services. This expansion prompted increased governmental intervention, particularly during the decade of the 1930's. During the Golden Era of the 1920's, business associations, in the words of a public relations counselor of the period, pursued the following objectives:

> First, to reduce the volume of legislation that interferes with business and industry; second, to minimize and counteract political regulation of business that is hurtful; third, to discourage radicalism by labor organizations and all sorts of agitators; fourth, . . . [to] fight for reasonable taxation by state, city and county government; fifth, [to promote] a scientific educational campaign against all socialistic and radical propaganda of whatever nature.[18]

Corporations, both independently and through associations, opposed rate regulation and antitrust enforcement, fought the growth and public acceptance of labor unions, supported high protective tariffs, and sought to force the government to sell its wartime facilities to private enterprise. In large measure, these efforts were successful.

Indeed, the atmosphere of the 1920's was favorable to business interests. The prevalent attitude of the decade was reflected by Presidents Warren G. Harding and Calvin Coolidge, who expressed views to the effect that what was needed in America was to take politics out of business and put business into politics. The sentiments of a large portion of the corporate community were expressed by a prominent business leader who, anticipating Charles E. Wilson's famous statement of a generation later, asserted:

> The welfare of business, especially of big business, the product of intense individualism, necessarily means the *public* welfare. The two are inseparable! . . . No citizens . . . were so well qualified to steer legislation and government as its top-notch business and professional men; none had such great interests at stake; none could judge of effective organization and transaction of public business so well as they.[19]

The failure of the business community to prevent the Depression destroyed the faith that many Americans had placed in such assertions during the 1920's and contributed to the election of President Franklin D. Roosevelt. Although corporate political effort continued unabated, corporate political influence reached its nadir during the New Deal. Significantly, the lack of influence is in part attributable to the failure of business leaders after the first hundred days to respond to the President's calls for cooperation. Corporate political response took the form largely of opposition to the New Deal legislative program by means of the usual trade-association activity and massive public relations campaigns designed to convince the public of the evils confronting them. Also new groups such as the American Liberty League were organized to oppose President Roosevelt. As indicated earlier, corporations poured large sums of money into electoral efforts to defeat "that man in the White House." Significantly, during the first Roosevelt administration, the Supreme Court served as a buffer between the business community and the administration's legislative program. During 1935 and 1936 alone, the Court declared seven major New Deal acts unconstitutional.

Among the pieces of New Deal legislation that have traditionally been considered "antibusiness" are the National Recovery Act, the Fair Labor Standards Act, the Securities Act of 1933, the Holding Company Act, the Securities Exchange Act of 1934, the TVA Act of 1933, the several Banking Acts of 1933 and 1934, the Social Security Act, and the National Labor Relations Act of 1935 (Wagner Act). Tradition notwithstanding, only the Wagner Act interfered significantly with classic corporate prerogatives. Termed by a liberal historian as "probably the most bluntly anti-corporation legislation the United States has ever accepted,"[20] the act authorized governmental supervision of two key aspects of business activity—cost and authority. Significantly, the impact of the Wagner Act was, in large measure, mitigated a decade later with the passage of the Taft-Hartley Act in 1947.

Ironically, the increased governmental regulation of the economy during the 1930's, which was partially a response to a multiplication in the number and importance of business groups, engendered an acceleration in corporate political endeavors. The reason is plain enough. "Wherever government controls a business, it becomes inevitable that the business should try to control the government."[21] With increased areas of direct contact between the federal government and industry, business associations and individual firms were compelled to redouble their political efforts.

THE POLITICAL USES OF PUBLIC RELATIONS

Business firms learned at an early date that "the medium is the message." World War I experience revealed the power of propaganda; and with further development of techniques of media exploitation, public relations became a valuable political tool for individual corporations and for business associations. Companies such as American Telephone and Telegraph and Du Pont attempted through printed and radio media to create an environment favorable to their corporate interests. Messages to the consumer, particularly favored by public utilities, strove to impress upon the public the benevolence of the enterprise and to forestall governmental attempts to interfere with its operations. The importance of business public relations in corporate political participation has, if anything, been enhanced since the advent of television. We shall consider this aspect of participation in greater detail when we examine present-day corporate political behavior.

Trade associations used the media extensively for political purposes. During the 1920's, local chambers of commerce enlisted the assistance of other business groups, including the National Association of Manufacturers and the American Bankers Association, to spread the gospel of the American Plan, which consisted primarily of opposition to the closed shop and to collective bargaining. Annually, hundreds of thousands of dollars were spent on mailings and on radio broadcasts beamed across the nation. Syndicated articles and "canned" editorials emanating from trade association offices were disseminated as news and as fact in newspapers and on radio. The fact that network broadcasting was virtually monopolized by two companies, which were themselves large corporations, guaranteed that views sympathetic to business would prevail. Participation by businessmen in civic associations was another technique for enhancing the public image of the business community. Virtually every available technique was utilized in the public relations effort. When asked "do you know any means of publicity that has been neglected by your organization?" the director of the Information Department of the National Electric Light Association responded, "Only one, and that is sky writing. I don't believe that we have tried that with airplanes."[22] In time, this technique was also utilized.

The public relations program begun in the 1920's was stepped up in the 1930's as opposition among businessmen to the Roosevelt administration mounted. After World War II, the campaign continued, with concentration on promoting the virtues of "free enterprise" while opposing the "welfare state" and big government. By 1950, however, the anachronistic character of the message had become so patent that a major *Fortune* feature inquired, "Is Anybody Listening?"[23] There has since been a shift in the business public relations effort from emphasis on the long-dead issues of the 1920's to reflection of the changed nature both of contemporary American society and of the business corporation. This shift will be examined in Chapter Five.

THE CO-OPTATION OF CORPORATE LEADERSHIP INTO GOVERNMENT

Events in both World Wars contributed to the involvement of corporate leaders in governmental decision making. Through the War Industries Board of World War I, industry groups determined for the firms within their industries standards of production and pricing, which then became formal governmental policy. Moreover, because of the scarcity within the government of experienced managerial personnel with understanding of economics, American mobilization during World War I was, to a large extent, planned and executed by businessmen who were in temporary federal government service. The integration of economic and military institutions during the process of mobilizing industry for the war effort was the foundation for what President Dwight D. Eisenhower later designated "the industrial-military complex."[24]

Business political activity of World War I included the service by some corporate managers as WOC's (without compensation) or as dollar-a-year men. These leaders contributed substantially to the war effort, while enhancing the positions of their companies through the contacts they developed and through their ability to influence national policies toward compatibility with the needs of industry. The above remarks are not, however, intended to suggest that businessmen who served in government were guilty of nefarious or corrupt behavior on behalf of their firms—their activities were based on the belief that they could most effectively aid the war effort by protecting and stabilizing industry. "They believed that it was their patriotic duty to pursue vigorously some of the same goals which they had sought for industry before the war and which they would continue to seek for industry in the postwar years."[25]

During World War II, the same pattern of business participation was evident, on a vastly increased scale. Corporate efforts were co-opted into governmental decision making through the establishment of innumerable industry advisory committees under the auspices of the Office of Production Management and the Office of Price Administration and through the use by the federal government of business executives in paid and unpaid capacities. As in World War I, the problem of dual loyalties was present. In a sense, the conflict is inevitable, since businessmen who come from private corporations and intend to return to them have tended to follow ingrained response patterns when confronted with issues for which the "public interest" is not abundantly clear. Bias, not corruption, was the real problem. Notwithstanding the limitations inherent in this scheme of business political participation, it was more effective in meeting the needs of the war effort than any alternative that could readily be devised.

Significantly, since World War II, a number of executive departments, most notably Commerce, Interior, and Defense, have continued to use business advisory committees. The continuing existence of such committees is in part due to the sustained state of undeclared war, which has required close governmental-industry relationships. Another factor is the increasing delegation to private corporations of such governmental activities as space exploration, the development and production of defense systems, and urban redevelopment. Finally, the pattern of advisory committees has proved helpful to the government in mobilizing industry support for governmental programs, and to the business community in influencing the formulation and implementation of governmental policy. Such advisory committees appear to be permanent fixtures on the Washington scene. We shall have occasion to examine them in greater detail in succeeding chapters.

SUMMATION

This historical review has indicated that both governmental and electoral activities of corporations have been part of American political history from the very beginnings of this country. Neither form of activity can be considered a novel development that has arisen only since World War II. Indeed, we are justified in considering corporate involvement in both arenas as an inherent characteristic of a pluralistic industrial democracy.

NOTES

[1]Charles A. Beard, *An Economic Interpretation of the Constitution of the United States* (New York: The Free Press, 1965), p. 188. Originally published in 1913.

[2]Robert Green McCloskey, *American Conservatism in the Age of Enterprise, 1865–1910* (New York: Harper & Row, Publishers, 1964), p. 6.

[3]McCloskey, *American Conservatism . . .*, pp. 6, 15.

[4]William Leggett of the New York *Post*, quoted in Richard Hofstadter, *The American Political Tradition* (New York: Vintage Books, Random House, Inc., 1954), p. 58, n. 10.

[5]For accounts of the Bank Veto fight, see Arthur M. Schlesinger, Jr., *The Age of Jackson* (Boston: Little, Brown and Company, 1950), pp. 74–114, 334–49; Hofstadter, *The American Political . . .*, pp. 45–67; and Alpheus Thomas Mason and Richard H. Leach, *In Quest of Freedom* (Englewood Cliffs, N.J.: Prentice-Hall, Inc., 1959), pp. 258–82.

[6]*Santa Clara County v. S. Pac. R.R. Co.*, 118 U.S. 394 (1886).

[7]The lurid tale of the struggle for control of the Erie Railroad is reported in Charles Francis Adams, Jr., and Henry Adams, *Chapters of Erie* (Ithaca, N. Y.: Great Seal Books, Cornell University Press, 1956). The political activities of the Southern Pacific are treated in Matthew Josephson, *The Robber Barons* (New York: Harvest Books, Harcourt, Brace & World, Inc., 1934), pp. 216–230, 347–74. Probably the best single account of the relationship between business corporations and municipal government is found in Lincoln Steffens, *The Autobiography of Lincoln Steffens* (New York: Harcourt, Brace & World, Inc., 1931).

[8]Quoted in Matthew Josephson, *The Politicos* (New York: Harvest Books, Harcourt, Brace & World, Inc., 1938), p. 118.

⁹Thomas C. Cochran and William Miller, *The Age of Enterprise* (New York: Harper & Row, Publishers, 1961), p. 171.

¹⁰William Allen White, *Masks in a Pageant* (New York: The Macmillan Company, Publishers, 1928), p. 79.

¹¹Louise Overacker, *Money in Elections* (New York: The Macmillan Company, Publishers, 1932), pp. 112–13.

¹²Richard Hofstadter, *The Age of Reform* (New York: Vintage Books, Random House, Inc., 1955), pp. 215–71.

¹³Louis D. Brandeis, *Other People's Money* (Philadelphia: Frederick A. Stokes Company, 1932).

¹⁴Robert H. Wiebe, *Businessmen and Reform* (Cambridge, Mass.: Harvard University Press, 1962), p. 212. See also Paul W. Glad, "Progressives and the Business Culture of the 1920s," *The Journal of American History*, LIII (June 1966), 75–89.

¹⁵Gabriel Kolko, *The Triumph of Conservatism* (New York: The Free Press, 1963), p. 3.

¹⁶Dwight Waldo, *The Administrative State* (New York: Ronald Press Co., 1948), p. 42.

¹⁷Louise Overacker, *Presidential Campaign Funds* (Boston: Boston University Press, 1946), p. 16.

¹⁸Corporate public relations counselor, E. Hofer, quoted in Cochran and Miller, *The Age of Enterprise*, p. 343.

¹⁹Charles N. Fay, vice-president of the National Association of Manufacturers, quoted in Mason and Leach, *In Quest of Freedom*, p. 440.

²⁰Eric F. Goldman, *Rendezvous with Destiny* (New York: Vintage Books, Random House, Inc., 1956), p. 284.

²¹Paul H. Douglas, *Ethics in Government* (Cambridge, Mass.: Harvard University Press, 1952), p. 32.

²²Cochran and Miller, *The Age of Enterprise*, p. 341.

²³William H. Whyte, Jr., and the editors of *Fortune, Is Anybody Listening?* (New York: Simon and Schuster, Inc., 1952).

²⁴See Paul A. C. Koistinen, "The 'Industrial-Military Complex' in Historical Perspective: World War I," *Business History Review*, XLI (Winter 1967), pp. 378–403.

²⁵Robert D. Cuff, "A 'Dollar-a-Year Man' in Government: George N. Peek and the War Industries Board," *Business History Review*, XLI (Winter 1967), p. 420.

Chapter Four

The Post-World War II Era: An Altered Political Economy And New Patterns of Participation

The official cessation of hostilities in 1946 marked the beginning of an era characterized by a hitherto unprecedented degree of governmental involvement in the economic sphere, particularly on the part of the federal government. This new pattern of involvement has been designated by many terms, including *mixed economy, pluralist economy, American economic republic, industrial state, positive state,* and *interdependent economy.* Whatever term is used to indicate the new relationship between the public and private sectors, the post-World War II political economy has been highlighted by a number of developments that are relevant to an understanding of the changes in recent patterns of corporate political participation.

RECENT DEVELOPMENTS IN AMERICAN
POLITICAL ECONOMY

GOVERNMENTAL RESPONSIBILITY FOR ECONOMIC STABILITY

The assumption of responsibility by the state for the smooth operation of the economy began during the crisis conditions of the Great Depression. The Employment Act of 1946 explicitly declared the continuing policy and responsibility of the government of the United States

> to coordinate and utilize all its plans, functions, and resources for the purpose of creating and maintaining, in a manner calculated to foster and promote free competitive enterprise and the general welfare, conditions under which there will be afforded useful employment opportunities, including self-employment, for those able, willing, and seeking to work, and to promote maximum employment, production, and purchasing power.[1]

Apart from capping the New Deal legislation of the 1930's, the real significance of the Employment Act stems from the assumption by the federal government of a positive economic role. The act constitutes a bench mark in the relations between government and business, since for the first time the federal government was given a mandate to monitor the economy in order to facilitate economic stability and growth and to enhance the "general welfare." Government was no longer limited to a regulatory or negative function but was to assume a role in economic planning. Although this planning role is limited when compared to the degree of governmental planning found in many European countries, it nevertheless represents a clear departure from previous national policy. Not unexpectedly, the legislation was opposed by many corporate leaders and by such business groups as the National Association of Manufacturers and the United States Chamber of Commerce.[2]

The Employment Act is also significant because it requires that the President deliver an annual economic report to Congress and because it established the Joint Economic Committee of Congress and the Council of Economic Advisers. The purpose of the President's report is to make known the economic health of the nation and to propose legislation to maintain and enhance the economy. Since the Joint Economic Committee has been of limited importance, its role will not be considered here.

The Council of Economic Advisers "is the nerve center of the American planning operation."[3] Its functions are to analyze, interpret, and forecast economic developments; to give policy advice to the President; to educate the President, the Congress, and the public; and to adapt and translate highly refined and purified economic concepts into workable public policy.[4] The Council has concerned itself with such sweeping matters as wage-price guideposts, employment levels and stability, deficits in the American balances of payments, competition and market structure, economic growth, fiscal and monetary policies to prevent inflation and recession, international economic policy, and foreign affairs. It has become increasingly influential in the formulation of national economic policy, and its recommendations have been of great importance to virtually every segment of the corporate community.

The institutional innovations of the Employment Act and its underlying mandate of positive governmental action have resolved the issue of the legitimacy of federal involvement in the economic sphere. Except for the most adamant opponents of state action, the question is no longer whether government should be an economic participant, but what the nature and extent of that participation should be.[5]

THE COLD WAR, MILITARY EXPENDITURES, AND FOREIGN AID

National military requirements have also contributed to the post-World War II pattern of federal economic activity. The involvement of the United States in the Cold War (with interspersed hot conflicts) has necessitated continuous cooperation between the federal government and industrial corporations to the needs of national defense. This collaboration has taken many forms.

First, the pattern of consultation between governmental departments and industry groups, established during two world wars, has been maintained during the Cold War era. A survey released by the House Committee on Government Operations indicates that during the mid-1950's there were between 5,000 and 6,000 industry advisory committees.[6] A number of government departments have continued the use of businessmen as WOC's. For the government, these consultative mechanisms serve to integrate with national requirements, the productive resources of America's most important industrial corporations. As will be seen subsequently, consultation also enables corporate leaders to influence governmental policy.

Second, because of the military requirements associated with extended American involvement in Europe, Korea, and Vietnam and with America's post-World War II policy of maintaining a virtually world-wide defense perimeter, the federal government has become the largest single purchaser of industrial goods and services. While some military equipment is produced in government-owned plants (frequently operated by large corporations), the traditional pattern of government reliance on private industry for satisfaction of its needs has continued. In addition to the traditional production and supervisory tasks, business firms have assumed new functions, for example, personnel contracting—selling to governmental agencies through "support contracts" the services of persons listed on the company payroll.

The over-all reliance of government upon the private sector is hardly surprising, since most of this nation's productive capacity as well as a substantial proportion of its technological expertise are found in industrial corporations. Moreover, governmental utilization, as opposed to governmental assumption, of business operations is ideologically preferable to many Americans.

As is stated in a 1965 Congressional report, "it is impossible to portray the scope of Federal procurement."[7] The Department of Defense alone annually issues approximately 10 million contract actions. The net value of military procurement actions in the fiscal period 1960 to 1964 (before the intensification of the U.S. commitment in Vietnam) totaled more than $123 billion. In fiscal 1967, the value of contracts let exceeded $40 billion. Over-all, in that fiscal year, more than 80 per cent of the federal government's purchases of goods and services (net of government sales) were for national defense, which includes actual military plus defense-related activities—a total of $74.3 billion. The trend, moreover, is an upward one. For fiscal 1969, the Pentagon budget proposals called for expenditures of $79.8 billion, which approached the peak annual expenditure of World War II.[8]

Some companies—notably in the aerospace industry—are almost totally dependent on government contracts for their economic survival. During the fiscal years 1961–1967, prime military contracts constituted more than 70 per cent of the total sales of the following defense contractors: Thiokol, 96 per cent; Newport News Shipbuilding, 90 per cent; Lockheed Aircraft, 88 per cent; AVCO, 75 per cent; McDonnell Douglas, 75 per cent; and Ling-Temco-Vought, 70 per cent. Each of the above companies received in excess of $1.3 billion in prime contracts during the seven-year period. Lockheed Aircraft led in the dollar amount of contracts awarded with more than $10.6 billion.[9]

The federal government's function as an allocator of strategic materials and natural resources has complemented its role as a military purchaser. In part because of its military need for vital raw materials, the federal government stockpiles large amounts of minerals and chemicals. Portions of this stockpile are sold to private industry in accordance with defense priorities.[10] Similarly, business firms are franchised by the federal government to tap the natural resources located in public lands and waterways. Timber rights, oil and gas drilling contracts, and mining concessions that run to billions of dollars annually are awarded to corporations by various federal agencies. Once again, business and governmental needs are intermeshed.

Finally, business firms are involved in governmental foreign aid operations. The international activities of a number of large corporations are, in part, subsidized indirectly by the United States government. During the first four and a half months of 1968, for example, more than $25 million in exports to underdeveloped countries of nine major American companies (including Ford, United States Steel, International Harvester, and Caterpillar Tractor) were financed by Agency for International Development (AID) moneys. As an incentive to American business to locate in underdeveloped areas, AID also insures private American investments in developing nations against economic and political risks. In mid-1968, almost $7 billion of such insurance was in effect. United States foreign policy and corporate needs are thus integrated in the AID program.[11]

TECHNOLOGICAL DEVELOPMENTS

The dramatic technological advances of the post-World War II period also contributed to increased governmental involvement in the economy. The huge costs associated with modern technology and its far-reaching social implications have necessitated collaboration between the public and private sectors to an unprecedented degree. For example, the entire aerospace venture, ranging from missile systems to communication satellites and moon exploration, has been a joint public-private enterprise. There has been a continuous increase in the number and importance of government research and development contracts for projects concerned with new forms and uses of communications, information retrieval and analysis systems, transportation resources, and nonmilitary applications of atomic energy.

These developments have activated the question of the social control of the fruits of the new technology. Among the issues of concern are the impact of automation on employment, the possible invasion of privacy by unrestricted use of new electronic devices and informational systems, and the influence of news media on the political and cultural life of the country. Just as social controls in the form of administrative guidelines, statutory standards, and licensing requirements affected the out-

standing technological developments of the pre-World War II
era—including the automobile, airplanes, radio, and television—
the new communications and information systems are being subjected to public regulation. Thus the technological advances
of the post-World War II era have resulted in two forms of governmental economic activity: (1) sponsorship of and active participation in the research and development efforts that have led
to significant advances; and (2) public supervision of the products and uses of these advances.

INCREASED EXPECTATIONS OF SOCIAL GROUPS

America's development into a highly urbanized, industrial
nation has created many social problems. The heightened expectations and the demands of a large sector of the public that
the government help alleviate these problems is another reason
for intensified and sustained governmental involvement in the
economic sphere. Often these demands are voiced by social
groups which, until quite recently, were considered outside the
pale of American life. The changing social role of the black
American presents a prime but not a unique example of these
problems. This social group has been engaged in a determined
struggle to enter the mainstream of life in the United States and
to experience the upward social and economic mobility historically associated with the "American Dream." Legal equality
has largely been achieved by invalidation of segregation laws
and by passage of civil rights legislation, and the efforts of blacks
are now directed primarily toward achieving economic equality.
Ironically, the accomplishments in the legal sector raised the
expectations of blacks in the economic sphere, thus heightening
the sense of relative deprivation, since these increased expectations have not been realized in accomplishments.[12]

Federal, state, and local governments have to greater or
lesser extent responded to demands that they employ their resources to alleviate unemployment and underemployment, sub-
standard housing, and inadequate educational and health re-

sources, which are the most pressing problems confronting large numbers of blacks. Response has been minimal, considering the extent of the needs, but government commitments to the solution of socioeconomic problems are the highest in our history. While a number of governmental programs are carried on in collaboration with private corporations—urban renewal and slum rehabilitation projects, on-the-job training, vocational education and job placement—the majority involve exclusively public efforts. With increasing frequency, however, business leaders have acknowledged a basic corporate obligation to use company resources, both unilaterally and in conjunction with governmental efforts, to assist blacks in raising their economic status.

Although a somewhat dramatic instance, governmental concern with the improvement of the condition of the black American is exemplary of the intensive post-World War II involvement of the public sector in fundamental social problems. The names of the three most recently established federal departments —Health, Education and Welfare; Housing and Urban Development; and Transportation—indicate the wide range of concerns that have become explicit areas of governmental interest. To a degree previously unknown in our national history, this social involvement has cast the federal government in the economic roles of consumer, producer, regulator, mediator, innovator, policy maker, and stabilizer. Because of the national scope and the deep-seated nature of many of this country's most pressing social problems, increased federal involvement in their resolution is inevitable. Ironically, a number of these problems (such as unemployment, pollution, and urban congestion and deterioration) have resulted from the tremendous technological advances of this century, which have affected the life styles of virtually all Americans. In essence, the federal government has actively acknowledged and has begun to fulfill its function as a backstop for the problems of American society.

It is significant that in the ten-year period between fiscal 1958 and fiscal 1967, total federal expenditures for nondefense purposes increased almost two and one-third times (from $36.7 billion to $83.1 billion), and federal purchases of nondefense goods and services more than trebled (from $5.3 billion to $17.3

billion). When these figures are added to expenditures for defense, the critical importance of federal expenditures to the economy can be appreciated. Equally important, by fiscal 1967, state and local governments had expanded their purchasing activities more than two and one-half times the 1958 dollar amount. In that ten-year period, combined federal, state, and local purchases averaged 20 per cent of the gross national product. The prognosis for the foreseeable future is that this percentage will increase, as all levels of government are called upon to satisfy the "guns and butter" needs of American society.[13]

•   •   •

In summation, the impetus for the expansion of the sphere of governmental economic activities since the conclusion of World War II has in large measure come from the legislative mandate contained in the Employment Act of 1946, the requirements of the Cold War and national defense, technological development, and the proliferation and intensification of social problems endemic to a complex urban industrial society in which people have become more interdependent and less self-sufficient. No other institution in what has been termed the "kaleidoscope of modern society" has experienced such a metamorphosis of social role as has government. The expansion in governmental activity is, to a great degree, an inevitable function of a capitalist system, for, as the late V. O. Key, Jr., suggested, "a private enterprise system must by its nature be also a system of state intervention."[14] Because of this expansion, a sharp line can no longer be drawn between governmental and nongovernmental organizations in defining functions as "public" and as "private." The critical distinction now is between degrees of publicness and privateness, and in a number of areas of social concern, the difference is increasingly difficult to ascertain.[15]

POSTWAR CORPORATE POLITICAL BEHAVIOR

The above discussion of the development of the mixed

economy after 1946 provides the necessary background against which to examine the nature of post-World War II corporate political involvement. Characterized more by changes in the scope and magnitude of business activities in the political sphere than by fundamental alterations, this pattern of involvement has several important dimensions.

PATENT, SELF-CONSCIOUS CORPORATE INVOLVEMENT

Political participation by corporations has become more patent and self-conscious than it had been—"patent" in that corporate leaders are much more willing than previously to acknowledge and discuss the political activities of their firms and "self-conscious" in that business leaders demonstrate an awareness of the actual and potential impact of their efforts and consciously seek to maximize their effectiveness. In the past, corporations and business associations followed a policy of "silence is golden"—either not acknowledging their political involvement or, at the very least, not advertising the fact that executives were concerning themselves with politics. While it is still very difficult for outsiders to obtain detailed information from company sources concerning particular aspects of corporate political policy and behavior, corporations are generally no longer reluctant to acknowledge that they have specific political interests, which they seek to further by active political participation.

There is a certain "rally-around-the-flag" quality associated with this change in political style. Articles such as "Politics—The Businessman's Biggest Job in 1958" and "Why Politics Needs Business in '66" exemplify this new spirit.[16] While much of this newly found corporate articulateness has been concentrated in the area of electoral involvement, exhortations by corporate sources concerning governmental activities have not been neglected. For example, in addressing a conference of corporate public affairs officers a few years ago, Henry Ford II remarked:

> There is widespread misconception that it is somehow wrong for corporations thus to attempt to influence legislation affecting

their interests. Nothing could be further from the truth. . . .
Things for which business may fight in self-interest may also
be very much in the national interest. . . . The problem with
"lobbying" activities is not to conceal their existence, nor to
apologize for them, but to make sure they are adequate, effective and impeccably correct in conduct.[17]

In recent years, corporate leaders have demonstrated a willingness to publicly champion views on a wide range of issues—from
such old chestnuts as tax, fiscal, and tariff policies to current
problems including civil rights, urban renewal, foreign affairs,
and medical care for the aged.

Business associations and trade groups have encouraged
both electoral and governmental endeavors by corporations. For
example, the Chamber of Commerce of the United States and the
various state chambers of commerce have assembled and distributed to corporations hundreds of thousands of pamphlets and
packets informing business firms and their managers how and
why they should become more active in politics. By 1960,
Action Course in Practical Politics, a textbook compiled by the
United States Chamber, had been adopted for employee political
education courses by more than a hundred corporations throughout the nation, including Alcoa, Boeing, Du Pont, Esso, Ford,
General Electric, and United States Steel.

Corporate political efforts have also been spurred by two
groups that were organized after the war. The Business-
Industry Political Action Committee (BIPAC) was formed by
the National Association of Manufacturers (NAM) in 1963 "to
serve as the political action arm of the national business community."[18] The organization, which is administratively separate
from its parent, engages in two types of activities: (1) political
education, which consists primarily of the publication of a pe-
riodical in which trends and developments in politics are discussed; and (2) political action, which consists of providing
direct financial support in the form of campaign contributions to
candidates for Congress who have the recommendation and support of the businessmen of their state or district.[19] While the
publication is sold on a subscription basis to corporations and is

paid for from company funds, contributions for political action are accepted only from individuals, in order to comply with federal legislation (18 U.S.C. § 610 [1951]) prohibiting corporate campaign contributions. Since, as will be discussed in Chapter Five, company moneys frequently reach political candidates in the form of individual contributions, it is safe to suggest that, on occasion, corporate funds probably have been received by BIPAC. In 1964, BIPAC contributed $203,000 to Republican and Democratic candidates for 86 House and 12 Senate seats, including some primary contests. Candidates supported by BIPAC won in 34 House contests (40 per cent) but in only one Senate race.[20]

The activities of the other new organization, Public Affairs Council, The Effective Citizens Organization, Inc. (ECO), have been of even greater importance in energizing corporations to political action. In 1954, ECO was founded on the belief that "political effectiveness is [so] essential to business effectiveness . . . that no prudent person, especially the businessman, can afford to be 'above politics.' "[21]

Although individual memberships are available, ECO is specifically geared to corporations, with membership fees ranging between $500 and $5,000. In early 1968, ECO had nearly 150 members. The organization takes no position or action on its own behalf concerning political issues; the heart of ECO's activities is the provision of information and expertise to corporations for the establishment of corporate public affairs programs. A company program consists typically of four essential elements: (1) Issuance by the company of policy statements encouraging employee political participation; (2) sponsorship of political and economic education courses for employees; (3) communication with the employees on issues which, in the opinion of the company, directly or indirectly affect either its or the employees' well-being; and (4) designation of a public affairs officer who is charged with the responsibility of conducting the program.[22]

Additionally, ECO assists corporations in their public affairs activities through seminars and workshops on local, state, and national government; research and consultation with companies concerning their public affairs endeavors; extensive library facilities relating to the conduct of public affairs; and numerous publications reporting on matters of political interest. The organization has also served as a forum for discussions among corporate public affairs officers. In 1968, ECO broadened the scope of its operations to encourage and assist its corporate members and affiliates in their efforts to help resolve the economic and social problems associated with the urban crisis. As of the end of 1967, compared with approximately 50 in 1960, more than 400 companies had established public affairs programs based on the ECO format. By 1968, ECO officials estimated that nearly 1,000 firms had participated in ECO-sponsored activities. Directors of the organization have included representatives of the United States Steel, Minnesota Mining and Manufacturing, Humble Oil, National Biscuit, Weyerhauser, General Electric, Ford, Boeing, Chase Manhattan, and Chrysler, as well as many other firms listed in the "*Fortune* Directory."

Since the early 1950's, corporations have established public affairs or governmental relations departments with increasing frequency, thereby formally recognizing and centralizing their organizational political activities. This trend is attributable, in part at least, to ECO efforts. The July 1966 edition of the *Directory of Public Affairs Officers*, published by ECO, shows that by 1966 nearly 350 companies had either organized departments or had designated individuals to handle public affairs activities.[23] To name but a few of the larger firms, Ford, General Electric, Gulf Oil, Monsanto Chemical, and Kaiser Aluminum and Chemical had established such departments. By its emphasis upon *corporate* political activities, ECO has contributed to the increasing independence of business firms from their traditional reliance on trade associations for political leadership.

CORPORATE POLITICAL SELF-RELIANCE

A second change in the pattern of corporate political participation since the end of World War II was touched upon in the preceding paragraph—the tendency for corporations to "go it alone" in their political involvement rather than to rely predominantly on trade and business associations. Increasingly, companies are delegating to their newly established governmental relations and public affairs departments the responsibility for promoting the interests of the firm by activities that previously were handled by general business associations, such as the NAM or the United States Chamber, or by industry groups. The tendency is particularly marked, though not surprisingly, among larger enterprises.

Among the activities of public affairs and governmental relations departments are: (1) political education and action, (2) governmental and legislative information and action, and (3) economic education. The principal objectives of these departments include professional coordination of diffuse company political activities, achievement of better corporate-community rapport, contribution to the over-all status and influence of the company, and improvement of corporate-governmental relations.[24] Frequently, firms assign to Washington and state capitals high-level officials who have the responsibility of conducting these activities on the major political battlegrounds. The activities of corporate Washington representatives will be examined in Chapter Five.

These developments do not threaten such well-established associations as the NAM, the United States Chamber of Commerce, the American Iron and Steel Institute, the American Petroleum Institute, or the Association of American Railroads, which are in no danger of going out of business. The overwhelming majority of corporations (nearly 90 per cent), including even the largest firms, rely upon these organizations to provide them with much of their information concerning national and state legislative issues.[25] Instead, the trend is to retain primary political policy initiative and implementation within the company rather than to trust it to external associations.

There are several plausible explanations for this switch in emphasis from collective to unilateral activity. One reason is that corporations often have political interests sufficiently limited and funds sufficiently ample that they need not be unduly committed to associational policies.

Second, because of government contracts, subsidies, licenses, and franchises, a given company may have specific individual political interests that are in direct opposition to those of other firms in the industry, and these interests cannot be pursued by reliance on trade association activities. This diversity among companies in terms of particular policies and needs makes individual action imperative. Moreover, because business associations must represent the views of a wide range of constituents, they must necessarily take positions of consensus on general issues, and such a position often does not meet the political needs of specific companies.

A third reason for increased corporate autonomy in political matters is the feeling on the part of some officials of large companies that business organizations do not adequately represent the political interests of large corporate constituents. Business associations frequently take positions on issues that have little long-term significance for corporations ("right-to-work" legislation and medical care for the aged legislation have been cited as examples by corporate managers) and neglect or omit matters of greater importance (for example, federal guideposts on wages and prices and restrictions on foreign investment).

Fourth, some corporate managers are disenchanted with the unremittingly negative stances that have been assumed by many associations. Recurrent expressions of dissatisfaction on the part of executives have no doubt had their effect; and since 1962, the National Association of Manufacturers, under its fulltime president, Werner P. Gullander, has made strong efforts to project a more positive image in the field of public affairs.[26]

Finally, the success of many business associations in accomplishing their political objectives has been debatable. While the effectiveness of pressure groups is difficult to measure with any degree of precision, available studies indicate that such groups are not nearly so effective as they lead their supporters to believe—or their opponents to fear. The nearly 2,000 trade associations differ substantially in size, resources, and effectiveness. For example, a few years ago one commentator raised the question, "NAM: Influential Lobby or Kiss of Death?" and concluded that the NAM's political failures far exceeded its successes.[27] Probably the potential political effectiveness of a well-coordinated effort by a large corporation frequently exceeds that of an association, which must represent a multiplicity of interests. As V. O. Key, Jr., pointed out,

> While in the field of political and legislative action it is the business association that is most visible, it is probably comparatively insignificant in its social power alongside the 100 to 150 giant corporations that dominate American business.[28]

In two areas, however, corporations continue to rely on the political activities of business associations. On the one hand, they depend on national business organizations to formulate policy concerning broad issues where their corporate interest is only tangential. On the other hand, in areas of specific industry-wide problems—such as tariff or taxation needs, the threat of hostile legislation, or the opposition of competing industries—industry trade associations continue to bear the brunt of conducting political action. Independent corporate political activity is most likely in competitive industries and in companies with individualized needs.

INCREASING CORPORATE BIPARTISANSHIP

A third change in the political participation patterns of corporations and corporate managers is the increasing degree of bipartisanship. For example, while corporate funds that find their way directly or indirectly into campaign coffers are still concentrated primarily on the Republican side of the rostrum, the Democrats have come into increasing favor. A postelection article in *Fortune* proclaiming "The Switch in Campaign Giving" indicated that in the 1964 presidential election, President Lyndon B. Johnson had been treated more favorably by members of the influential Business Council than had his opponent, Senator Barry Goldwater.[29] Another *Fortune* survey indicates significant changes in the partisan voting behavior of corporate managers. Of a sample consisting of one hundred ranking officers—either the chairman or the president—drawn from three hundred of the largest U.S. corporations, nearly one-third (29) had shifted party loyalties between 1960 and 1964. While in 1960, 89 officers had voted for Vice-President Richard M. Nixon and only 11 for Senator John F. Kennedy, in 1964 only 60 voted for Senator Goldwater while 40 supported President Johnson (there were no switches to the Republican side).[30]

Although this change in 1964 was perhaps more a function of the candidates involved than a radical switch in party commitment, it appears likely that the almost monolithic quality of Republican support by business circles has been broken, unless current policies of the Democratic Party should be so drastically reversed as to utterly antagonize corporate interests.

Significantly, in 1968, despite the electoral victory of Republican Presidential candidate Nixon over the Democratic hopeful, Vice-President Hubert H. Humphrey, Mr. Humphrey had significant support from corporate leaders. While Mr. Nixon received the votes and financial contributions of a large majority of business managers, nearly 1,000 businessmen, including the top executives of some of the nation's largest corporations, were members of Businessmen for Humphrey.[31] Notable among Mr. Humphrey's supporters were Henry Ford II, chairman, Ford Motor Company; Thomas J. Watson, Jr., chairman, International Business Machines; Edgar F. Kaiser, chairman, Kaiser Industries; G. William Miller, president, Textron; James J. Ling, chairman, Ling-Tempco-Vought; former Commerce Secretary, John T. Connor, president, Allied Chemicals; C. Peter McColough, president, Xerox; and Robert E. Slater, president, John Hancock Insurance. At least one of these pro-Humphrey executives had supported Mr. Nixon in 1960. The extent of corporate support for Mr. Humphrey—particularly by corporate leaders who had backed President Johnson in 1964—is all the more impressive when it is recalled that before becoming Vice-President, the Democratic nominee had the reputation of being an "extreme liberal," and many of his political positions aroused the antipathy of virtually the entire business community. On the other hand, his rival, Mr. Nixon, had been closely aligned with business throughout his political career. The 1968 White House race suggests that the departure of some leading corporate executives from Republican ranks in 1964 was more than a one-election defection and that the era of virtual fealty by big business to Republicanism had ended.

This conclusion is reinforced by the growing interdependence in the American economy, discussed earlier, which has confronted businessmen with the necessity of living and working with national administrations which, until the narrow Republican victory in 1968, had been—except for the eight-year Eisenhower hiatus—Democratic since 1932. As Robert Engler points out in *The Politics of Oil,*

> despite . . . partisan leanings, the integrated [oil] companies have a long view of politics as one of the instruments of business. They appreciate the worth of maintaining good relationships with each of the major parties.[32]

Moreover, during recent presidential elections, there have been examples of the top executives of a given company "pairing" their political support—one officer favoring the Democratic candidate while the other assisted the Republican nominee. Illustrative of this pairing in either 1964 or 1968 were officials of Ford, Aero-Jet General, Ling-Tempco-Vought, Textron, and John Hancock Insurance. The existence of divided political loyalties among corporate leaders is, of course, not unprecedented. In 1928, for instance, although the large majority of the business leaders of the nation—including many General Motors executives—supported Republican candidate Herbert Hoover, John J. Raskob and Pierre S. Du Pont of G.M. contributed heavily to the presidential campaign of Democrat Alfred E. Smith.[33] Indeed, between 1928 and 1932, Raskob was chairman of the Democratic National Committee. Similarly, top officers of Union Carbide were divided in their political loyalties in 1928. While still not a commonplace, such split allegiances among corporate leaders appear, however, to be more frequent today than at any previous point in our national history.

It has been suggested that, since 1960, the federal government under the Democratic Party, with collaboration of large corporate interests, has embarked upon a "New Economic Policy," which features planned governmental deficits, strong business growth, and no recessions. The consequence of this detente is that "a significant sector (still a minority) of national corporate power has now joined in responsible national government, accepting the Democratic party as the vehicle."[34]   This acceptance exists primarily among managers of large, Eastern, national firms, while the heads of smaller, regionally based firms (particularly outside the East) have retained their traditional Republican commitments.   This dichotomy is in substantial measure a result of the intimacy of the relationship between the federal government and large corporations, frequently to the disadvantage of smaller companies.

Two other factors may still further enhance the increasing bipartisanship on the part of business leaders.   One is the increasing frequency with which positions of corporate leadership are being assumed by men whose political proclivities were, in large measure, shaped by memories of their adolescent or young adult experience with the Great Depression.   Although evidence on this point is limited, managers within this age group appear more favorably disposed toward the Democratic Party than were their fathers.   Since young people who are currently starting their business careers were born during the Second World War and have lived under Democratic administrations most of their lives, affiliation with the Democratic Party by business leaders of the 1980's and 1990's may well be accepted then as a normal state of affairs.   Moreover, while there is disagreement among sociologists regarding the rate of social mobility present in American society, there is little question that technological training has increasingly become a prerequisite for business leadership and that individuals of lower socioeconomic origins have tended toward such training.[35]   As highly trained individuals with more diverse origins assume positions of leadership, they are likely to be more flexible in their political attitudes than are the present generation of business leaders, who are, however, in turn, politically more flexible than their predecessors.

A second factor has contributed to the growth of business bipartisanship—the conscious efforts made in recent years by Democratic administrations for rapprochement with the corporate community.   Unlike the policies of either guarded neutrality or muted hostility toward business that characterized Democratic administrations earlier in this century, both President Kennedy and President Johnson actively solicited business support. Indeed, one of the ironies of the 1962 steel price increase controversy was that President Kennedy had striven to achieve cordial relations with industry. For example, on one occasion during the early days of his administration, the President remarked to the National Industrial Conference Board,

> We know that your success and ours are intertwined—that you have facts and know-how that we need. Whatever past differences may have existed, we seek more than an attitude of truce, more than a treaty—we seek the spirit of a full-fledged alliance.[36]

Although the appointments of Robert S. McNamara (president of Ford) and Douglas Dillon (Dillon, Read and Company) to the cabinet were in partial measure motivated by this desire, subsequent events destroyed the brief interlude of cordiality that President Kennedy enjoyed with business. Upon assuming office, President Johnson sought to mend the administration's political fences in the industrial sector. His efforts were so successful that *Fortune* quotes one Wall Street man as describing the President as "the first President during my lifetime who really understands business."[37]

One manifestation of this increased corporate bipartisan emphasis warrants special mention—the sponsorship by companies of nonpartisan (as a practical matter, bipartisan) electoral activities. In recent years, many firms have participated in nonpartisan political campaign fund-raising activities designed to encourage employees to contribute to political parties and candidates. An ECO survey of 114 leading corporations indicates that 45 firms had such programs in 1964 as opposed to 22 in 1960.[38] Among the participating firms were Atlantic Refining, Boeing, American Telephone and Telegraph, Chase Manhattan Bank, Ford, General Electric, and Union Carbide. Aerojet General, a subsidiary of General Tire and Rubber, has been a leader in nonpartisan fund raising. In 1964, the company raised more than $136,000 for parties and individual candidates, up from

$60,000 in 1960. Contributions were divided almost equally between the two major parties.[39]

While political fund raising is the primary nonpartisan activity carried on by corporations, some firms also conduct voter-registration drives and sponsor plant and office visits by political candidates. Although the number of firms participating in nonpartisan activities will probably increase, many firms will continue to shy away from such participation because of an unwillingness to assist people who are not likely to support the company's interests. This latter prospect cannot, however, detract from the fact that by the mid-1960's, more corporations were engaging in nonpartisan ventures than would have been considered possible at the close of World War II.

The developments discussed in this section are significant because they indicate that both the Democratic leadership and influential segments of the business community have become willing to accept the necessity to abandon the stereotyped thinking that had contributed to a seemingly congenital hostility between the Democratic Party and industry during most of this century. As a result, corporate political activity has become less ideological and more pragmatic.

INTRACOMPANY ACTIVITIES

The final trend associated with corporate political involvement since the end of World War II (and particularly after the mid-1950's) has been the concerted emphasis placed by firms upon intracompany political activities, notably political education programs. These internal activities include formal political instruction through meetings and seminar courses, communications to employees by means of company house organs and other written media, encouragement of employees to seek public office, and the organization and conduct of the nonpartisan activities that were discussed in the previous section. Such programs are designed to impart political lore, to inform employees of the issues, and to energize employees to political endeavors—particularly at the grass-roots level, where such endeavors may help to create a favorable political environment for the firm. In most companies, the coordination of internal activities has been a primary responsibility of governmental relations or political affairs departments, and often constitutes between a quarter and a half of the work load of these units.

While intracompany political activities are not completely novel—a generation ago Robert Brady noted the existence of corporate endeavors in the area of political education[40]—the magnitude and variety of current efforts are unparalleled. A study of corporate public affairs activities released by the National Industrial Conference Board in mid-1968 indicates that 53 per cent of 1,033 companies surveyed offer some form of political education program. The 553 firms that provided political education were almost equally divided among those presenting formal in-plant courses (278) and those relying upon informal instruction conducted by means of printed materials and occasional oral or film presentations (275). Of the corporations that had formal programs, 77 conducted them on a "continuous basis"; 109, a "couple of times" yearly; and 90, "once during the past two years."[41] In most instances, company political education activities are of recent origin. Of 76 (out of 113) corporations which responded affirmatively to an ECO inquiry regarding whether they "have a political education program," 64 firms indicated that they had begun their programs since 1958.[42]

Significantly, business firms no longer view such intracompany activities as surreptitious ventures, but, rather, as legitimate pursuits to be acknowledged to shareholders and to citizenry alike. This new feeling of legitimacy associated with corporate internal political endeavors is probably due in part to the concerted efforts of organizations such as the United States Chamber of Commerce and ECO, which urge upon corporate leaders the civic duty of companies to engage in such activities. Thus a feeling of community responsibility has been coupled with an underlying sense of political necessity to convince managers of the need for intracorporation political activities.

Managers who are entrusted with the direction of political education programs are quick to reject the suggestion that the programs are designed to sell employees a company bill of goods;

however, they are generally and admittedly based on the hope
and the intention that the efforts will incline employees toward
sympathy with the firm's positions on public matters (particularly taxes and government spending) and, thereby, will create
a more favorable political environment for corporate operations.
The emphasis of these programs is, therefore, on local grass-roots
issues and participation. The benefits potentially accruing to a
firm as a result of its political education activities were recently
suggested by one corporate leader. He reported:

> For a long time at Caterpillar [Tractor Co.], we have encour-
> aged our people who may be so inclined to participate in poli-
> tics. As a result, we have among our employees, mayors of
> several different communities, a great many members of city
> councils and school boards, a state representative, and many,
> many others directly participating in government. Surely there
> is no better way to have the businessman's voice heard than for
> the businessman himself to be the politician.[43]

Although company programs usually are assertedly nonpartisan,
the tone and format of some have cast doubt upon the credi-
bility of this claim. Some programs have had a distinct bias
favoring the Republican Party; for example, a film presented
in one program began with a talk by the then Vice-President
Richard M. Nixon explaining the necessity for political involvement. Firms also vary in policy as to which employees are eli-
gible to participate in these programs. While most corporations
permit employees on all levels of the work force to participate,
some restrict attendance to supervisory and salaried personnel.[44]
Presumably, in these situations, the company considers employees in higher positions to be either more receptive to the
positions asserted in the program or more influential in the community at large. Although there are, of course, exceptions, internal political efforts have been noticeably unsuccessful in mo-
tivating middle-level management to actual political endeavors
on the local or state level.[45] Probably the primary contribution
of these education programs has been to develop on the part of
white-collar and managerial-level employees a greater appreciation of and identification with company interests.

SUMMATION

In this chapter we have examined four salient characteristics of corporate political participation since the conclusion of World War II. These are (1) the patent and self-conscious nature of corporate involvement, (2) the increase in corporate emphasis upon independent political activity and the attendant decrease in reliance upon general business and trade organizations, (3) the growth in the bipartisan emphasis of corporate political activities, and (4) an unprecedented concentration of attention on intracompany political activities designed to create a favorable environment for the company in the political arena. These changes in the pattern of corporate involvement must be considered in the context of the significant development discussed in the first half of this chapter—the emergence of a mixed or interdependent political economy in the United States in which the federal government has become the single most important economic participant and in which business corporations, in virtually all aspects of their operations, must deal with government.

Underlying each of the four changes in corporate political activity is the desire on the part of business managers to deal more effectively with public authority. No other single factor has functioned more effectively to necessitate and to legitimate corporate political involvement than the growth in size and importance of all levels of government. The irony in this situation will not be lost upon those persons who are opposed to the corporate presence in the political arena.

NOTES

[1] 15 U.S.C. § 1021 (1946).

[2] The political history of the Employment Act is found in Stephen

Kemp Bailey, *Congress Makes a Law* (New York: Columbia University Press, 1950). Business opposition to the act is discussed particularly in Chap. 7.

[3]Arthur Selwyn Miller, *The Supreme Court and American Capitalism* (New York: The Free Press, 1968), pp. 87–88.

[4]Walter W. Heller, *New Dimensions of Political Economy* (New York: W. W. Norton & Company, Inc., Publishers, 1967), pp. 16, 17.

[5]A perceptive analysis of the development and future of governmental economic planning in the United States is found in Eugene V. Rostow, *Planning for Freedom* (New Haven, Conn.: Yale University Press, 1959).

[6]*Hearings, Amendment to the Administrative Expense Act of 1946*, U.S. Congress, House of Representatives, Committee on Government Operations, 85th Cong., 1st Sess. (Washington: U.S. Government Printing Office, 1957), p. 2.

[7]*Report, Economic Impact of Federal Procurement*, U.S. Congress, Subcommittee on Federal Procurement and Regulation of the Joint Economic Committee, 89th Cong., 1st Sess. (Washington: U.S. Government Printing Office, July 1965), p. 1.

[8]The figures and statistics given in this paragraph were drawn from the following sources: *Background Material on Economic Impact of Federal Procurement—1965*, U.S. Congress, Subcommittee on Federal Procurement and Regulation of the Joint Economic Committee, 89th Cong., 1st Sess. (Washington: U.S. Government Printing Office, 1965), p. 10 (Table 8); President of the United States, *Economic Report of the President, Together with the Annual Report of the Council of Economic Advisers* (Washington: U.S. Government Printing Office, 1968), pp. 209 (Table B-1), 280–281 (Table B-60); Federal Reserve Bank of San Francisco, "Pentagon Faces '69," *Monthly Review* (March 1968), pp. 59–63; *The Federal Budget—Its Impact on the Economy* (New York: National Industrial Conference Board, Inc., 1967), pp. 14–18; and "Defense Orders Start to Peak Out," *Business Week*, October 28, 1967, pp. 44–46.

[9]*Legislators and the Lobbyists*, 2d ed. (Washington, D.C.: Congressional Quarterly, Inc., 1968), p. 56.

[10]The role of the federal government as an allocator of raw materials is examined in Glenn H. Snyder, *Stockpiling Strategic Materials* (San Francisco: Chandler Publishing Company, 1966).

[11]The figures in this paragraph were drawn from "Totting Up

the Cost of Foreign Aid Cuts," *Business Week*, August 3, 1968, pp. 26–27.

[12]For a discussion of the concepts of "relative deprivation" in the context of Negro expectations, see Thomas Pettigrew, "White-Negro Confrontations" in Eli Ginzberg, *The Negro Challenge to the Business Community* (New York: McGraw-Hill Book Company, 1964), pp. 40–41.

[13]The figures and the statistics given in this paragraph were drawn from President of the United States, *Economic Report* (1968), pp. 209 (Table B-1), 280–281 (Table B-60).

[14]V. O. Key, Jr., *Politics, Parties, and Pressure Groups*, 5th ed. (New York: Thomas Y. Crowell Co., 1964), p. 84.

[15]For an interesting scalar representation of the allocation of social functions among public and private organizations in various countries, see Robert A. Dahl and Charles E. Lindblom, *Politics, Economics, and Welfare* (New York: Harper & Row, Publishers, 1953), pp. 3–24. See also the comments of Harlan Cleveland's "Introduction," in Harlan Cleveland and Harold D. Lasswell, *Ethics and Bigness: Scientific, Academic, Religious, Political and Military* (New York: Harper & Row, Publishers, 1962), p. xxv.

[16]L. R. Boulware, "Politics—The Businessmen's Biggest Job in 1958," *Labor Law Journal*, IX, No. 8 (August 1958), 587–94, and "Why Politics Needs Business in '66," *Nation's Business* (June 1966), 42–45, 76, 78, 80, 82.

[17]Reprinted from an address by Henry Ford II, delivered at the Presidents Conference on Public Affairs, Chamber of Commerce of the United States, Detroit, Michigan, January 5, 1961.

[18]Statement of Robert L. Humphrey, President, Business-Industrial Political Action Committee (BIPAC), *Hearings*, on H.R. 15317 and related bills, U.S. Congress, House of Representatives, Subcommittee on Elections of the Committee on House Administration, 89th Cong., 2d Sess. (Washington, D.C.: U.S. Government Printing Office, 1966), p. 119.

[19]*Hearings*, on H.R. 15317 . . . , pp. 119–20.

[20]Herbert E. Alexander, *Financing the 1964 Election* (Princeton, N. J.: Citizens' Research Foundation, 1966), p. 99.

[21]Reprinted from *Let's Look at ECO* (Washington, D.C.: Effective Citizens Organization, Inc., n.d.), p. 3. Before late 1966,

ECO was known solely as "The Effective Citizens Organization, Inc." In that year, the Board of Directors passed a resolution prefixing "Public Affairs Council" to the former name. In explaining its action, the Board stated:

> The reasons for this change are obvious: businessmen generally are in agreement that they must be "effective citizens"; public affairs is accepted as a new dimension of corporate responsibility; and ECO—as the motivational and educational organization for this corporate activity—should clarify its function to the business community.

(Reprinted from *Program*, Public Affairs Council, Effective Citizens Organization, Inc., Roundtable for Public Affairs Officers, November 28–29, 1966, The Mayflower Hotel, Washington, D.C., p. 3.)

[22]From *Program*, Public Affairs Council, Effective Citizens Organization, Inc., Roundtable for Public Affairs Officers, November 28–29, 1966, The Mayflower Hotel, Washington, D.C., p. 5.

[23]*Directory of Public Affairs Officers*, 7th ed. (Washington, D.C.: Effective Citizens Organization, Inc., 1966).

[24]David J. Galligan, *Politics and the Businessman* (New York: Pitman Publishing Corporation, 1964), pp. 103–15.

[25]*The Role of Business in Public Affairs*, Studies in Public Affairs, No. 2 (New York: National Industrial Conference Board, Inc., 1968), p. 8.

[26]For accounts of these activities, see Frank J. Prial, "A 'New' NAM?" *The Wall Street Journal*, May 31, 1966, p. 1, col. 6; and "NAM Is Playing by a New Set of Rules," *Business Week*, December 17, 1966, pp. 114–18.

[27]Richard W. Gable, "NAM: Influential Lobby or Kiss of Death?" *Journal of Politics*, XV, No. 2 (May 1953), 254–73.

[28]Key, *Politics, Parties . . .* , p. 98.

[29]Herbert E. Alexander and Harold B. Meyers, "The Switch in Campaign Giving," *Fortune*, LXXII, No. 5 (November 1965), 170.

[30]Edmund K. Faltermayer, "What Business Wants from Lyndon Johnson," *Fortune*, LXXI, No. 2 (February 1965), 122, 125.

[31]The information in this paragraph is drawn from the following sources: "Nixon and Business," *The Wall Street Journal*, October 16, 1968, p. 1, col. 6; "Humphrey Forces List Edgar Kaiser," *Oakland Tribune*, September 24, 1968, p. 6, cols. 5 and 6; "Businessmen in the News: Who Is for Whom in the Election," *Fortune*, LXXVII, No.

5 (October 1968), 46; "Businessmen Vote for Nixon," *Business Week,* October 5, 1968, pp. 31–33; and "Business 'Angels' Place Their Bets," *Business Week,* May 18, 1968, pp. 108–10, 112. See also, Terry Robards, "Poll of Executives Puts Nixon Ahead," *The New York Times,* October 27, 1968, p. 1, col. 2.

[32]Robert Engler, *The Politics of Oil* (Chicago: Phoenix Books, The University of Chicago Press, 1967), p. 366.

[33]Louise Overacker, *Money in Elections* (New York: The Macmillan Company, 1932), p. 157.

[34]David T. Bazelon, "Big Business and the Democrats," *Commentary,* XXXIX, No. 5 (May 1965), 39, 44.

[35]See, for example, Seymour Martin Lipset and Reinhard Bendix, *Social Mobility in Industrial Society* (Berkeley, Calif.: University of California Press, 1964), Chaps. 3, 4; *The Big Business Executive 1964: A Study of His Social and Educational Background* (New York: Scientific American, Inc., 1965), pp. 2–4; and Joseph Ben David, "The Growth of the Professions and the Class System," in Reinhard Bendix and Seymour Martin Lipset, *Class, Status and Power,* 2d ed. (New York: The Free Press, 1966), pp. 459–72.

[36]Quoted in Grant McConnell, *Steel and the Presidency, 1962* (New York: W. W. Norton & Company, Inc., Publishers, 1963), p. 51.

[37]Quoted in "Editorial: The Big Man with a Little Voice," *Fortune,* LXXI, No. 2 (February 1965), 115, 116.

[38]Public Affairs Survey" (Washington, D.C.: Effective Citizens Organization, Inc., June 1965), p. 5 (mimeographed).

[39]Alexander, *Financing the 1964 Election,* p. 105.

[40]Robert A. Brady, *Business as a System of Power* (New York: Columbia University Press, 1943), p. 301.

[41]*The Role of Business . . . ,* p. 22.

[42]Reprinted from "Public Affairs Survey" (Washington, D.C.: Effective Citizens Organization, Inc., June 1965), pp. 3–4.

[43]Reprinted from William H. Franklin, "Government—with or without Business" (Speech delivered before the Illinois State Chamber of Commerce, Chicago, Illinois, October 21, 1966).

[44]The 1968 National Industrial Conference Board study indicates that of 278 firms offering formal political education programs, 161 offer them to all employees; 73, to supervisory employees; 65, to salaried employees; and 1, to hourly employees. (Responses totaled

more than 278 because of multiple answers by some respondents.)
The Role of Business . . . , p. 22.

[45]Andrew Hacker and Joel D. Aberbach, "Businessmen in Politics," *Law and Contemporary Problems*, XXVII, No. 2 (Spring 1962), 266–79. Compare Galligan, *Politics and* . . . , pp. 67–102.

Chapter Five

Nature and Extensiveness of Corporate Political Activities

E arlier in this book, we differentiated *governmental* from *electoral* corporate political activities. The line between the two types of political involvement is imprecise, since occasionally a specific political activity by a corporation fits equally well into either category; however, the distinction is not without analytical utility. Governmental activities, it will be recalled, include both political involvement intended to influence the formulation and execution of policy by governmental decision makers and efforts designed to create a public opinion favorable to the corporation's political goals. Electoral activities center around the selection and support of candidates or of issues that come before the public.

CORPORATE EMPHASIS ON
GOVERNMENTAL POLITICS

While corporations participate actively in both categories of activities, primary attention today, as in the past, is given to governmental politics. Of the three reasons for this emphasis, the principal one is based on the episodic nature of the electoral process. Although the selection of public officials is of great importance to business firms, elections for the many different local, state, and national offices take place only periodically—at specified times. Consequently, while electoral activity may assume great importance during certain periods of the years, at other times there is little to be done.

On the other hand, the wide range of governmental operations is continuous. Legislative bodies meet, administrative agencies oversee business operations, governmental units award contracts, courts decide cases, public officials threaten investigations, competing social interests pursue their objectives, and public opinion must be cultivated throughout the year. The governmental process is ongoing and, as we saw in the preceding chapter, affects many aspects of corporate activity in our mixed economy. Since most political decisions that are of importance to the corporation occur outside the electoral process, business firms naturally concentrate their activities in the much broader arena of governmental politics.

The second reason for the emphasis on governmental politics is that corporations have historically been more effective in accomplishing their governmental objectives than in achieving their electoral goals. In the electoral arena, corporations must compete with many and various social interests—including ethnic and religious groups, membership organizations, and labor unions—which command varying degrees of support as a result of a network of voter loyalties. "Members" of the corporation do not, in the same fashion, identify with the political goals of the firm; for shareholders and employees, the importance of corporate affiliation is usually secondary to other forms of self-identification. Thus corporations, unlike traditional interest groups, cannot hope to deliver the vote, which also explains the relative lack of influence they have had with the political power brokers who historically have controlled the selection of candidates in many large urban centers.

On the other hand, organization, financial resources, access and prestige, economic hegemony, and social patronage—assets that corporations possess in ample degree—are quite effective in the area of governmental politics where votes are not crucial. Moreover, in their efforts to influence particular aspects of governmental decision making, business firms often encounter a narrower range of competition than in the electoral arena. While the matter of airline routes is of great importance to United Air Lines, it is of little concern, for example, to the Ancient Order of Hibernians or the Anti-Defamation League. The likely competitor is a clearly recognizable industry opponent or consumer organization whose hostility can be predicted and against whom the corporation can concentrate its political energies in a narrowly defined "sphere of influence." Accordingly, governmental politics offers opportunity for greater political efficacy than is possible in the more diffuse realm of electoral activity.

The final reason for concentration on governmental activities relates to the existence of legal restrictions upon corporate electoral participation. Corporations are prohibited by Section 610 of the United States Criminal Code from making contributions or expenditures in connection with federal primary or general elections.[1] More than half the states have adopted similar legislation banning corporate moneys in state elections. Accordingly, significant aspects of potential corporate electoral involvement have been declared illegal, and some business leaders are reluctant to engage their companies even in those activities that are clearly permissible (for example, expressing partisan views to members of the "corporate family" and advertising in political journals). Some corporate managers tend, moreover, to be highly secretive in their individual electoral activities in order to forestall possible criticism of their organizations. While legal restrictions have been largely ineffective in that corporate electoral involvement has been not eliminated but merely driven underground, such involvement is nonetheless surrounded by an unfortunate aura of illegitimacy.[2]

Since corporate governmental activities are subject to virtually no legislative restrictions—with the minor exception of registration of full-time lobbyists under the Federal Regulation of Lobbying Act of 1946[3]—corporations are far less circumscribed in their governmental politics than in electoral pursuits. Moreover, this involvement does not suffer the taint of illegitimacy discussed above. It is considered proper for corporations, along with other social groups, to use the pluralistic political process to pursue their legislative or administrative interests, as long as they abide by the recognized rules of the political game.

The net result of these three factors is that corporations have emphasized and, for the foreseeable future, will continue to emphasize governmental over electoral political activities (although the latter category of endeavors has hardly been neglected). We shall now examine in detail the forms of corporate governmental and electoral politics.

CORPORATE GOVERNMENTAL POLITICS

Corporate governmental politics includes a wide variety of activities which involve business firms with diverse aspects of the public decision-making process and span the executive, legislative, administrative, and judicial branches of government. Corporate governmental endeavors are also directed at the nurturing of a favorable political climate among the general public through the use of the mass media for public-relations purposes. Some of the more important forms of corporate governmental activities are examined in this section.

TRADE-ASSOCIATION ACTIVITIES

While, as mentioned earlier, over-all corporate dependence on business and trade associations has declined, business firms continue to maintain membership in, contribute to, and provide leadership for business and trade associations. These organizations represent corporate interests before governmental bodies, and they attempt to create a favorable public image for the business community. Broad-gauged groups such as the Chamber of Commerce of the United States, the National Association of Manufacturers (NAM), and the Committee for Economic Development (CED) concern themselves with such public issues of a general business interest as taxation, fiscal and monetary policy, inflation, governmental regulation, and labor relations. Corporations tend to rely on these groups primarily for general back-up support in political areas where they do not choose to participate actively on a unilateral basis. Business associations serve valuable functions in providing firms with background materials on a myriad of issues and by acting as the *"advance guard* for the business community in areas which need to be tested."[4] We have already examined the important role in energizing corporations to individual political action of general-purpose business associations, particularly the Chamber of Commerce of the United States, and of newer, functionally specific organizations, such as the Public Affairs Council, Effective Citizens' Organization, Inc. (ECO), and the Business and Industry Political Action Committee (BIPAC).

Frequently designated as the "liberal" business group, the CED has in many respects been unique among national business associations. The purpose of the CED, which was established during World War II, is

> to arrive through conscientious and objective study at economic policies within the framework of our free enterprise system and our democratic form of government which will redound to the benefit of the general welfare through maintaining high employment and economic stability.[5]

In pursuing these objectives, the CED has, in the opinion of most observers, successfully eschewed partisanship and has emphasized research on the crucial economic issues of the day. Its policy statements, which are frequently the result of CED-sponsored studies conducted by nationally recognized independent scholars, are attentively read by public officials of both parties. The organization restricts its lobbying activities to the issuance of these statements and to testimony by its officers. Alone among business groups, it favored passage of and suggested several provisions in the Employment Act of 1946. The

CED has not concerned itself either with activating corporations to political involvement in the manner of the United States Chamber and ECO or with developing a favorable public opinion of the business community. The importance of the CED is enhanced by its trustees—never exceeding 150 during the first 15 years of its existence, and of them, 38 have held high elective or appointive offices in the federal government, many during the Eisenhower administration.[6]   Not surprisingly, the leadership of CED has consistently included representatives of such large national concerns as Crown Zellerbach, Studebaker, Eastman Kodak, Ford, B. F. Goodrich, and Procter and Gamble.

Turning now to the activities of the narrowly based industry trade associations, groups such as the American Iron and Steel Institute, the National Electrical Manufacturers Association, the American Petroleum Institute, and the National Association of Retail Druggists seek to promote specific industry interests.   These associations are particularly effective in presenting to governmental bodies a united front on issues of public policy.   Their tasks include promoting legislation favorable to the industry, influencing the enforcement of existing legislative and administrative standards, safeguarding the industry from hostile activities by competing social and economic groups, and molding public opinion.   A few examples of industry-group activities will illustrate their functions.

For years, the American Textile Manufacturers' Institute has striven to narrow the import quotas on foreign textiles.   The Institute's campaign has included public relations programs as well as lobbying within Congress to encourage the passage of legislation limiting imports.

The Pharmaceutical Manufacturers' Association has taken up the cudgels for the drug industry against the Food and Drug Administration (FDA) by opposing federal efforts to regulate the quality and the cost of drugs.   A recent FDA Commissioner, Dr. James L. Goddard, paid the organization a backhanded compliment regarding its efforts in opposition to the agency's regulatory attempts when he remarked that the "PMA is a very effective lobby group in my opinion.   They make their presence felt."[7]   The Association's efforts attracted particular attention in early 1968, when it lobbied against FDA efforts to remove from the market drugs that were of little or no medical value.

Another industry group, the Association of American Railroads, has long been engaged in a bitter conflict with the truckers (primarily the American Trucking Association), water transport carriers, and the airlines. At issue are alleged inequities in the pattern of federal financial support of non-rail carriers and attempts by these carriers to capture shares of the transportation market that have traditionally been held by the railroads.

The conflict between the truckers and the railroads became particularly bitter during the early 1950's. The Eastern Railroads Presidents Conference, a regional organization, conducted an extensive public relations campaign in Pennsylvania designed to prevent the passage of certain highway legislation. The bill, favored by the Pennsylvania Motor Truck Association, would have increased the weight limits of trucks using state highways. While the ostensible purpose of the campaign was to protect highways from surface damage resulting from continual usage by heavy motor vehicles, the real concern of the railroads was the concerted attempt by the truckers to increase their share of the profitable long-distance freight-hauling business. Although the governor vetoed the bill passed by the Pennsylvania legislature, three and a half years later his successor signed similar legislation into law. The dispute eventually reached the United States Supreme Court, which refused to support contentions of the truckers that the railroads' public relations campaign constituted a conspiracy to destroy their long-haul freight business, in violation of the Sherman and Clayton anti-trust acts. The Court was of the opinion that to restrict public relations activities by trade associations (or others) would interfere with the normal political process and with the constitutional right of a citizen to petition the government.[8]

Most trade-association activities are undertaken by organizations that have been on the scene for a number of years. Occasionally, short-lived industry groups are formed, principally to represent member corporations on a single pressing issue. When Congress was considering the renewal of the Reciprocal Trade Act in 1953, a number of ad hoc groups emerged, only to disappear when the legislative controversy had died down.[9] On occasion, ostensibly industry-wide groups may be merely façades, behind which a few corporations pursue their political interests.

LEGISLATIVE AND ADMINISTRATIVE CONTACTS

Company officials or their representatives often testify before governmental bodies and before officials who make decisions affecting the firm. Legislative and administrative hearings are a major point of contact between the corporation and these decision makers. Such a hearing provides an opportunity for business firms to present their case to the appropriate public officials and serves as a forum in which a company may seek to enlist public opinion and support for its position.

In addition to activities before governmental bodies, corporations devote considerable effort to contacting individuals who occupy legislative, administrative, and executive positions. This process, which the public ordinarily calls lobbying, consists of presenting a company's position on given issues; attempting to obtain support for those positions; providing to sympathetic officials information that will be helpful in obtaining favorable action; convincing the disinclined of the error of their ways; and selling the firm's goods and services in such a manner as to facilitate the awarding of a critical contract, license, or subsidy. The wide range of corporate dealings with individual governmental officials constitutes basically a process of communication —communication intended to generate favorable governmental decisions. Generally, the emphasis of these contacts is on information and advocacy, not pressure. At least in the legislative context, governmental officials generally view these efforts as being helpful.[10]

PUBLIC RELATIONS: THE "NEW LOBBY"

Corporations attempt to generate public support for governmental action favorable to their interests through modern communications media. Firms continually seek to enhance their "image," in order to make the public more favorably disposed toward positions taken in the companies' relations with government. The older notion of "the public be damned" has clearly given way to an attitude of "the public be cultivated."[11] A number of years ago, this type of activity was explained as follows:

> When a destructive bill is pending in a legislature it has to be dealt with in a way to get results. I am not debating that. But to depend, year after year, upon the usual political expedients for stopping hostile legislation is shortsightedness. In the long run isn't it better and surer to lay a groundwork with the people back home who have the votes, so that proposals of this character are not popular with them, rather than depend upon stopping such proposals when they get up to the legislature or commission?[12]

Public utilities have long followed this advice with great success. Among the earliest of these corporate practitioners was the Bell system. Realizing even before World War I the inevitability of governmental regulation, the Bell management under the leadership of Theodore N. Vail sought to reduce the potential negative effects of regulation by enlisting public support.

> Through steady emphasis on efficient and economical service and through frequent reports to its shareholders, it strove to demonstrate a conviction on the part of management that, "We feel our obligation to the general public as strongly as to our investing public, or to our own personal interests."[13]

The efforts of "Ma Bell" have been so successful that in 1965 when the Federal Communications Commission (FCC) started its first investigation of the rate structure of American Telephone and Telegraph Company (the parent company of the Bell system) in 27 years, there was considerable public opposition to the FCC's action.

Similarly, private power and light companies have engaged in extensive public relations activities to obtain support for their rate increase requests and to prevent the spread of publicly owned power. For example, Northern California customers of the Pacific Gas and Electric Company receive with their billings a monthly newsletter, which frequently extols the virtues of private power, reports on services to the public that it renders through its activities, and bemoans its tax burden to the federal, state, and local governments. Reference has already been made to the battle royal between the Eastern Railroad Presidents Conference, under the leadership of the Pennsylvania Railroad, and the Pennsylvania Motor Truck Association over the permissible weight of trucks on state roads. Both sides engaged New York public relations firms to conduct campaigns which involved the extensive use of mass media, the drumming up of grass-roots support, and the planting of advertisements and articles supposedly originating from citizens' groups. It has been estimated that the fees paid by the combatants to their respective public relations firms reached an aggregate sum exceeding $1 million.[14]

Industrial corporations engage in similar public relations activities. For example, the automobile industry conducted an extensive publicity campaign protesting the standards proposed by officials of the Auto Safety Advisory Council in accordance with the National Traffic and Motor Vehicle Safety Act of 1966.[15] The attack was two-pronged: (1) an effort to convince the public that the industry had already undertaken the essential safety measures; and (2) the reiteration of charges that proposed standards would be economically disastrous to the automobile industry, since price increases would be inevitable, thereby placing domestic producers at a serious competitive disadvantage with foreign automobile makers. This attack impaired the efforts of the Council to effect some of its proposed safety standards.

Similarly, members of the lumber industry have opposed through extensive newspaper advertising the efforts of conservationist groups to secure passage of legislation setting aside lumber-rich acreage along the California coast for a Redwood National Park. Proclaiming "Yes, America's majestic redwoods have already been saved!" a full-page *The Wall Street Journal* ad sponsored by the Georgia-Pacific Company, the nation's second largest lumber firm, castigated the arguments of supporters of the redwoods park as "distortions and innuendo."[16]

Thiokol Chemical Corporation, a maker of aerospace products, surveyed public opinion on the subject of the government's program to land a man on the moon by 1970. In explaining the company's reason for the survey, a Thiokol spokesman stated, "The future of the space program hinges on public reaction, and we want to keep our finger on the pulse of the public."[17] The results of the survey were distributed to the press and to interested persons in Washington.

In addition to the practices discussed above, corporations engage in other forms of public relations activities. Frequently used techniques of public indoctrination include public-service advertising that contains selected maxims of political and economic thought and the dissemination of literature to schools, churches, and customers. The enlisting or manufacturing of grass-roots communications to public officials by employees, shareholders, or townspeople is another form of public relations activity. Finally, corporate leaders make policy statements regarding matters of public concern which, while private and individual in character, carry the imprimatur of company involvement.

V. O. Key, Jr., referred to the extensive utilization of public relations techniques by corporations for political purposes as the New Lobby.[18] The term is appropriate since, in essence, mass media are used for political purposes in an effort by business firms to inform and to influence the public at large, just as they have sought to inform and to influence governmental officials and bodies through the use of more traditional lobbying techniques. On occasion, corporations have been accused of being overzealous in their political proselytizing. For example, the American Broadcasting Company received unfavorable press comment for allegedly attempting to control the news, in connection with its ill-fated merger negotiations with International Telephone and Telegraph Company. Such criticism, is, however, relatively rare. On the whole, corporations have been almost as successful in selling their political views as they have been in merchandising their products. Their job is made easier because the publishing and broadcasting firms operating the mass media are themselves large corporations and thus generally are sympathetic to business viewpoints. Consequently, the political tone of the media does not even approximately reflect the distribution of attitudes and opinions in the society as a whole.

GOVERNMENT SERVICE BY
BUSINESS LEADERS

Another type of corporate governmental activity takes the form of service by corporate leaders in official governmental posts, either on a leave basis or while actively involved in company activities. At the federal cabinet level, the Departments of Commerce; Defense; Health, Education and Welfare; and the Treasury have been headed in recent years by former corporate executives on leave from their companies. At a lower level, corporate managers serve in staff or line positions in executive and administrative departments. This form of participation is also pronounced within state government, although the firms represented tend to be both smaller and locally based. For example, Governor Ronald Reagan of California relied heavily on business executives when he filled cabinet and subcabinet positions and appointed heads of important state administrative agencies at the beginning of his term of office in 1967.

We have already mentioned the services rendered by corporate officials as part-time governmental consultants and advisers. The wartime practice of utilizing businessmen either as uncompensated consultants to administrative and executive departments or as members of the numerous advisory committees is now a firmly established aspect of the Washington scene. Ranging from the new autonomous Business Council (formerly called the Business Advisory Council), which was originally formed as an advisory group to the Department of Commerce, on down through the elaborate structure of committees in the Departments of Commerce, Defense, Treasury, and the Interior, to the various administrative agencies, business leaders are called upon as consultants, advisers, and, occasionally, part-time administrators. The Business Council includes the most important business leaders in the country; among others, Ralph J. Cordiner of General Electric, Albert L. Nickerson of Mobil Oil, and Roger

Blough of U.S. Steel have served as chairmen. In a recent year, its approximately 160-man membership included the chairman or president of the top two automobile makers, of two of the three leading steel firms, of two of the Big Three in chemicals, and of two of the top four rubber producers.

Between 5,000 and 6,000 committees in the federal government are concerned with virtually every aspect of governmental activities that relate to industry. Many advisory committees are called on during emergency situations; for example, the Interior Department summoned industry members of the Foreign Petroleum Supply Committee to a meeting in Washington during the Arab-Israeli conflict of 1967. The committee, consisting of representatives of twenty American-owned international oil companies, was asked to develop emergency plans for increasing domestic oil output if necessary as a result of the hostilities.

Former Secretary of Commerce Sinclair Weeks ably presented the rationale underlying the use of advisory committees in an explanation of the functions of the Business and Defense Services Administration within his department. The agency was intended to

> see to it that, while private business, of course, cannot dictate Government policy and plans, it be placed in a position where it can effectively approve or disapprove of the implementation of such policy and plans from the standpoint of their practical workability in everyday industrial operation.[19]

Members of advisory committees have been drawn primarily from the larger firms in given industries; and the committees have been criticized for tending, in their operations, to favor Big Business, because of the unconscious or conscious bias of the business executives. In any event, through participation on such committees, corporate managers and, indirectly, their firms, have been in a position to influence governmental decision making in areas relevant to their operations.

In addition to serving within regular government departments, business managers serve on innumerable federal task forces and commissions. For example, Charles B. Thornton, board chairman of Litton Industries, was a member of the National Advisory Commission on Civil Disorders (the Kerner Commission) appointed by President Johnson, which placed primary blame for domestic racial tensions on white racism. Indeed, in late 1967, President Johnson formed the National Alliance of Businessmen, consisting exclusively of corporate leaders from throughout the nation and headed by Henry Ford II, chairman of Ford Motor; the President's specific objective was the direct involvement of the business community in national efforts to obtain employment for minorities.

A somewhat less publicized type of politically significant relationship between corporate employees and governmental officials results from the collaboration between the federal government and business firms in utilizing science and technology for public purposes. Scientists and engineers from aerospace, electronic, and communication companies work closely—often on a daily basis—with their counterparts in federal agencies such as the National Aeronautics and Space Administration (NASA), the Atomic Energy Commission (AEC), and the Defense Department in planning and developing the spacecraft, satellites, defense systems, and nuclear hardware that seemingly have become integral parts of the American way of life. Through their joint efforts on scientific and technological projects, these corporate and governmental technocrats make important decisions affecting the annual expenditure of billions of dollars of public moneys, as, for example, by determining what programs to present to Congress and by tailoring project specifications to the capabilities of particular private contractors. In addition, certain assumptions about long-term governmental policy are built into these technical decisions. When reified into expensive technological systems, these assumptions become constraints upon public officials determining future domestic and foreign policies.

On the state levels, Governor Reagan of California instituted an interesting, albeit rather unusual, use of corporate executives as governmental consultants and advisers. Early in his administration, the Governor established a task force, consisting of executives of major corporations operating in California, to investigate the operations of state agencies and to recommend changes to improve governmental efficiency. Known as the Governor's Survey on Efficiency and Cost Control, the task force included representatives lent by approximately 250 companies, including such national concerns as Aerojet-General, Atlantic Richfield, Bethlehem Steel, General Motors, and Xerox, and such California-based companies such as Bank of America, California Packing, Crown Zellerbach, Southern Pacific, Pacific Gas and Electric, Kaiser Aluminum and Chemical, and Standard Oil of California.[20] A novel aspect of this task-force operation was that it was financed entirely from private funds, primarily those of the participating firms. The Survey received considerable criticism because of the partisan composition of the task force, the potential conflict of interest posed by the fact that some participants came from corporations closely regulated by the state, and the fact that a number of its major proposals proved unworkable or unwise.

Although this discussion has emphasized the governmental participation by businessmen in administrative or executive capacities, in recent years men who have risen to prominence as corporate leaders have served as members of Congress, particularly of the Senate. Notable examples are Senators Robert S. Kerr, president of Kerr-McGee Oil Industries (Oklahoma); Charles H. Percy, a former board chairman of Bell & Howell (Illinois); Wallace F. Bennett, former president of the National Association of Manufacturers (Utah); and Ralph Flanders, a Vermont toolmaker and Boston banker (Vermont).

CORPORATIONS AND ADMINISTRATIVE AGENCIES

The maintenance of a continuous liaison with governmental agencies charged with the regulation of business activities is an essential form of corporate governmental involvement. It is crucial that cordial agency-corporate relationships be maintained, because of the extensive decision-making authority of regulatory bodies over the firms in a regulated industry with regard to rate making, production allotments, licenses, certificates of convenience, and franchises. Accordingly, corporations devote considerable time and energy in an attempt to cultivate and to constrain their regulators.

Starting with the establishment of the Interstate Commerce Commission (ICC) in 1887, administrative agencies were intended to restrict business practices considered contrary to the "public interest." Historically, however, vigorous regulation has been both transitory and sporadic; and many observers have noted the short-lived periods of regulatory zeal on the part of personnel of an agency, the rapid development of an agency-client relationship between the regulators and the regulated, and the need inherent within the administrative process of accommodation between an agency and its constituents.[21] Indeed, as early as 1892, Attorney General Richard Olney, a prominent corporation lawyer before he became the head of the Justice Department, wrote to a railroad president who had expressed concern over the newly created Interstate Commerce Commission:

> The Commission, as its functions have now been limited by the courts, is, or can be made, of great use to the railroads. It satisfies the popular clamor for a governmental supervision of railroads, at the same time that that supervision is almost entirely nominal. Further, the older such a Commission gets to be, the more inclined it will be found to take the business and railroad view of things. It thus becomes a sort of barrier between the railroad corporations and the people and a sort of protection against hasty and crude legislation hostile to railroad interests. . . . The part of wisdom is not to destroy the Commission but to utilize it.[22]

Olney proved to be a prescient analyst of the ICC's future.

Accommodation may occur from the agency's inception when it attempts to co-opt, or absorb, elements of the client group into the leadership of the policy-determining structure of the agency in order to avert threats to its existence or stability. Examples of this co-optation are found in the relationship between the communication carriers and the Federal Communications Commission, the railroads and the Interstate Commerce Commission, and the airlines and the Civil Aeronautics Board.[23]

In other instances, the influence of constituents over the agency increases with the passage of time. This process has been characterized as a life cycle divided into four periods: gestation, youth, maturity (the process of devitalization), and old age (debility and decline). The first two stages are marked respectively by a public enthusiasm and demand for governmental regulation of an industry and by vigorous efforts on the part of the newly established agency. Subsequently, the following characteristics develop: gradual identification between the administrators and their clientele, consultation with this clientele prior to appointment of high-level administrative officials, service by business executives in tours of duty as regulators, and cooperation between the agency and its clients in securing legislation appropriations for the agency's work.[24] Both the regulators and the regulated often join forces to oppose threatened encroachments by other industry groups or government agencies. For example, the power and jurisdiction of the newly created Department of Transportation were limited partly as a result of collaborative opposition by existing federal agencies and by industry representatives concerned with various aspects of transportation.

The relationship between the recently established National Traffic Safety Agency and the automobile industry provides an interesting case study of the process of agency-business accommodation. Created in 1966 by the National Traffic and Motor Vehicle Safety Act, which unanimously passed both houses of Congress despite strenuous industry opposition, the Agency has from the outset been strongly criticized by the automobile makers. In December 1966, when the Agency issued 23 proposed regulations for industry comment, the automobile producers bitterly attacked the suggested rules on the grounds that production lines might be forced to close down because they could not meet the standards for 1968 cars. When the final standards were announced on January 31, 1967, the Agency withdrew 3 of the 23 proposed standards, modified 8 others, and gave the industry more time to comply with the requirements. At this juncture, the Agency's head safety engineer resigned, terming the new standards "totally inadequate," a mere rubber-stamping of what the industry would have done in the absence of federal standards. Still, industry complaints continued, and several months later the Agency agreed to take under consideration modification of one of the most controversial and significant safety standards—that relating to the construction and padding of car interiors. The automobile industry also instituted a suit challenging the 1968 standards. The Agency, moreover, gave tacit approval to a price increase which would reimburse the manufacturers for the safety equipment.[25]

While the safety-standards controversy was raging, President Johnson named the members of the Auto Safety Advisory Council. In compliance with the requirements of the 1966 act, a bare majority of the members of the Council came from the general public but the remainder were drawn from the ranks of the automobile manufacturers, the car-equipment industry, and the automobile dealers.

While there is evidence that the Agency is currently persisting in its efforts to push the automobile makers into incorporating safety changes more rapidly than they would like, the initial standards were, in the opinion of most observers, disappointingly unrigorous. Hence, although the pattern of industry-agency relations is still in the process of formation, thus far the automobile manufacturers have been able to deal effectively with the new regulatory body.

The accommodation process affords corporations access to and impact upon regulatory agencies concerned with their operations. The extent of this access and impact varies. The size and prestige of a company contribute to a corporation's political efficacy before an administrative body. The influence of a given company or industry group on agency policy is often proportional to the homogeneity of the agency's constituency. Thus, the fewer the combatants and the more uniform their interests, the greater the opportunity for company success. Indeed, because of the inverse relationship between the number, identity of purpose, and strength of the constituents and the consequent independence of the agency, regulatory bodies often attempt to nurture conflict among their clients to prevent any single constituent from becoming too powerful.

In one area of agency activity—rule making—many administrative bodies are required by statute (1) to inform interested parties of the intended issuance of administrative rulings so that they can present their views on the matter, and (2) to receive petitions for the issuance, amendment, or repeal of rulings. The Federal Administrative Procedure Act of 1946, for example, gives to groups affected by the rulings an opportunity to submit their positions to the agency, thus injecting them formally into the rule-making process.[26] Agencies frequently request client groups to comment on proposed rules even before they are officially announced; they also attempt to formulate standards acceptable to their clients in order to forestall lengthy legal challenges. The benefits of this procedure for large corporations have been described as follows:

> Legislation is put into practice through a series of administrative steps and . . . at each stage in the administrative process, an interested party may have the right to ask adaptation of the decision in such a way as to avoid injury to him. Big companies have the legal resources and administrative contacts to take advantage of such rights; small companies do not. And for big companies, this activity in the administrative sphere is far more attractive; it usually avoids the publicity which may spotlight the attempt to participate in the legislative process and is less apt to demand the time of top management; government administrators would often prefer to deal with the specialist in the corporation who knows the most about the topic, whereas senators or legislative committees are often believed to be more accessible to prominent people.[27]

In performing their rule-making functions, executive departments—which are also covered by the Administrative Procedure Act—are similarly mindful of the wishes of their clients. For example, in 1967, the Department of Commerce announced that it would publish a proposed revision of certain lumber standards because of "significant and substantial" opposition within the industry based on the results of a Department-sponsored poll of lumber producers and users.[28]

As a result of the importance of clientism within govern-

mental bodies, the regulation of business firms was characterized
a few years ago as one of "the symbolic uses of politics," since

> it is one of the demonstrable functions of symbolism that it in-
> duces a feeling of well-being: the resolution of tension. Not
> only is this a major function of widely publicized regulatory
> statutes, but it is also a major function of their administration.
> Some of the most widely publicized administrative activities
> can most confidently be expected to convey a sense of well-
> being to the onlooker because they suggest vigorous activity
> while in fact signifying inactivity or protection of the "regu-
> lated."[29]

There is reason to believe, however, that the regulatory system
has had more than merely symbolic value in constraining corporate activity. Robert E. Lane points out that, although economic factors are a minor reason for the traditional opposition
of business to regulation, the primary cause is the deep-seated
hostility that exists among businessmen because of the psychic
costs resulting from the activities of administrative bodies. These
costs originate from the fact that public regulation challenges
the manager's belief systems, questions his judgments, deprecates
the importance of the business role, limits his autonomy of behavior, and creates anxiety by introducing new uncertainties into
an already unpredictable environment.[30]   Lane also suggests that
the process of accommodation discussed above can never be
complete because government administrators and businessmen
share different occupational traits and value systems and belong
to differing reference groups. While scholars may disagree, most
businessmen do not consider public regulation to be moribund.
Accordingly, there is evidence indicating that the administrative
arena is still a real corporate political battleground rather than
simply the scene of inevitable triumphs by business.

CORPORATE LEGISLATIVE ACTIVITIES

Another type of corporate political involvement of a governmental character is the drafting of legislative and administra-

tive proposals which support the interests of the firm and the positions it favors. We have already dealt with the process, institutionalized under the Administrative Procedure Act, whereby companies suggest the content of administrative measures. A more informal, but comparable, process takes place on the legislative front. Corporation representatives often suggest or "plant" legislation with congressional or state representatives, doing much of the spade work by way of preparing speeches, lining up witnesses for hearings, and providing necessary data. Sometimes corporate legislative involvement, particularly at the state level, takes the form of intergroup negotiation. This process has been described as follows:

> An act of a legislature may be in reality only the ratification of an agreement negotiated by the representatives of those private groups with an interest in a specific question. The legislative body, far from being pressured into conversion of private understandings into the law of the land, may act with an alacrity that comes from the pleasure of avoiding the agony of deciding a dispute between groups.[31]

Indeed, in Illinois the terms of numerous legislative proposals affecting both the mine operators and the unions were fixed by a type of collective bargaining, with both labor and management supporting the consensus bill before the legislature.[32] Similarly, within an industry, firms are likely to "clear" with their corporate colleagues proposed legislation of industry-wide interest before submission to legislative bodies.

CORPORATIONS AND THE JUDICIAL PROCESS

A final form of corporate governmental endeavor involves the use of the legal process to challenge legislation and administrative or executive rulings that are viewed as adverse to company interests. The purpose of corporate legal action is to obtain maximum flexibility for company activities; and by threatening the use of legal procedures, a company may be able to forestall unfavorable governmental activity. While resort to the courts and judicial decision making have traditionally been viewed purely as legal matters, in recent years both lawyers and political scientists have explicitly recognized the political nature of the judicial process.[33]

There are several aspects to corporate political involvement in the judicial and legal context. As do other interest groups, companies attempt to influence the selection of judges. Corporate attorneys or outside counsel who are often active members of important bar association committees frequently make their judicial preferences known to official bodies and officials who are charged with the recommendation and appointment of members of the bench in the hope that these preferences will be followed. David Truman considers "influencing the selection of judges" to be "much the most important indirect means of access to the judiciary."[34]

The history of public involvement in the economic sphere has been marked by the attempts of business firms to challenge such involvement by means of litigation.[35] The process of judicial review, which is the heritage of *Marbury* v. *Madison,* has provided a mechanism for corporations to contest governmental action.[36] Between 1886 and 1937, for example, the Supreme Court gave powerful support for business interests, consistently invalidating federal and state legislative efforts that established minimum-wage and maximum-hour standards as well as legislation that strengthened the position of labor unions.[37] The legal doctrines of economic and substantive due process, which gave rise to these decisions, were largely discarded by the Court in 1937; since then, the Court has been almost entirely permissive regarding new forms of economic regulation.

Yet the courts remain the most important forums in which corporations attempt to obtain favorable interpretations of legislation and to test the powers of administrative agencies. There is, for example, always a steady volume of cases arising under the antitrust acts; and there are continual challenges of the criteria by which regulatory bodies establish utility rates and award certificates of convenience. At times, moreover, the legal challenge is against competitors, either in the same industry (for example, private antitrust suits) or in competing industries (for example, the litigation between the railroads and truckers in Pennsylvania).

Where they are not direct combatants, corporations sometimes assist other beleaguered companies by seeking access to the courts through *amicus curiae* status, which permits them to submit briefs or to join in the oral argument of a critical issue. Corporate counsel also "lobby through law reviews":[38] through publication in legal journals of articles concerning matters in which their clients are involved, corporate counsel attempt to establish a favorable environment in which to handle cases by advocating legal interpretations helpful to them. The success of such technique is, however, open to serious doubt, since the identity of counsel and the interests they represent are usually known within the profession.

Corporate action in the judicial sphere also may serve to delay (often for many years) the application of unfavorable rulings or the enforcement of legislation, may permit the interested party to attempt to shape the interpretation of such matters, and often may provide a weapon for negotiation, since an opponent—whether private or governmental—often desires to avoid protracted litigation. Moreover, judicial decisions by an appellate court often require interpretation and enforcement by inferior courts or by other branches of government. Thus corporations may attempt, once again, to forestall an unfavorable result through legal procedures. Because all these legal activities are costly, the financial resources of the corporation provide it with an asset of political significance in combating opponents. Lawyers are familiar with the not uncommon courtroom scene of a single young government attorney pitted against a battery of experienced corporate practitioners. However, ample corporate legal resources do not necessarily ensure corporate legal success.

Accordingly, the courtroom is an important political arena for corporations. A generation ago, Mr. Justice Owen J. Roberts gave the following description of the function of the Supreme Court:

> When an act of Congress is appropriately challenged in the courts as not conforming to the constitutional mandate, the judicial branch of the Government has only one duty—to lay the article of the Constitution which is invoked beside the statute which is challenged and to decide whether the latter squares with the former. . . . The only power it has if such it may be called is the power of judgment.[39]

This interpretation of judicial review as a passive and apolitical function no longer carries weight among students of the legal process. The Supreme Court and lower Federal and state tribunals are now recognized as forums in which important political decisions are made.

THE WASHINGTON REPRESENTATIVE

On the federal level, corporations increasingly entrust the development of the strategy and tactics of company governmental activities to a relatively recent arrival on the national scene —the Washington representative. The "company's man in Washington" is frequently a high-level corporate official, to whom are delegated the responsibilities of selling the company and its products, of serving as a two-way informational conduit between the company and the government, and of just plain "politicking" on Capitol Hill and within executive departments and administrative agencies. Due to the cost of sustaining a full-time representative and the fact that it is the larger firms which have the most extensive relations with the federal government, the great majority of corporations that employ Washington representatives are large national firms.[40] The 1968 study of 1,033 corporations conducted by the National Industrial Conference Board indicated that while 17 per cent of all respondents maintained branch offices in Washington, 34 per cent of large companies (more than 5,000 employees) had such offices. Only 7.5 per cent of medium (1,000 to 4,999 employees) and 2 per cent of small (500 to 999 employees) maintained Washington offices.[41] Although the task of marketing the company's products continues to occupy the bulk of most Washington representatives' time, political activities assume increasingly greater importance. A survey of corporate public-affairs officers, published in 1965 by the Effective Citizens Organization (ECO), disclosed that the proportion of time which public-affairs officers devote to "legislative and/or governmental relations" was "up sharply since [the] previous survey" (conducted in 1961 and 1962) and took more time than any other single activity.[42] While most of the public-affairs officers surveyed by ECO are not Washington representatives, there is evidence that the increased attention paid to governmental relations at the headquarters level is reflected in activities in the nation's capital.[42a] Taxation, labor policies, regulatory provisions, ownership of natural resources, governmental budgetary policy, tariff restrictions, acquisition of contracts and licenses, levels of foreign aid, subsidies, and civil rights legislation constitute the spectrum of policy issues that are of concern to the more than 300 Washington representatives and their companies.

Similar activities are conducted by company representatives on the less dramatic but very significant local and state levels, which in the opinion of some corporate observers are now the most important arenas for business political endeavors. Relatively few companies (fewer than 6 per cent of the firms surveyed by the National Industrial Conference Board) maintain branch offices in state capitals.[43] Instead, most firms tend to depend either upon home-office personnel or branch management located within the geographical area for their information concerning local and state political issues. Locally and state-wide, problems of zoning, real estate assessment, urban renewal, taxation, school construction, wage-and-hour legislation, and bond proposals assume significance, in addition to some of the areas of governmental concern mentioned in the preceding paragraph. Corporate governmental involvement on the nonfederal level will probably increase, because state and local spending has been rising by nearly 10 per cent a year and by 1968 would have exceeded federal outlays but for the big increases in defense expenditures as a result of the Vietnam war.[44]

• • •

If used in a broad, nonpejorative sense, the term *lobbying* would subsume much of the corporate governmental activities discussed in this section. In all instances, these activities are intended to influence governmental decisions through the process of communications with appropriate public officials. As suggested earlier, it is in the sphere of governmental or policy politics that business corporations have historically concentrated their activities and have achieved their most notable successes. While the drama of electoral activities catches the public fancy, the great majority of critical decisions are made in day-to-day governmental politics.

CORPORATE ELECTORAL ACTIVITIES

Corporate electoral activities, similarly, cover a wide spectrum. There are, however, some critical differences between corporate involvement in governmental politics and company electoral activities. Because, as mentioned in an earlier section of this chapter, the federal criminal code prohibits corporate contributions or expenditures in federal elections, companies either (1) conceal their electoral activities, with the exception of those which are unquestionably nonpartisan in character; or (2) conduct them in the name of company personnel, who are viewed, presumably, as acting in an individual capacity.

NONPARTISAN PROGRAMS

Turning first to permissible, basically nonpartisan (in reality, bipartisan) corporate activities, we have referred to company political education programs, which are designed primarily to secure a favorable political climate for the firm. Complementing such programs are voter registration and campaign contribution drives. The number of companies that conduct such activities has increased significantly since the mid-1950's. Partisanship may, however, be introduced, at times, into these activities, which are normally organized on a bipartisan basis to meet the rigors of legal restrictions. For example, it has not been unknown for a corporate executive to send to a subordinate a letter indicating that he (the executive) had made a campaign contribution to a particular party and suggesting that the employee make a donation to "the party or candidate of his choice," then report this fact to a designated superior.[45] Similarly, the content of political education programs can be tailored to emphasize partisan viewpoints. Corporations tend, however, to be reasonably circumspect about engaging in overt partisanship in order to avoid possible employee antipathy and legal action.

CAMPAIGN CONTRIBUTIONS AND EXPENDITURES

Corporations use various techniques as they engage in partisan electoral politics.[46] Corporate campaign contributions, made either directly or indirectly through managerial employees, constitute a significant form of electoral involvement.

Direct corporate contributions assume many forms: purchases by executives (often in the name of subordinates) of blocks of tickets to fund-raising dinners; gifts or loans of company facilities, products, or personnel; assignment of media time or advertising space; the siphoning of money to candidates or parties by means of inflated fees for legal, industrial-relations, or public-relations services; cash contributions to trade-association campaign funds; release of employees for political campaigning and seeking political office (at times retaining the individual on the company payroll); and advertisements in convention or anniversary booklets published by candidate or parties. The last-mentioned practice has proved highly profitable for both major parties. For example, the 1965 Democratic publication, *Toward an Age of Greatness*, is estimated to have grossed approximately $1 million, with net proceeds of nearly $900,000. Many of the advertisers were corporations either regulated by or doing business—particularly as defense contractors—with the federal government.[47]

In an effort to discourage the stratagem of full-page advertisements (often costing $15,000 apiece) placed by corporations in partisan publications, Congress, in 1966, enacted a provision prohibiting the deduction of the cost of such advertisements as a business expense if "any part of the proceeds directly or indirectly inures (or is intended to inure) to or for the use of a political party or a political candidate."[48]   In 1968, the section was amended to restore tax deductions for the costs of advertisement in the programs of the national political party presidential conventions if (1) the proceeds of the program are used solely to defray the expenses of conducting the convention or a subsequent convention; and (2) the amount paid or incurred for the advertising is "reasonable" in light of the business which the advertiser expects to gain from the advertisement.[49]   The amendment was designed to distinguish between advertising expenditures that are commensurate with ordinary commission rates and serve a legitimate business purpose and those that are inflated in amount and actually constitute indirect campaign contributions.   It is too early to judge the effectiveness of these measures in reducing the amount of corporate advertising in party publications.

Corporations also participate in electoral politics indirectly through their officers and directors.   Corporate executives occasionally occupy important positions in state or national political circles—not infrequently connected with party financing.   Some recent instances of business leaders serving in partisan capacities are Edgar F. Kaiser, board chairman of Kaiser Industries, as the California Republican Party treasurer; Ralph J. Cordiner, formerly chairman of General Electric, as national Republican finance committee chairman; Matthew G. McCloskey, president of McCloskey Construction, as Democratic national treasurer; Arthur B. Krim, president of United Artists, as national Democratic finance committee chairman; and Charles H. Percy, chairman of Bell and Howell, as chairman of the Republican committee on program and progress.

Partisan participation also assumes other forms.   In their study of the national party committees, Cornelius P. Cotter and Bernard C. Hennessy found that "corporation executive" was the second most prevalent occupational category ("lawyer" was first) among national committee members of both parties between 1948 and 1963.   Corporation executives constituted 12.1 per cent of the Democratic National Committee and 16.2 per cent of the membership of the Republican National Committee for an aggregate of 14.14 per cent during the 15-year period—nearly one-half the representation of lawyers.[50]   Corporate executives also serve as delegates to state and national party conventions.

Company funds frequently find their way into partisan coffers in the form of donations by executives.   Bonus or salary arrangements, padded expense accounts, and the distribution of firm moneys in individual names (on occasion without the knowledge of the "contributor") are common devices.   The names of corporate executives frequently appear on the lists of large contributors to party funding groups.   For example, during the 1964 campaign, a contribution of $1,000 or more to the Democratic Party made the donor a member of the "President's Club" (which was purely a fund-raising device with no organizational identity or purpose) and gave him the opportunity to attend a club dinner with President Johnson.   Since the days of the Eisenhower administration, Republican givers have had an opportunity to join the "Republican Congressional Boosters Club" at an identical price.   Occasionally, corporate executives pool their individual contributions through executive-level company committees, thereby increasing the company's political impact on the recipient.   Donors to such committees can either designate a party or a specific candidate or leave the distribution of the moneys to the discretion of the committee.   Such committees apparently seek unpledged contributions to enhance the company's flexibility and independence in distributing the funds and thereby garner greater political credit for the firm.

While the exact magnitude of contributions by corporate executives is unknown, some revealing data are available.   In 1957, a Senate committee reported that 199 officials from many of the nation's 225 largest firms contributed nearly $2 million in amounts of $500 or more to interstate committees during the 1956 campaign.   This sum, more than 18 per cent of the total value of known gifts of $500 or more, was distributed between the major parties as follows: Republican, $1,816,597; Democratic, $103,725.[51]

Although, as the above figures indicate, the Republican Party has customarily received the lion's share of contributions made by corporate officials, there are signs that the pendulum has begun to swing in the opposite direction. Comparative figures give some of the details of this development. In 1956, members of the Business (Advisory) Council contributed nearly $270,000 to President Dwight D. Eisenhower's campaign, and $4,000 to that of Democratic challenger Governor Adlai E. Stevenson. Although BAC bipartisanship increased slightly in 1960 (Senator John F. Kennedy received a little more than $35,000, compared to more than $240,000 for Vice-President Richard M. Nixon), the 1964 election marked the first time that a Democratic candidate received more than minimal support from the group. President Lyndon B. Johnson collected $135,450 as compared with $87,100 for Senator Barry Goldwater.[52] In 1968, notwithstanding the anticipated victory of former Vice-President Richard M. Nixon over Vice-President Hubert H. Humphrey, the Democratic candidate had the financial backing of some corporate leaders. While it is virtually certain that Mr. Nixon was more generously favored by BAC members than was Mr. Humphrey (the figures are not presently available), it is highly unlikely that the great disparities in the amounts of BAC contributions received by the presidential contenders in 1956 and 1960 will be replicated when the 1968 figures are released. As suggested in the last chapter, the almost monolithic structure of Republican support by corporate circles is being eroded.

Although such donations are technically the individual activities of the donor rather than formal corporate action, they nevertheless enhance the political access enjoyed by the company. In the opinion of Alexander Heard, largesse by corporate officials "increases the importance of the corporate community and of individual companies in the financial constituencies of officeholders."[53]

Some of the techniques employed by corporations in the area of governmental politics are also used in the electoral sphere. These include support (financial and otherwise) of trade-association activities; use of "public-service" advertising for the benefit of a particular candidate or party; distribution of "educational" political literature to shareholders, employees, customers, or suppliers; and the announcement by leading company officials of private positions on candidates or issues.

CORPORATIONS AND THE GOVERNORS' CONFERENCE

An interesting example of corporate political action that is neither wholly governmental nor totally electoral is the practice among business firms of assuming the expenses of the annual national Governors' Conference. Companies lend or donate products and facilities and make manpower available in order to fulfill the requirements of this important political meeting. The roster of businesses bearing the costs of the 1966 conference in Los Angeles ranged from General Motors, Aerojet-General, and Alcoa to the California Wine Growers Association and Walt Disney Productions.[54] This activity constitutes yet another source of contact with public officialdom, thereby enhancing the political access of the participating companies.

EXTENSIVENESS OF CORPORATE POLITICAL INVOLVEMENT

The above description of governmental and electoral political activities engaged in by corporations and their managers is by no means exhaustive. It does not suggest, moreover, the wide variations in the extent of political involvement among business firms. Corporate political activity varies significantly in both scope and magnitude. *Scope* refers to the spectrum or breadth of issues with which a political participant is concerned, while *magnitude* pertains to the intensity or depth of involvement within a given scope.[55] Some companies seek to exercise influence over a wide scope of political problems, and they engage in a high magnitude of activity in many areas of politics. At the other extreme, some firms restrict their efforts to perhaps a single issue, which involves sporadic contacts with a limited number of governmental units. For example, because of its nationwide operations, Ford Motor concerns itself continuously with a wide variety of political issues on the federal level and in many states and local communities (ranging from federal defense expenditures to local zoning policies). On the other hand, the sole political action of a local food-processing company may consist of desultory efforts to modify the local health-standards ordinance that affects its operations. Scope and magnitude, moreover, vary over time according to the political needs of the firm. Thus, while political activity is common to corporations in general, the nature and extent of this activity vary significantly.

Because of the scarcity of both quantitative and qualitative data pertaining to political activities of individual firms, it is difficult to calculate either the scope or the magnitude of aggregate corporate political activity. Indeed, a prime area of potentially fruitful research would involve case studies of the overall political activities of individual corporations. Such research would reveal the totality of a company's political activities both within the firm and in the variety of political areas in which it is active, rather than merely concentrate on a single issue (e.g., tariffs) concerning which various interest groups have sought to influence public policy.[56] Observation of the firm's political endeavors from an internal perspective would make possible a more accurate gauge of the scope and magnitude of corporate activity.

One of the few available sources of information concerning the extent of corporate political participation is the survey of corporate public activities released by the National Industrial Conference Board in mid-1968. Several findings by the NICB provide rough measures of company political involvement. The study indicates that nearly all of the 1,033 respondent firms review federal (98 per cent), state (97 per cent), and local (93 per cent) legislative issues. Of the large (more than 5,000 employees) companies, 53 per cent pay "continuous" attention to federal legislation, as opposed to approximately 35 per cent of both the medium (1,000 to 4,999 employees) and the small (500 to 999 employees) firms. On the state and local levels, however, the differences in the frequency of review of legislation by corporations of different sizes diminish significantly. Indeed, a greater percentage of small companies than of large or medium-sized firms continuously review local legislative issues. The survey indicates, moreover, that for all three levels of government, most companies (never less than 63 per cent, irrespective of size) engage in a "continuous" or a "frequent" review of legislation, rather than simply an "occasional" review.[57]

Another measure of aggregate corporate political activity is furnished by the NICB statistics on company communications with public officials concerning legislation. Most respondents reported that, in the two-year period preceding the survey, they had made oral or written presentations of company views on legislative issues to federal (90 per cent), state (90 per cent), and local (82 per cent) legislators or officials. While for all levels of government a higher percentage of large firms communicated with officials than did medium or small firms, differences among the three categories were very slight—generally a few percentage points—and in the case of the "small" and "medium" classifications, almost negligible. Large companies tended to present their legislative views somewhat more frequently than did smaller companies, except at the local level where small companies demonstrated the greatest rate of frequency. Of the companies reporting that they presented their legislative views to officials, approximately 50 per cent indicated that they had done so "somewhat more often" than "once or twice" during the two years preceding the survey and approximately 20 per cent "much more frequently."[58]

More than 85 per cent of the corporate communications to public officials of all levels of government, reports the NICB, were in opposition to proposed legislation. In nearly two-thirds of the instances, however, companies that opposed legislation also proposed alternatives. Large companies were particularly inclined toward making suggestions. Relatively few companies (less than 5 per cent) advanced wholly new legislative approaches without prior solicitation from government.[59]

One additional finding of the NICB is particularly relevant. Political involvement was more pronounced among nonmanufacturing than among manufacturing companies, particularly at the local and state levels. For example, in response to the query concerning the frequency of company review of legislative issues, 57 per cent of nonmanufacturers as compared with 36 per cent of manufacturers indicated that they conducted "continuous" review. On the state level, the difference between the two categories was particularly striking with 68 per cent of nonmanufacturers maintaining a "continuous" review as opposed to only 35 per cent of manufacturers. Similarly, nonmanufacturing firms presented their views on legislative issues to public officials somewhat more frequently than did manufacturers, particularly at the state level, where there was an almost 2:1 ratio between the two classifications.[60] The likely reason for the great attention given by nonmanufacturers to state politics is that more than 70 per cent of the firms represented in this category were in industries subject to extensive state regulation—banking, utilities, and insurance.

Although helpful in gauging some of the broad dimensions of corporate political activity, the NICB report makes no attempt to evaluate the quality of participation among the companies studied or to ascertain, except in very general terms, specific areas of political involvement. Despite the paucity of sophisticated data in the NICB study and in other research pertaining to corporations, several generalizations concerning aggregate corporate political involvement are warranted.

First, as indicated by the above statistics, almost all business corporations, even those which are small, engage in *some* form of political activity.

Second, the scope and the magnitude of corporate political involvement are functions of (1) the size of the firm, (2) the degree of regulation of the enterprise by the government, and (3) the extent to which company business and well-being depend upon governmental decisions. The larger the firm and the greater the importance of governmental decisions to its operations, the greater the scope and the magnitude of corporate involvement. Of the three factors, however, size—standing alone —appears to be least important.

A third generalization is that in recent years, there has been an increase in the scope and the magnitude of corporate political activities. This fact is reflected both by the greater number of firms that have established offices in Washington and in state capitals and in the expanded institution of public-affairs or governmental-relations departments at the headquarters level. This trend has also resulted in an increasing dependence by corporations on political specialists who can bring expertise to bear on the company's behalf. This greater emphasis upon political activities will probably continue as the multifaceted involvement with local, state, and federal governments increases. Significantly, more than one-half of the respondents to the NICB survey indicated that they expected company interest in local and state issues to expand over the ensuing five years and nearly two-thirds expressed the same opinion concerning federal legislation. Less than 1 per cent of those responding expected their interest to decline at any level of government.[61]

An interesting dimension of any discussion of the extensiveness of corporate political involvement is the contrary views held by business managers and nonbusinessmen concerning the extent of this involvement. A typical business view of the extent of corporate political activities in the mid-1960's was expressed by Harold Brayman, a former director of public relations of Du Pont:

> Generally speaking, business has less contact with people in government than does any other major section of our society. Certainly it has far less than do the labor people who cultivate government officials intensely; or agriculture whose contacts are very great in the field of government; or several of the professions, notably teaching, which maintain constant and continuous pressures upon government.[62]

In a 1968 survey conducted among businessmen by the *Harvard Business Review,* executives described past business political activities as follows: very extensive, 3 per cent; fairly extensive, 16 per cent; moderate, 36 per cent; somewhat limited, 30 per cent; and very limited, 15 per cent. Thus, the overwhelming majority of the respondents (who totalled more than 2500) considered the extent of business political activity to be either limited or moderate. In response to a question as to what the extent of business political activity *should be*, executives replied: very extensive, 19 per cent; fairly extensive, 43 per cent;

moderate, 28 per cent; somewhat limited, 6 per cent; and very limited, 4 per cent.[63]   An almost identical study published by the *HBR* four years earlier yielded similar findings.   While 1964 respondents (totalling approximately 1700) thought that the past political activity of business was somewhat less extensive than did executives queried in 1968—the responses were: very extensive, 2 per cent; fairly extensive, 11 per cent; moderate, 31 per cent; somewhat limited, 34 per cent; and very limited, 22 per cent—their views concerning how extensive that activity should be were virtually the same as those given by managers in the latter study.[64]   Hence, in both years, the large majority of businessmen saw a need for increased business involvement in politics.

Interestingly, respondents in both polls evaluated past business political activity as more ineffective than effective.   In the 1968 survey, 26 per cent of those replying considered business efforts either very effective (3 per cent) or fairly effective (23 percent), while 43 per cent termed them either very ineffective (8 per cent) or fairly ineffective (35 per cent).   The remaining 31 per cent rated the effectiveness of business political activities as "half and half."   These findings almost replicate the 1964 figures.

It is significant that only 6 per cent of the 1968 *HBR* respondents had replied to the 1964 survey.   Accordingly, despite an almost completely different sample for the two years, the results were quite similar.   This fact suggests that businessmen share a high degree of consensus concerning the actual and desired extensiveness of business political activity and the effectiveness of such activity.

On the other hand, nonbusinessmen tend to see the shadow of corporate involvement covering all political activities.   Labor unions have traditionally held this view and numerous scholars have concluded that economic elites are omnipresent, especially in the area of community politics.   For example, Robert and Helen Lynd reported that

> Middletown [Muncie, Indiana] has . . . at present what amounts to a reigning royal family.   The power of this family has become so great as to differentiate the city today somewhat from cities with a more diffuse type of control.   If, however, one

views the Middletown pattern as simply concentrating and personalizing the type of control which control of capital gives to the business group in our culture, the Middletown situation may be viewed as epitomizing the American business-class control system. . . . The business class in Middletown runs the city.[65]

While the validity of the business political control thesis—particularly as it relates to the large corporation in the national political context—will be analyzed in Chapter Eight, it is well to point out that there exists a great diversity of opinion among informed observers regarding both the extent and the effectiveness of political activity by economic interests. It is likely that business political involvement is neither as limited as the *Harvard Business Review* survey leads one to believe nor as ubiquitous as the Lynds' study suggests. Managers probably underestimate the extent of corporate political participation as a result of (1) a lack of personal involvement in company political activities; (2) a tendency to take a narrow view of the nature of politics; and (3) a propensity toward equating extensiveness with effectiveness. On the other hand, those who overestimate the political activities of business have often tended to do so for either philosophical or methodological reasons that are based on the implicit assumption of the primacy of economic factors in all political relationships.

SUMMATION

This chapter has centered on an examination of the nature of corporate political behavior. For purposes of analysis, a distinction has been made between *governmental* and *electoral* political activities. Corporations pay primary attention to governmental politics because of the continuous nature of governmental operations as opposed to the episodic character of electoral activity, the history of greater business effectiveness in governmental politics, and the fact that the most important political decisions are made in the governmental area. Important forms of corporate governmental activities include supporting trade-association activities, establishing and maintaining legislative and administrative contacts, utilizing public relations techniques on a continuous basis, serving in governmental posts by corporate managers, maintaining a continuous liaison with administrative agencies, drafting and promoting favorable legislation and rulings, and utilizing the legal process to accomplish political objectives. Increasingly, corporations are entrusting these governmental activities to specialists who operate out of Washington and the state capitals.

While corporations do engage in some nonpartisan electoral activities, most electoral involvement is partisan. A primary activity is the channeling of corporate funds to candidates and parties through corporate managers and by a wide variety of techniques. Corporate executives also engage in electoral politics by holding important posts in state and national party circles.

The paucity of available information makes difficult any accurate estimate of the scope and the magnitude of corporate political involvement. While business managers tend to underestimate the extensiveness of corporate activities, nonbusiness observers are inclined to overestimate it. It appears, however, that political involvement by business firms, while virtually universal and probably growing in scope and magnitude, varies with the size of the firm, the extent of public regulation, and the importance of governmental decisions to its operations.

NOTES

[1]18 U.S.C. § 610 (1951).

[2]The subject of the effect of federal restrictions on corporate electoral activities has been treated most recently in Edwin M. Epstein, *Corporations, Contributions and Political Campaigns: Federal Regulation in Perspective* (Berkeley: Institute of Governmental Studies, University of California, Berkeley, 1968).

[3]2 U.S.C. § § 261–270 (1946).

[4]Reprinted from David J. Galligan, *Politics and the Businessman* (New York: Pitman Publishing Corporation, 1964), p. 67.

[5]Karl Schriftgiesser, *Business Comes of Age* (New York: Harper & Row, Publishers, 1960), p. vii.

[6]Schriftgiesser, *Business* . . . , p. 162.

[7]Quoted in David Sanford, "Drugs: Dr. Goddard's Guesstimate," *The New Republic*, CLVIII, No. 8 (February 24, 1968), 16.

[8]For a comprehensive treatment of the dispute between the truckers and the railroads, see Andrew Hacker, "Pressure Politics in Pennsylvania: The Truckers vs. The Railroads," in Alan F. Westin (ed.), *The Uses of Power* (New York: Harcourt, Brace & World, Inc., 1962), pp. 323–76. See also *Eastern Railroad Presidents Conference, et al. v. Noerr Motor Freight, Inc., et al.*, 365 U.S. 127 (1961), *reversing* 155 F.Supp. 768 (1957).

[9]See Raymond A. Bauer, Ithiel de Sola Pool, and Lewis Anthony Dexter, *American Business and Public Policy* (New York: Atherton Press, 1964).

[10]Helpful discussions of these points are found in Lester W. Milbrath, *The Washington Lobbyists* (Chicago: Rand McNally & Company, 1963), p. 20 and Chap. 15; Bauer, Pool, and Dexter, *American Business* . . . , Chaps. XII, XXIV; and Donald R. Matthews, *U.S. Senators and Their World* (New York: Vintage Books, Random House, Inc., 1960), Chap. 8.

[11]Accounts of this change in managerial philosophy are found in Earl F. Cheit, "Why Managers Cultivate Social Responsibility," *California Management Review*, VII, No. 1 (Fall 1964), 3–22; R. Joseph Monsen, Jr., *Modern American Capitalism* (Boston: Houghton Mifflin Company, 1963); Francis X. Sutton, *et al.*, *The American Business Creed* (New York: Schocken Books, 1962); and Clarence C. Walton, *Corporate Social Responsibilities* (Belmont, Calif.: Wadsworth Publishing Company, Inc., 1967).

[12]B. J. Mullaney, a director of the utility interests' Illinois information committee during the 1920's, quoted in Stanley Kelley, Jr., *Professional Public Relations and Political Power* (Baltimore: The Johns Hopkins Press, 1956), pp. 12–13. For a recent discussion of the necessity of corporate public relations, see Harold Brayman, *Corporate Management in a World of Politics* (New York: McGraw-Hill Book Company, 1967).

106 NATURE OF CORPORATE POLITICAL ACTIVITIES

13Morrell Heald, "Management's Responsibility to Society: The Growth of an Idea," *Business History Review*, XXXI, No. 4 (Winter 1957), 378.

14Hacker, in Westin (ed.), *The Uses of Power*, p. 372.

1515 U.S.C. § § 1381–1425 (1966).

16*The Wall Street Journal*, December 20, 1967, p. 13.

17Frederick C. Klein, "More People Prefer . . . ," *The Wall Street Journal*, September 25, 1967, p. 1, col. 6.

18V. O. Key, Jr., *Politics, Parties and Pressure Groups*, 5th ed. (New York: Thomas Y. Crowell Co., 1964), p. 131.

19Former Secretary of Commerce Sinclair Weeks quoted in *Interim Report on WOC's and Government Advisory Groups*, Pursuant to H. Res. 22, U.S. Congress, House of Representatives, Committee on Judiciary; Antitrust Subcommittee. 84th Cong., 2nd Sess. (Washington, D.C.: U.S. Government Printing Office, April 24, 1956) p. 8.

20*Summary Report and Recommendations* (Sacramento, Calif.: Governor's Survey on Efficiency and Cost Control, February 1968), pp. 147–49.

21See, for example, Marver H. Bernstein, *Regulating Business by Independent Commission* (Princeton, N.J.: Princeton University Press, 1955); Walton Hamilton, *The Politics of Industry* (New York: Alfred A. Knopf, Inc., 1957); and Philip Selznick, *TVA and the Grass Roots* (New York: Harper Torchbooks, Harper & Row, Publishers, 1966); Walter Adams and Horace M. Gray, *Monopoly in America* (New York: The Macmillan Company, Publishers, 1955), pp. 54–58; and Murray Edelman, *The Symbolic Uses of Politics* (Urbana, Ill.: University of Illinois Press, 1967). Compare Louis L. Jaffe, "The Independent Agency—A New Scapegoat," *Yale Law Journal*, LXV (June 1956), 1068–76.

22The Olney letter is quoted in Matthew Josephson, *The Politicos* (New York: Harcourt, Brace & World, Inc., 1938), p. 526.

23See, for example, Victor G. Rosenblum, "How to Get into TV: The Federal Communications Commission and Miami's Channel 10," in Westin (ed.), *The Uses of Power*, pp. 173–228; Louis L. Jaffe, "The Scandal in T.V. Licensing," *Harper's Magazine*, CCXV, No. 1288 (September 1957), 77–84; and Louis J. Hector, "Problems of the CAB and the Independent Regulatory Commissions," *Yale Law*

Journal, LXIX (May 1960), 931–64. Selznick discusses the concept of co-optation in *TVA and the Grass Roots,* especially pp. 13–16; 259–61.

[24]The "life-cycle" theory of regulatory history is best explained in Bernstein, *Regulating Business . . . ,* Chap. 3.

[25]The material for this paragraph and the succeeding two paragraphs is drawn from the following sources: *Berkeley Daily Gazette,* December 15, 1966, p. 5, cols. 1 and 2; *San Francisco Chronicle,* December 16, 1966, p. 14; *San Francisco Sunday Examiner and Chronicle,* January 1, 1967, Sec. 1, p. 12, col. 1; *San Francisco Chronicle,* January 7, 1967, p. 2, cols. 7 and 8; *The Wall Street Journal,* February 1, 1967, p. 3, cols. 1 and 2; *San Francisco Chronicle,* February 3, 1967, p. 11, cols. 3–8; "Car Safety Measures Lose Their Sharp Bite," *Business Week,* February 4, 1967, pp. 30–31; *San Francisco Chronicle,* March 21, 1967, p. 10, cols. 1 and 2; *The Wall Street Journal,* March 21, 1967, p. 3, cols. 2 and 3; *Consumer Reports,* April 1967, pp. 190–94.

[26]5 U.S.C. § § 551–559 (1967).

[27]Lewis Anthony Dexter, "Where the Elephant Fears to Dance Among the Chickens: Business in Politics? The Case of du Pont," *Human Organization,* XIX (Winter 1960), 190.

[28]*San Francisco Sunday Examiner and Chronicle,* April 30, 1967, Sec. 1, p. 7, cols. 7 and 8.

[29]Edelman, *The Symbolic Uses of Politics,* p. 38.

[30]Robert E. Lane, *The Regulation of Businessmen: Social Conditions of Government Economic Control* (New Haven, Conn.: Yale University Press, 1954), pp. 1–35.

[31]Key, *Politics, Parties and . . . ,* p. 145.

[32]This process is described in Gilbert Y. Steiner, *Legislation by Collective Bargaining* (Urbana, Ill.: University of Illinois, 1951).

[33]For examples of political analyses of the judicial process by lawyers, see Alexander M. Bickel, *The Least Dangerous Branch* (Indianapolis: The Bobbs-Merrill Co., Inc., 1962); Robert H. Jackson, *The Supreme Court in the American System of Government* (New York: Harper Torchbooks, Harper & Row, Publishers, 1963); Arthur Selwyn Miller, *The Supreme Court and American Capitalism* (New York: The Free Press, 1968); and Fred Rodell, *Nine Men* (New York: Vintage Books, Random House, Inc., 1964). Relevant works by political scientists include Theodore L. Becker, *Political*

Behavioralism and Modern Jurisprudence (Chicago: Rand McNally & Company, 1964); Edward S. Corwin, *American Constitutional History* (New York: Harper & Row, Publishers, 1964); Walter F. Murphy and C. Herman Pritchett, *Courts, Judges, and Politics* (New York: Random House, 1961); Victor G. Rosenblum, *Law as a Political Instrument* (New York: Random House, Inc., 1955); Glendon Schubert, *Judicial Policy-Making* (Glenview, Ill.: Scott, Foresman & Company, Educational Publishers, 1965); Glendon Schubert (ed.), *Judicial Decision-Making* (New York: The Free Press 1963); Clement E. Vose, "Litigation as a Form of Pressure Group Activity," *Annals of the American Academy of Political and Social Science*, CCCXIX (September 1958), 20–31; Henry J. Abraham, *The Judiciary* (Boston: Allyn and Bacon, Inc., 1965), pp. 97–104; and Robert G. McCloskey, *The American Supreme Court* (Chicago: The University of Chicago Press, 1960).

[34]David B. Truman, *The Governmental Process* (New York: Alfred A. Knopf, Inc., 1951), p. 489.

[35]1 Cranch 137 (1803).

[36]Exemplary cases are *Ashwander v. TVA*, 297 U.S. 288 (1936); *Houston, East & West Texas Ry. Co. v. United States* [The Shreveport Rate Case], 234 U.S. 342 (1914); *Railroad Retirement Board v. Alton Railroad Co.*, 295 U.S. 330 (1935); *Carter v. Carter Coal Co.*, 298 U.S. 238 (1936); *National Labor Relations Board v. Jones and Laughlin Steel Corp.*, 301 U.S. 1 (1937); *Electric Bond & Share Co. v. SEC*, 303 U.S. 419 (1938); *Steward Machine Co. v. Davis*, 301 U.S. 548, 57 S.Ct. 883 (1937); *Bibb v. Navajo Freight Lines, Inc.*, 359 U.S. 520 (1959); *Dean Milk Co. v. City of Madison*, 340 U.S. 349 (1951); *General Motors Corp. v. Washington*, 377 U.S. 436 (1964); *Brotherhood of Locomotive Engineers v. Chicago, R. I. & P.R. Co.*, 382 U.S. 423 (1966); *Associated Industries of New York State, Inc. v. Ickes*, 134 F.2d 694 (2d Cir. 1943); *Youngstown Sheet & Tube Co. v. Sawyer*, 343 U.S. 579 (1952).

[37]For further discussions of this period, see Miller, *The Supreme Court and . . .* , Chaps. 2, 3; and Robert Green McCloskey, *American Conservatism in the Age of Enterprise* (New York: Harper & Row, Publishers, 1954), Chap. 4.

[38]This expression was coined by Congressman Wright Patman. See 103 *Congressional Record* 14758 (daily ed.), August 27, 1957, reprinted in Murphy and Pritchett, *Courts, Judges and Politics*, pp. 308–11.

[39]*United States* v. *Butler*, 297 U.S. 1, 62–63 (1936).

[40]The activities of corporate Washington representatives are discussed in Paul W. Cherington and Ralph L. Gillen, *The Business Representative in Washington* (Washington, D.C.: The Brookings Institution, 1962); and Richard Austin Smith, "The Company's Man in Washington," *Fortune*, LXXIII, No. 4 (April 1966), 132–35, 186–97.

[41]*The Role of Business in Public Affairs*, Studies in Public Affairs, No. 2 (New York: National Industrial Conference Board, Inc., 1968), p. 8.

[42]From "Public Affairs Survey" (Washington, D.C.: Effective Citizens Organization, Inc., June 1965), p. 3 (mimeographed).

[42a]See Cherington and Gillen, *The Business Representative . . .* , especially pp. 114–25.

[43]*The Role of Business . . .* , p. 8.

[44]President of the United States, *Economic Report of the President, Together with the Annual Report of the Council of Economic Advisors* (Washington, D.C.: U.S. Government Printing Office, 1968), p. 209 (Table B-1).

[45]See, for example, *Hearings, 1956 Presidential and Senatorial Campaign Contributions and Practices*, U.S. Congress, Senate Subcommittee on Privileges and Elections of the Committee on Rules and Administration, 84th Cong., 2d Sess., 1956, pp. 558–59. In the instance cited, however, the letter from the chief executive of the company did go on to state that the employee's signature was not required on his memorandum of action.

[46]The material in this section is drawn primarily from Epstein, *Corporations, Contributions and . . .* , Chap. 6. While parts of the following discussion are specifically footnoted, readers who desire additional documentation are referred to my earlier work. The most comprehensive general discussions of electoral financing in the United States are found in Alexander Heard, *The Costs of Democracy* (Chapel Hill, N.C.: The University of North Carolina Press, 1960), and the series of research monographs published by the Citizens' Research Foundation under the general editorship of Herbert E. Alexander.

[47]*Congressional Quarterly Weekly Report. Special Report: 1964 Political Campaign Contributions and Expenditures*, No. 3, Part I of 11 Parts, January 21, 1966, pp. 57–240. See pp. 60–66.

[48]Int. Rev. Code of 1954, §§ 276 (a) and (b).

[49]Int. Rev. Code of 1954, § 276 (c).

[50]Cornelius P. Cotter and Bernard C. Hennessy, *Politics Without Power* (New York: Atherton Press, 1964), Table 4, p. 52.

[51]The statistics are drawn from *Report, 1956 Presidential and Senatorial Campaign Contributions and Practices*, U.S. Congress, Senate, Subcommittee on Privileges and Elections of the Committee on Rules and Administration, 85th Cong., 1st Sess. (Washington, D.C.: U.S. Government Printing Office, 1957), Exhibits 25 and 26, as cited in Heard, *The Costs of Democracy*, pp. 114–15.

[52]Herbert E. Alexander, *Financing the 1964 Election* (Princeton, N.J.: Citizen's Research Foundation, 1966), pp. 90–95; and Herbert E. Alexander and Harold B. Meyers, "The Switch in Campaign Giving," *Fortune*, LXXII, No. 5 (November 1965), 170–71.

[53]Heard, *The Costs of Democracy*, p. 112.

[54]*San Francisco Chronicle*, July 5, 1966, p. 19, cols. 1–5.

[55]The analytical relevance of the distinction between "scope" and "magnitude" is developed further in Robert A. Dahl, "Business and Politics: A Critical Appraisal of Political Science," in Robert A. Dahl, Mason Haire, and Paul F. Lazarsfeld, *Social Science Research on Business: Product and Potential* (New York: Columbia University Press, 1959), pp. 34–38.

[56]Examples of valuable research studies of this character are Bauer, Pool, and Dexter, *American Business and Public Policy*; Earl Latham, *The Group Basis of Politics; A Study in Basing-Point Legislation* (Ithaca, N.Y.: Cornell University Press, 1952); Joseph Cornwall Palamountain, Jr., *The Politics of Distribution* (Cambridge, Mass.: Harvard University Press, 1955); Robert Engler, *The Politics of Oil* (Chicago: Phoenix Books, The University of Chicago Press, 1967); Aaron Wildavsky, *Dixon-Yates: A Study in Power Politics* (New Haven, Conn.: Yale University Press, 1962); and O. Garceau and C. Silverman, "A Pressure Group and the Pressured: A Case Report," *The American Political Science Review*, XLVIII (September 1954), 672–91.

[57]The statistics in this paragraph are drawn from *The Role of Business* . . . , p. 8.

[58]The statistics in this paragraph are drawn from *The Role of Business* . . . , p. 10.

⁵⁹*The Role of Business* . . . , p. 10.

⁶⁰The statistics in this paragraph are drawn from *The Role of Business* . . . , pp. 8, 10.

⁶¹*The Role of Business* . . . , p. 8.

⁶²Reprinted from Harold Brayman, *Corporate Management in a World of Politics* (New York: McGraw-Hill Book Company, 1967), p. 68.

⁶³Stephen A. Greyser, "Business and Politics, 1968 (Special Report)," *Harvard Business Review*, XLVI, No. 6 (November–December 1968), 10.

⁶⁴Stephen A. Greyser, "Business and Politics, 1964 (Problems in Review)," *Harvard Business Review*, XLII, No. 5 (September–October 1964), 28.

⁶⁵Robert S. Lynd and Helen Merrell Lynd, *Middletown in Transition* (New York: Harcourt, Brace & World, Inc., 1937), p. 77.

Chapter Six

The Managerial Whys and Wherefores of Corporate Political Involvement

Although, as we have seen in the preceding chapters, corporate involvement has long been a fact of American political life, until recently little attention was given to analysis of the rationale underlying this involvement. As the business-in-politics movement gained momentum after the mid-1950's, corporate managers, with an occasional helping hand from the scholarly community, have offered a variety of explanations of and justifications for corporate political activity. From this large and diverse list, the following rationales warrant serious discussion:

1. The interests of the corporation and of society are coterminous. Accordingly, business managers should and do act in a trusteeship capacity to safeguard the public interest.

2. Corporations are disenfranchised and, thus, unlike individuals, do not possess an inherent polit-

ical identity. Therefore, corporate managers must consciously and deliberately establish an appropriate political role for the firm. A corollary to this proposition, which is occasionally advanced by business executives, is that electoral activity constitutes the primary route by which corporations can achieve political influence and, hence, should be the focus of company involvement.

3. Corporate political involvement is as much a result of the personalities and prerogatives of top corporate managers as it is a consequence of pragmatic political necessities.

4. A fundamental purpose of the corporate presence in the political arena is to counterbalance the great power of labor unions which constitutes a threat to the survival of private enterprise.

5. The impact of the "political climate" on corporate decisions has become all the more intense in an era characterized by an explicit, unavoidable, and ever-increasing interdependence between business and government. The creation and maintenance of a favorable governmental environment is a prerequisite to the successful conduct of business activities. Accordingly, political participation serves a corporate need for "reluctant self-protection."

The remainder of the chapter will be devoted to an analysis of these five managerial explanations of corporate political involvement.

CORPORATE INTEREST EQUALS NATIONAL INTEREST

Charles E. Wilson, a former president of the General Motors Company and Secretary of Defense in the Eisenhower administration, once stated to a Senate committee, "For years I thought what was good for our country was good for General Motors, and vice versa."[1] In this sentiment, he succinctly expressed a reason frequently advanced by business executives to explain corporate political involvement—that the interest of the nation is identical with the interest of business and that, accordingly, corporations and their managers are admirably situated to satisfy public needs through political as well as economic leadership. This company interest–national interest rationale for corporate political activity has three bases.

President Calvin Coolidge best expressed the first basis, which is ideological in character, when he asserted that "the business of America is business." While this thesis has never gone unchallenged and business values have had to compete with other cultural influences, it has been "the business principle [which] has given a synthetic cohesion to the far-flung diversity of American life."[2]   Accordingly, the necessity for creating an environment congenial to "America's business" is widely accepted by both corporate managers and the general public.   In ideological statements concerning capitalism, as well as in the minds of many members of the public, social and political freedoms are considered derivatives of economic freedom.   A complementary contention advanced is that as the interests of corporate enterprise are enhanced, the national interest is maximized.   This thesis has its theoretical foundations in the classical economics of Adam Smith, who considered that the public good would be promoted if each person—led by the inexorable "invisible hand" —pursued his own interest.

A second possible explanation is attributable to the managerial role, particularly in the era of large-scale organizations, which differ greatly from the traditional models of capitalistic enterprise.   In order to justify to himself and to others the power which he possesses as a result of his organizational position, the manager rationalizes his own social role and that of his organization as maximizing the interests of the community.   Harold D. Lasswell provides a valuable insight into this psychological mechanism by his analysis of the political personality.   In *Power and Personality*, he suggests that the "political type" is characterized by an intense craving for deference, which is ungratified by his ordinary interpersonal relationships.   This craving is "displaced upon public objects (persons and practices connected with the power process)" and rationalized in terms of "public interest."   Lasswell summarizes the development of motive in the political personality as follows: (1) Private motives (2) displaced on public objects (3) rationalized in terms of public interest.[3] Arguably, as a consequence of his psychological needs the corporate executive subconsciously develops a sincere belief in the convergence of public and corporate interests. His perspective of public necessity convinces him that by pursuing corporate objectives he is acting in the best interests of society.[4]

A third explanation for the "company interest–national interest" rationale involves much the same motivation as the recent ideological emphasis placed by business managers upon social responsibility as a basic requirement of corporate activity—that is, the desire to preserve for the corporation the greatest degree of autonomy from constraint by other social interests. The concentration of extensive social and economic power in the hands of corporate executives has created the necessity of emphasizing the identity of corporate and community social interests. Similarly, the existence of corporate political power has required managers to assure the public of the commonality of corporate and national interests.[5]

CORPORATE AND NATIONAL INTERESTS
NOT IDENTICAL

Business leaders who attempt to justify corporate political action on the basis of identity of interest or selfless public service demonstrate a fundamental lack of understanding of the basic character of the political process. Implicit in their position is the assumption that there exists a single, unitary conception of *the* public interest about which all men of good will agree. Such is not the case.[6] Those who espouse this view fail to appreciate the inherently ambiguous nature of the public interest, which, in essence, derives from an amalgam or pragmatic consensus of the conflicting views of diverse social interests. Basically, advocates of this position fail to recognize that diversity of interest is fundamental to a pluralistic society. Basic to democracy is the achievement of a dynamic equilibrium among competing interests in a way that meets the needs and desires of the broadest possible segment of the citizenry and enables that citizenry to participate in the decision-making process.

The difficulties inherent in attempts to equate the interests of any single group with the public interest are suggested by the comments of Wayne A. R. Leys:

> There are three meanings which can reasonably be attributed to "the public interest" as a set of criteria for judging proposed governmental actions. Ideally, governmental action will
>
> (1) maximize interest satisfactions (utility)
> (2) be determined by due process
> (3) be motivated by a desire to avoid destructive social conflict (good faith).
>
> In judgments of specific policy issues, it is seldom possible to find an alternative that satisfies all three criteria equally well. It is seldom possible to eliminate entirely all but one alternative as claiming to meet the demands of "the public interest." A pragmatic attempt to define the nature of the problematic situation sometimes reduces our uncertainty as to which of the "public interest" criteria is most relevant. But in the end the existentialists are correct: there is a leap of faith, a commitment, an engagement.[7]

The above discussion does not suggest that the corporation and the broader society do not share common goals. Indeed, when viewed within a comprehensive social context, the corporation is simply an important structural arrangement of American society, designed to fulfill economic functions that are necessary to any industrial civilization.[8] A distinguishing characteristic of the political economy of the United States has been the delegation to business corporations of most of the responsibility connected with the production and distribution of goods and services. In performing these tasks, however, business corporations are acting on behalf of the total society.

For example, the total volume of sales by General Motors in 1965 accounted for more than 2 per cent of the gross national product. Indeed, GM's net operating revenues that year exceeded the 1964 gross national product of any nation, below the top nine, in the non-Communist world. GM's 1965 federal income tax represented 1.87 per cent of the federal government's receipts for the year and 6.83 per cent of all corporate income taxes paid during the period. Since any significant policy decision by General Motors regarding capital expenditures, foreign investment, or production levels has great impact on the national economy, company officials must consider the economic health of the country while furthering the best interests of the firm. Conversely, governmental officials cannot take actions inimical to the long-run welfare of General Motors or of the other automobile firms without adversely affecting national economic stability. The importance of the industry becomes all the more apparent when one considers that, in 1966, the Big Three automobile makers occupied, in terms of sales, three of the top five positions among the 500 largest American industrial corporations; employed nearly 2 per cent of all civilian, nonagricultural workers (and over 10 per cent of the aggregate labor force of the 500 leading industrials); and possessed over 8.5 per cent of the assets of the top 500 industrial firms.[9] More generally, "so strategic is their economic position and so dependent upon them are thousands of persons that what happens to any one of the giant firms is of the greatest moment to the entire population and, perforce, to the makers of public policy."[10]

Even in the economic sphere, however, the interests and objectives of any single company, including General Motors, are not and cannot be coterminous with the "public interest," as was made abundantly clear in GM's case during the debate over the National Traffic and Motor Vehicle Safety Act of 1966.[11] Antitrust policy is predicated on the assumption that what may be good for an economically dominant firm may not benefit competition in the national economy. Moreover, corporate executives have conceptions of the desirability of advertising regulations, depreciation write-offs, foreign-investments restrictions, and wage-and-price guidelines that differ from those of representatives of other social interests. Indeed, within any business firm, managers may disagree about what constitutes the corporate interest. For example, in the case of large corporations such as Du Pont, "there is very real difficulty in discovering what [the company's] 'interest' is," because of the diversity of organizational activity and accordingly, Du Pont has a "wide variety of interests and orientations."[12] Since goal conflict or diversity is a basic characteristic of all large-scale organizations, the same can be said of virtually any enterprise represented in the annual *"Fortune* Directory."

In the early 1950's, a *Fortune* article nominated corporations as the champions of the American Federal Republic and suggested that the relationship between the Presidency and the corporation was one of "dependence . . . not unlike that of King John on the landed barons of Runnymede, where Magna Carta was born."[13] The assertion is valid, considering this country's reliance upon business corporations for the fulfillment of the economic tasks of society. However, if it is considered as a suggestion for the foundation of public policy, the dangers inherent in the above description are apparent. Notwithstanding increasing corporate sensitivity to what has been termed the public consensus,[14] even in the area of economic policy, the community of interest between business firms and other political participants in our society is, at best, imperfect. Emmette S. Redford pithily summarized the point when he concluded:

> Business can never be government, nor be like government *in the most significant sense* because neither the traditional corporation, seeking profits, nor the metrocorporation, seeking a social role, nor corporate management, serving as agent for some interests and broker among others, can have the breadth of view ("public-interest" perspective) required of government, and because corporate management will not be as representative of and responsive to the total interests served ("democracy") as government under the American political constitution can claim to be.[15]

BUSINESS RATIONALITY AND GOVERNMENTAL EFFICIENCY

As a subsidiary to the corporate interest–public interest thesis discussed above, managers occasionally assert that corporate political involvement is necessary to further the public good by introducing rational business values and skills into government. This argument is based upon several assumptions. Because of the necessity for testing business performance by the measure of profitability, corporate operations are assumed to be rational and practical, thus resulting in cost efficiencies. Accordingly, business managers are presumably levelheaded individuals who do not make decisions in an unbusinesslike manner. Thus, runs the argument, if governmental decisions were made by businessmen, rationality and efficiency would abound and the public interest would be served. Efficiency and rationality are, therefore, presumed to be norms that are equally operative for all public institutions, including welfare agencies, universities, and hospitals, as well as federal departments. This subthesis fails on three counts.

In the first place, as an increasing number of scholars have recognized, the operations of large-scale business organizations do not conform to the profit-maximization model assumed by business managers and classical economic theory alike to be in effect. Galbraith terms the theory of profit-maximization "the approved contradiction" since it does not comport with managerial motivations of large-scale firms.[16]   R. Joseph Monsen and Anthony Downs view corporate managers of large-scale organizations as basically profit satisfiers, rather than maximizers, in that while managers attempt to maximize their own lifetime incomes, they do not seek to maximize profits for the firm. Instead they seek a level of profits that will satisfy the various groups making claims upon the corporation (including shareholders, labor unions, government officials, and the public at large). The essentially political task of satisfying multiple publics has replaced the presumably simpler task of an earlier era— that of maximizing the interests of the shareholder.[17] Monsen and Downs point out, moreover:

> Inefficiencies are inherent in all *large* organizations. Hence they will exist not only in large managerial firms with diffused ownership, but also in large non-profit organizations, large owner-managed firms, and even large government agencies. Therefore, even if we agreed with traditional theory that the owners of a firm wish to maximize profits (and we do agree in the case of

owner-managed firms), we would contend that the difference between *owner* motivation and *managerial* motivation will cause systematic deviations from profit-maximizing behavior as long as the firm is large enough so that the owners themselves cannot supervise all facets of its activities.[18]

Second, the image of business organizations as the major loci of rationality has largely been destroyed by the emergence of systems analysis, which was developed almost entirely within the public sector, particularly in conjunction with the "McNamara Revolution" in the Department of Defense during the early 1960's. Instead of contributing organizational know-how to government, significantly and ironically, business corporations have adapted to their own operations the knowledge acquired in the development of such techniques as cost-benefit analysis, systems analysis, and program budgeting. Reflecting these techniques are such innovations as Program Planning and Budgeting System (PPBS) and Program Evaluation Review Technique (PERT), which are used by the military and other governmental agencies. Indeed, the necessity for governmental units to develop criteria of cost efficiency comparable to that of business profitability has provided a prime impetus to this development of systems analysis in governmental economy. Also, the public has become increasingly aware that private-sector organizations are not immune from bureaucracy and uneconomical decisions. Witness, for example, the quarter-billion-dollar mistake made by the Ford Motor Company in designing and marketing the Edsel or the operations of some of the eastern railroads (most notably the New Haven and the Long Island), which pushed them to the point of bankruptcy. Frequent articles in *Fortune* magazine point out examples of managerial mistakes and lost corporate opportunities.[19]

Moreover, in those areas where governmental decision making has explicitly been delegated to private corporations (administration by contract), the resulting efficiencies have hardly been overwhelming. Consequently, in recent years, government officials have been utilizing incentive contracts, in which the contractor assumes the risk of making reasonable estimates and performing efficiently, if he is to make a profit, rather than contracts—such as the now prohibited cost-plus-fixed-fee or cost-plus-percentage-of-cost contracts—in which the government bears the risk. The rationale for the emphasis on the incentive contracts is to increase the efficiency of contracting firms.

Finally, although the line between governmental and nongovernmental organizations is blurring, distinctions in function can nonetheless be drawn. These differences relate primarily to the unique character of the political process, in which the terms *efficiency* and *rationality* have somewhat different meanings than in the business setting. The determination of social priorities—an important ingredient of governmental decision making—is based upon value choices. Values are not objective, and thus they do not lend themselves well to the calculus of cost-benefit analysis.

Accordingly, the implementation of a program of rational cost savings may be dysfunctional in political terms because of an incompatibility with fulfillment of various social needs. For example, further study of a proposed welfare program directed toward minority groups might be more "economical" than immediate action; however, in a community in which racial tensions are heightened, to wait until the most efficient program costwise has been worked out before taking any steps apparent to the minority group might result in conflagration. Similarly, dollar values cannot be the only concern of governmental decision makers in locating new facilities. Experts in the governmental budgetary process recognize that the federal budget is a compromise in the allocation of public resources, with the purpose of maintaining an equilibrium among diverse social interests. Business values alone are insufficient criteria for determining the over-all social costs of governmental policies. A rational economic decision may not be a rational political decision, and vice versa. In the words of Aaron Wildavsky,

> The encroachment of economics upon politics is not difficult to understand. Being political is viewed as bad while being economical is acclaimed as good. . . . Studies based on efficiency criteria are much needed and increasingly useful. My quarrel

> is not with them as such at all. I have been concerned that a
> single value, however important, would triumph over other
> values without explicit consideration being given to them. . . .
> Economic rationality, however laudable in its own sphere, will
> swallow up political rationality unless it also finds talented de-
> fenders.[20]

Accordingly, the justification of a corporate political role on the
grounds of enfusing the governmental sector with good, rational,
and efficient business values as compared with bad, irrational,
and inefficient standards commonly ascribed to public agencies
is neither accurate nor realistic.   Indeed, it is arguable that
one consequence of corporate political involvement is that certain
inefficiencies result from the fact that firms receive special benefits
that are not economically justifiable. Just as the corporate interest
—national interest thesis is a gross oversimplification of a complex
relationship, so too the corporate rationality—public inefficiency
formula is misstated. Neither reason constitutes a sufficient explanation of our justification for corporate political action.

THE DISENFRANCHISED CORPORATION
AND ELECTORAL POLITICS

A second rationale frequently given to explain business
firms as active political participants is that, inherently, corporations as such are "disenfranchised and are without political identity."[21] This unhappy state of affairs is viewed as a consequence
of the fact that "strictly speaking, the corporation, being an
artificial person, can have no . . . policy viewpoint of its own."[22]
The logical implication of this view is that since the corporation
is not officially accounted for in traditional political theory,
which emphasizes the role of a general constituency of individuals, it can never be a true political actor in the sense that a
human person can be. Some corporate managers fear, as an
inevitable consequence of this inherent lack of formal political
identity, a lack of political effectiveness resulting from an

absence of institutional mechanisms for the registering of corporate sentiment. These businessmen propose as a remedy that corporations develop a unique political role for themselves in order to achieve the political identity necessary for effective participation in a pluralistic democracy. As a subsidiary part of this thesis, electoral politics is seen as the primary road to political influence, and, therefore, firms and their managers should concentrate their energies on effectively representing corporations in the electoral sphere.

CORPORATE POLITICAL IDENTITY

Each of the above contentions appears to be based on misconceptions about (1) the nature and the impact of corporate participation in the political arena; and (2) the status of such participation in the context of widespread political involvement by groups and associations in American society. It is true that corporations are disenfranchised in the sense that organizational entities, unlike individuals, cannot vote or hold office—in the American political order, these prerogatives are accorded only to human persons. But, as we have seen, such activities constitute but one small element in the total pattern of political involvement. Although lacking "official" status in political theory, corporations have pursued their interests continually and effectively through a wide variety of governmental and unofficial electoral activities discussed in the preceding chapter, as well as through corporate managers' acting in their individual capacities. In reality, business firms have not been disenfranchised, except in the most formalistic sense of the word. As will be seen, moreover, while political theory may not recognize a corporate political role, public policy does.[23]

The theoretical horizon is not so bleak as those espousing the disenfranchisement theory assert. For nearly a century, corporations have been "persons" within the meaning of the Fourteenth Amendment. As Arthur S. Miller has noted, "the ramifications [of this development] have been considerable, for this almost casually accepted notion was the basis for corporate protection of liberty and property against violations of due process of law—but a process of law that had no historical antecedent."[24] Business corporations have been accorded the safeguards of the First or Fourteenth Amendments in cases involving communications, collective bargaining, libel,[25] and property.

This constitutional protection for the corporate personality has particular relevance to corporate political activity. For example, in the litigation arising out of the dispute between the railroads and truckers in Pennsylvania, which was discussed in the previous chapter, the Supreme Court noted that to ban the activity by the Railroad Conference would

> disqualify people from taking a public position on matters in which they are financially interested [and] would thus deprive the government of a valuable source of information and, at the same time, deprive the people of their right to petition in the very instances in which that right may be of the most importance to them.[26]

In using the term *people*, the Supreme Court was referring to the activities of railroad corporations.

This explicit recognition of the propriety of corporate political action is merely one indication of the acceptance of such action in American politics. We have already seen, for example, that the Administrative Procedure Act charges administrative agencies and executive departments with a duty to solicit the views of regulated firms—which are almost invariably corporations. Similarly, with the exception of the prohibition against corporate campaign contributions and expenditures (which also applies to the electoral activities of labor organizations), there are no statutory restrictions in the political area that are generally applicable to corporations. The Federal Regulation of Lobbying Act of 1946, for instance, does not distinguish corporations from other political participants.[27] Implicit in the judicial and statutory recognition of corporate political acts is an acceptance of the following political facts: (1) that, as a practical matter, corporations do possess organizational political viewpoints and interests; and (2) that, as was pointed out earlier, managers, in conducting corporate political activities, generally act in accordance with organizational rather than individual policies and seek to accomplish company as distinguished from personal objectives. Thus, as a matter of public policy, in almost all respects, corporations have been accorded precisely the same political status as other interest groups. Collective political activity is basic to the political process and has been an integral part of the American scene since the early days of this country. Although corporations may lack an inherent political identity, they constitute, as a class, a most important interest group. The search by business leaders for a unique political role is thus unnecessary.

ELECTORAL DISENFRANCHISEMENT AND
LEGISLATIVE EFFECTIVENESS

Turning briefly to the contention of some corporate leaders that business firms have been precluded from effective political participation as a result of electoral disenfranchisement, little need be said to lay this myth to rest. This alleged disenfranchisement is hardly complete since, as we have seen, corporations and their managers engage in a wide and effective variety of electoral activities.

Even accepting for the moment the contention that the business community has been unable to elect sympathetic representatives, particularly at the national level, this purported failure has not hindered corporate legislative and policy efforts. The demise in the 89th Congress of an AFL-CIO-supported measure that would have repealed the "right-to-work" proviso of the Taft-Hartley Act (Section 14(b)), which permits states to bar union-shop labor contracts, does not demonstrate a business constituency lacking adequate representation in Congress.[28] This example is made especially persuasive when it is recalled that in its 1964 platform the Democratic Party pledged a repeal of Section 14(b)—yet failed to deliver, notwithstanding large majorities in both houses of Congress and a Democratic President.

Similarly, the provisions of the federal income tax law relating to depletion allowances, depreciation write-offs, and investment credits do not sustain the conclusion of corporate political weakness. In addition to these general tax relief provisions, there are the numerous bills which, although cast in general language, provide relief for only one or a handful of companies.[29]

Passage of the Federal Bank Merger Act, which provided relief from the application of the antimerger provisions of the Clayton Act, is yet another example of corporate legislative effectiveness.[30] In 1967, the railroads were able to secure passage of legislation that required compulsory arbitration in the dispute between the carriers and the railway shop-craft unions, despite strenuous opposition from organized labor. On the state level, legislation to tighten the provisions of Workman's Compensation Acts has been sought and obtained by business firms in a number of states, with Pennsylvania being a notable example.

In the above discussion, we are not suggesting that corporations have piled success upon success in the legislative fields of battle. With the passage of the National Traffic and Motor Vehicle Safety Act, a lone author (Ralph Nader) prevailed over the Big Three of the automobile industry. Similarly, the Truth-in-Packaging legislation enacted during the 89th Congress was bitterly opposed by the food-processing industry. Other recent instances of acts passed by Congress despite opposition from industry groups include the Air Quality Act of 1967; the Water Qualities Standards Act of 1965; the Truth-in-Lending Act of 1968; and, in 1967, a bill applying stringent inspection standards to meat packers. While, in a sense, these measures exemplify corporate legislative failures, in each instance the statute, as ultimately enacted, was considerably weaker than the measures favored by the proponents. Conspicuous examples of this fact are the National Traffic and Motor Vehicle Safety Act, which includes no criminal sanctions and but minimal civil penalties for willful violation of standards, and the Truth-in-Packaging Act, which provides for voluntary compliance with industry guidelines rather than mandatory governmental standards.[31]

In an article entitled "Why Business Always Loses," Theodore Levitt expressed the opinion that, ever since 1887, when American business had its first important experience with government regulation in the form of the Interstate Commerce Act, business has been a persistent and predictable loser in all its major legislative confrontations with government and with the voting public.[32]

As the foregoing discussion indicates, the available evidence does not substantiate the claim that business does always lose. While some legislation opposed by industry groups is enacted into law, other measures desired by business interests are passed. Moreover, as we have seen, the mere passage of an "antibusiness" bill may have a negligible effect if the standards and enforcement provisions of the bill are weak. The actual content of an act is the critical determinant of whether business has really lost. Like any other social interest, business has its share of legislative victories, defeats, and compromises. It is neither a constant winner nor a chronic loser.

Additionally, the asserted failure of corporate electoral activity is exaggerated. For example, a few observers considered 1964 to be a fatal disaster for the business community since over two-thirds of the Congressional candidates backed by the AFL-CIO's Committee on Political Education (COPE) were elected. Such a view is unwarranted, however, particularly in light of the 1966 elections, in which only about half of the COPE-endorsed candidates for Congress and approximately a third of the COPE-endorsed gubernatorial candidates were elected. The 1968 results were but slightly better. By way of comparison, in the 1962 off-year election, two-thirds of COPE-sponsored congressional candidates and 60 per cent of COPE-backed gubernatorial aspirants were elected.[33]

Moreover, while the United States Senate no longer warrants the appellation "The Businessmen's Senate," which was applied to that body in the late nineteenth century, senators sympathetic to the needs of the business community still sit on both sides of the aisle. Such support in legislative halls is increasing at least in the sphere of national politics, since, as we have seen, the traditional antipathy between the corporate community and the Democratic Party appears to be lessening to a degree—particularly among larger firms—and since both parties now encompass viewpoints spanning along any liberal-conservative continuum. Therefore, the candidates supported or opposed by corporate interests are no longer automatically identifiable by party label, and thus the election of Democrats to office is not necessarily a sign of corporate ineffectiveness. This is particularly true since, with regard to matters of most direct corporate concern (for example, taxes and defense spending), the views of the two political parties tend more and more to approach each other.

Businessmen tend to forget a related factor—that is, all legislators desire to help their constituents, particularly significant ones. Accordingly, even a reputedly antibusiness congressman is accessible to spokesmen of important corporations located in his district. While a representative may not, in every instance, support the corporation's position, he will at least tend to be sympathetic to the company's needs and will, where possible, promote them, unless they are clearly antithetical to either the interests of his other constituents or his personal political philosophy. For example, Senators Mike Mansfield of Montana and John O. Pastore of Rhode Island, both having reputations as liberal Democrats, are also well known respectively for their representation of Montana copper interests and of Rhode Island textile manufacturers.

In summation of this point, while theoretically disenfranchised, corporations have a very real identity in American politics as a matter both of long-standing practice and of public policy. Moreover, although businessmen frequently assert the contrary, electoral activity is not the primary or even the best route to political influence. The most notable political accomplishments of American corporations have come not from attempts to elect candidates (in which activity, however, they have met with considerable success), but rather from their efforts through governmental politics in influencing the enactment and enforcement of the myriad of laws, rules, and regulations that directly and indirectly affect the operations of business firms. "Campaigns and elections, it may be repeated, are not the totality of politics. . . . The decisions taken between elections constitute the basic stuff of politics, the pelf and glory for which men and groups battle."³⁴

<h2 style="text-align:center">MANAGERIAL PERSONALITY
AND PREROGATIVE</h2>

Another reason for corporate involvement in politics is based as much on managerial personality and prerogative as on the requirements of *Realpolitik*. Corporate leaders who are deeply committed to political views frequently seek to implement their philosophical positions through their business activities. Such managers view their economic endeavors as a logical extension of political persuasion and, where feasible, formulate company policy and action in ways leading to the accomplishment of both economic and political objectives.

It is inevitable, for example, that a corporation of the size and importance of the Ford Motor Company be engaged in political activity. However, the degree of involvement in public (including political) affairs evidenced by the nation's second largest automobile maker during recent years is probably to a considerable extent a function of the interest which Henry Ford II has manifested in these matters. To take a more extreme and more partisan example, the political activities of the Lewis Food Company on behalf of certain conservative groups were a result of the proclivities of its late president and controlling stockholder, D. B. Lewis.³⁵ Another recent example of corporate political activity that, on the basis of the Congressional hearings and report, in large measure appears to be an extension of a manager's personal objectives was the involvement of the International Latex Corporation in the campaign of Senator Thomas J. Dodd, with the apparent objective of enhancing the prospects of the company's chief executive for an ambassadorship.³⁶

Corporate political activity that is predicated, in large measure, upon the political inclinations of company executives is more prevalent among small or medium-sized, closely held firms in which stock ownership is concentrated in the hands of the managers or a family group than in giant public companies. The phenomenon is not unknown, however, among larger companies where there are strong managerial personalities in positions of control. In addition to the Ford Motor Company and International Latex Corporation, publicly held corporations which have been politically active largely as a consequence of the propensities of their chief executives include Sun Oil Company, Pan American World Airways, Harvey Aluminum, and Eversharp.

The activities of Patrick J. Frawley, board chairman of Eversharp, Technicolor, and Schick Electric, illustrate this point. Frawley, through the companies he heads, has spent several hundred thousand dollars a year supporting anti-Communist and conservative political causes and combating the political "neutralization," which, in Frawley's opinion, has affected American businessmen. The political activities of the firms led by Frawley demonstrate the broad range of his political concerns. During the 1966 general elections, Schick paid for a ten-page political advertisement supplement which appeared in newspapers throughout California, urging the passage of a referendum that would restrict the distribution of allegedly pornographic literature; notwithstanding this support, the measure was defeated by the voters. While Frawley has expressed the opinion that corporate political involvement is "good for the country, good for the company, and good for the shareholders,"[37] he cast doubt on at least two-thirds of this assertion when he subsequently reported that a boycott by "left-wing radicals" was responsible for a 53 per cent decline in the net profits of Eversharp during 1967.[38] Indeed, in reporting the loss of profits by the Frawley-led companies, *Newsweek* pointed out the potential danger to business organization of highly ideological political activities, raising the question "Is 'Right' Wrong?"[39] The Eversharp experience suggests that while the public is willing to accept as proper business political participation that is related to usual company concerns, it may not similarly approve of corporate politics that are peripheral to the interests of the firm and involve very controversial issues.

While the case of Frawley and the companies he heads is hardly unique, personal managerial political philosophy is usually not the controlling motivation for corporate political activity. Rather, it is a factor complementary to and supportive of the other reasons that underlie political involvement. The political significance of managerial prerogative should, however, not be discounted.

COUNTERBALANCE UNION POWER: A PRIMARY CORPORATE POLITICAL MOTIVATION

Although each of the three reasons discussed above constitutes an important rationale for corporate political action, an even more basic motivation for such activity in recent years, particularly in the realm of electoral politics, has been the desire of business managers to counteract the political activity of organized labor. Many business leaders seemingly live in dread terror of a political takeover by organized labor, which would, presumably, imperil the American System. Invariably, electoral successes by labor-backed candidates arouse consternation among corporate managers, who view this as positive proof of political domination by trade unions. Indeed, one commentator suggested several years ago that a takeover of the Democratic Party had occurred, with organized labor emerging as a decisive political force which combined the assets of "money, organization, and a driving zest for the things that can be gained in politics."[40]   A corporate leader, Lemuel R. Boulware, formerly vice-president in charge of employee relations at General Electric, termed organized labor the "ideological competitors and intended executioners" of business.[41]   If one takes statements made by corporate managers at face value, then American business has been unable to equal labor's political efficiency, let alone to compete with its "limitless" slush funds.

Although declamations of peerless labor political power became less prevalent after the mid-1950's, they are not entirely of ancient vintage. The Chamber of Commerce of the United States has recently held that "political expenditures by labor organizations have such an impact upon our political institutions as to threaten basic human freedoms."[42]

In the context of contemporary politics, it would appear that, standing alone, counteracting organized labor is a singularly unpersuasive reason for corporate political action. The romance between labor and the Democratic Party has, of late, been undergoing noticeable strains. In early 1966, a rift developed between George Meany, president of the AFL-CIO, and the Johnson administration. Although a partial rapprochement was achieved prior to the 1966 congressional elections and the AFL-CIO strongly supported the presidential candidacy of Vice President Hubert H. Humphrey in the 1968 campaign, tensions persisted, particularly among the rank-and-file members, as a result of policy differences between the unions and the administration. If, as it is reasonable to expect, future Democratic administrations continue to cultivate ties with corporate interests, these strains will probably remain.

Moreover, labor's vaunted congressional strength has gained little for it in the way of substantial legislative successes. For example, the AFL-CIO has met with consistent failure in Congress to accomplish its most important legislative goal—the repeal of the "right-to-work" section (14[b]) of the Taft-Hartley Act— and in its endeavors to broaden the coverage of the federal minimum wage to the extent desired by union interests. In reviewing the record of the first session of the 90th Congress, President Meany accurately noted that the AFL-CIO could not "find much satisfaction in the record," which he said "can be summed up in five words—inadequate funding and unfinished business."[43] On the electoral front, the 1966 congressional election—with a substantial percentage of union-backed candidates, including a number of long-term union stalwarts, meeting defeat—has been characterized as one in which the "Unions Fail to Deliver the Goods."[44] There was only slight improvement in 1968.

In view of the declining number of union members, the growing disenchantment between the union leadership and the rank and file (manifested in the inability to translate leadership policy into members' votes), dissension among important union leaders, the increasingly white-collar composition of the work force, the latent hostility that organized labor has always experienced in American society, and the basically conservative ideological bias of union leaders, the fears of organized labor held by business leaders are exaggerated. While, given the financial and human resources of unions, it would be fallacious to argue seriously that organized labor is today without influence, it is equally erroneous to cast the unions in the role of an invincible juggernaut. Unquestionably, however, a primary labor political asset is a reputation for being powerful, "a *reputation* precariously sustained by the words of their leaders and the fears of their enemies."[45]

When measured in terms of electoral and legislative successes, the political effectiveness of organized labor has declined since the late 1940's, thus making unrealistic any corporate fears of union domination of American politics. Labor no more controls the political order of the United States than do business corporations. More will be said in Chapter Seven about the political role of organized labor.

NEED FOR A FAVORABLE
POLITICAL CLIMATE

The final reason frequently given to explain the need for corporate political activities is the direct and immediate impact of political factors upon managerial decisions resulting from the interdependence between government and business. At a time when, as we have seen, virtually every aspect of corporate activity is vitally affected by decisions made at all levels of government, business managers fear that corporate abstinence from political involvement would subject business firms to the hazards of lambs dwelling in a meadow also inhabited by wolves. Accordingly, they seek to assure a favorable political climate.

Corporations seek increased access to the realms of governmental decision making in order to influence public policies that affect their vital interests. Such policies include, among others, the awarding of contracts, the allocation of materials, the establishment of production standards, wage-and-price guidelines, antitrust enforcement, company capitalization requirements, tax and tariff structures, route and franchise licensing, labor relations, foreign capital investment limitations, safety standards, and environmental pollution controls.

*THE IMPACT OF ECONOMIC
INTERDEPENDENCE*

Proponents of the argument that corporate political activity is necessary to create a favorable political climate also stress that interdependence, while always present to some degree, is now *the* essential characteristic of the American political economy. Accordingly, business interests must ensure that governmental power and responsibility are in safe hands. In short, corporate political action is viewed as necessary (1) to neutralize, to the greatest possible extent, the impact of governmental constraints on business activities and (2) to obtain assistance for corporate activities from governmental sources.

This model of the changing political environment surrounding the contemporary corporation is substantially accurate. Greatly concerned with the social, political, and economic implications of this pattern of interdependence, John Kenneth Galbraith has outlined some of its dimensions. He describes the relationship between the federal government and the large corporation as follows: "The industrial system, in fact, is inextricably associated with the state. In notable respects the mature corporation is an arm of the state. And the state, in important matters, is an instrument of the industrial system."[46] While Galbraith's thesis has been properly criticized for presenting an exaggerated picture of the symbiotic relationship between the corporation and the state, the mutual dependence is beyond dispute. It could be argued that this development constitutes the pragmatic American response to the mid-twentieth century growth of socialism in many areas of the world. In contemporary society, the spread of large-scale industrialization inevitably requires a growth in government's participation in the economy. Corporate capitalism and state socialism constitute, therefore, two possible manifestations of the same general trend.[47] In any event, interdependence promises to be the essential characteristic of the American political economy during the foreseeable future.

Advocates of the favorable-political-climate argument tend to overestimate somewhat both the novelty and the extent of present governmental influence upon economic activities by not recognizing (1) that the state has always exercised some control over economic activity and (2) that a substantial proportion of business decisions are outside the purview of governmental control. Earlier discussion noted the close relationship between governmental units and corporations which dates back to the early nineteenth century when public authorities became involved in the operations of business firms as both promoters and regulators. Indeed, as Andrew Shonfield has pointed out, "the conventional view of a business community with a zero margin of tolerance for public intervention is false. Historically, American capitalism in its formative period was much readier to accept intervention by public authority than British capitalism."[48]

Second, despite the seeming omnipresence of governmental constraints, corporate managers actually make most of their operating decisions outside the scope of public scrutiny. For example, decisions relating to capital investment, product development, employment, pricing, and plant location are, in the main, made by businessmen without the necessity of obtaining any approval from a public agency. In certain dramatic instances, the federal government has exerted direct pressure on companies concerning a particular operating decision—for example, federal pressure on United States Steel in 1962 to rescind a price increase. These instances, however, are exceptions rather than the norm, a fact evidenced by the resultant surprise and outrage of many businessmen when they occur. It is noteworthy, parenthetically, that the business activities of the state are subject to a much greater degree of public supervision than that to which corporations are expected to submit. The above two observations, although seemingly contradictory, clearly point out that governmental involvement is neither as novel nor as ubiquitous as businessmen often suggest.

THE RELUCTANT PARTICIPANTS

As a subsidiary point to the political-climate explanation of corporate political participation, business managers often assert that such participation is contrary to their real wishes and is only reluctantly undertaken for the self-protection of the firm. Although corporations are frequently pictured as political intruders, upsetting the natural equilibrium of the governmental system by their importuning, business managers often view themselves as being pulled into the political arena much against their wishes and better judgment. They play the political game because a policy of noninvolvement would be harmful to their business operations. They also see politicians and public officials as expecting, and even demanding, their participation.

The validity of this view is limited, since it fails to recognize the inherently political character of business operations and overemphasizes the assertedly innate desire of corporate leaders for political passivity. It does, however, offer a valuable insight. Corporations occasionally are unwilling political participants, particularly in the area of electoral politics. In the crudest form of the game, corporations (via their executives) are solicited for campaign funds—used as "milk cows" in the view of businessmen[49]—with the unstated but implicit understanding that a failure to contribute might result in unfavorable governmental action in areas critical to the firm's activities. For example, in one southwestern state, it is reported that a dinner in honor of the incumbent member of a certain regulatory agency is held during the year in which he is running for re-election. Under the local custom, firms in the industry regulated by the agency are expected to buy tickets to the dinner for an amount determined by an "official" schedule based upon the firm's average annual volume of business in the state. The proceeds of the dinner, of course, are contributed to the campaign fund of the incumbent agency member. The lessons of Mark Hanna's policy of systematic assessments of corporations, which prevailed around the turn of the century, have not been forgotten!

While the mechanical efficiency of the dunning system described above is probably atypical, the pattern of explicit or tacit understandings of financial obligations owed by companies to candidates and parties is not. Even where overt and blatant pressure is not present, firms engaged in exchanging goods and services with governmental units appreciate the wisdom of ingratiating themselves with those who make governmental decisions of great business consequence. This is true on the local level, where zoning exemptions, municipal franchises and tax assessments are involved; on the state level, where "certificates of convenience" and utility rates are frequently at issue; and finally on the national level, where procurement contracts, labor relations, research subsidies, or depreciation allowances are of concern to business. In essence, corporate political involvement can be considered a type of insurance policy in which companies must necessarily invest in order to safeguard against risks at the hands of governmental decision makers.

Notwithstanding the criticisms that have been made of the political-climate thesis and of the subsidiary contention attributing corporate political involvement to reluctant self-protection, these rationales are far more convincing than the other reasons offered to explain the necessity for this involvement. This dual explanation, moreover, reveals a refreshingly frank acknowledgement by business leaders of the purpose of political activity—the necessity of obtaining access to areas of public decision making in order to attempt to effect certain goals—and has the virtue of viewing political participation in realistic terms. The explanation manifests an awareness of the fact that corporations exist in a pluralistic setting fraught with politics, and that, therefore, they must be political actors in order to survive against conflicting groups, including both other social interests and corporate competitors. Such a view, moreover, recognizes implicitly that a private enterprise system must by its very nature also be a system of state intervention, and, accordingly, business corporations must seek to structure the framework within which such intervention takes place.

SUMMATION

The analysis in this chapter has centered on the five major reasons offered by business leaders to explain corporate political involvement: (1) the identity between the corporate interest and the national interest; (2) the need to establish a political identity for the disenfranchised corporation, particularly through

electoral politics; (3) the managerial personality and prerogative; (4) the need to counteract the threatened political domination by organized labor; and (5) the fundamental importance
of a favorable political climate in an interdependent political
economy. All these explanations combine elements of political
fact with healthy dosages of political ideology. In discussing each
rationale, we have sought to distinguish these two ingredients.

Implicit in each of the five reasons given by managers is the
underlying premise of the legitimacy of political involvement by
business firms. Understandably, business leaders pay relatively
little attention to the knotty theoretical problems that this involvement poses for a democratic society. These problems are
not, however, neglected by others. As will be seen in the next
chapter, opponents of political activity by business firms raise a
number of serious objections.

While the issue of the legitimacy of corporate political involvement will be analyzed more fully later, it is appropriate to
point out that the political-climate rationale for this involvement
is fundamental to any theory of legitimacy. Elements of the
other four managerial explanations of corporate politics are of
theoretical interest. It is upon the fifth rationale, however, that
a theory of corporate political legitimacy must ultimately be
based—or, in the alternative, such legitimacy must ultimately
be found lacking.

NOTES

[1] Quoted in *The New York Times*, January 24, 1953, p. 8, col. 8.

[2] Max Lerner, *America as a Civilization* (New York: Simon and
Schuster, Inc., 1957), p. 312.

[3] All the quoted references to Lasswell are from Harold D. Lasswell, *Power and Personality* (New York: Compass Books, The Viking
Press, Inc., 1962), p. 38.

[4] Additional insights into this question are found in Francis X.

Sutton, Seymour E. Harris, Carl Kaysen and James Tobin, *The American Business Creed* (New York: Schocken Books, 1962), Chaps. 1, 17. See also Clifford Geertz, "Ideology as a Cultural System," in David E. Apter (ed.), *Ideology and Discontent* (New York: The Free Press, 1964), pp. 47–76; and David Riesman with Nathan Glazer and Reuel Denney, *The Lonely Crowd*, abridged ed. (New Haven, Conn.: Yale University Press, 1961), pp. 131–35. Compare Paul A. Samuelson, "Personal Freedoms and Economic Freedoms in the Mixed Economy," and Earl F. Chiet (ed.), *The Business Establishment* (New York: John Wiley & Sons, Inc., 1964), pp. 193–227.

⁵For additional discussion of this point, see Earl F. Cheit, "Why Managers Cultivate Social Responsibility," *California Management Review*, VII, No. 1 (Fall 1964), 3–22.

⁶The difficulties in discerning the "public interest" have been pointed out by Glendon Schubert and Frank J. Sorauf. For summaries of their positions, see their contributions to Carl J. Friedrich (ed.), *Nomos V . . . The Public Interest* (New York: Atherton Press, 1962), pp. 162–76 and 183–90. Also relevant are Herbert McClosky, "Consensus and Ideology in American Politics," *American Political Science Review*, LVIII, No. 2 (June 1964), 361–82; and Anthony Downs, *An Economic Theory of Democracy* (New York: Harper & Row, Publishers, 1957). Compare Walter Lippmann, *The Public Philosophy* (Boston: Little, Brown and Company, 1955), Chap. 4; Grant McConnell, *Private Power and American Democracy* (New York: Alfred A. Knopf, Inc., 1966), pp. 157–65 and 336–68; Henry S. Kariel, "The Corporation and the Public Interest," *Annals of the American Academy of Political and Social Science*, CCCXLIII (September 1962), 39–47; the views of C. W. Cassinelli, Gerhard Colm, and Wayne A. R. Leys in Friedrich (ed.), *Nomos V*, pp. 44–53, 115–28, 237–56; and Charner M. Perry and Wayne A. R. Leys, *Philosophy and the Public Interest* (Chicago: Committee to Advance Original Works in Philosophy, 1959).

⁷Wayne A. R. Leys, "The Relevance and Generality of 'The Public Interest,'" in Friedrich (ed.), *Nomos V . . .* , p. 256.

⁸Discussions of the relationship between economic institutions and society are found in Talcott Parsons and Neil J. Smelser, *Economy and Society* (New York: The Free Press, 1956); Neil J. Smelser, *The Sociology of Economic Life* (Englewood Cliffs, N.J.: Prentice-Hall, Inc., 1963); Wilbert Moore, *The Impact of Industry* (Englewood Cliffs, N.J.: Prentice-Hall, Inc., 1965); Manning Nash, *Primitive*

and Peasant Economic Systems (San Francisco: Chandler Publishing Company, 1966); and Karl Polanyi, *The Great Transformation* (Boston: Beacon Press, Inc., 1959).

[9]The statistics in this paragraph are drawn from the following sources: President of the United States, *Economic Report of the President, Together with the Annual Report of the Council of Economic Advisors* (Washington: U.S. Government Printing Office, 1968), pp. 234–35 (Table B-22); "The Massive Statistics of General Motors," *Fortune*, LXXIV, No. 2 (July 15, 1966), 298; and "The 500 Largest U.S. Industrial Corporations," *Fortune*, LXXV, No. 7 (June 15, 1967), 196–213.

[10]Morton S. Baratz, "Corporate Giants and the Power Structure," *Western Political Quarterly*, IX, No. 2 (June 1956), 411.

[11]15 U.S.C. § § 1381–1425 (1966).

[12]Louis Anthony Dexter, "Where the Elephant Fears to Dance Among the Chickens: Business in Politics? The Case of du Pont," *Human Organizations*, XIX (Winter 1960), 191.

[13]John Knox Jessup, "A Political Role for the Corporation," *Fortune*, XLVI, No. 2 (August 1952), 154.

[14]Adolph A. Berle, Jr., *Power Without Property* (New York: Harcourt, Brace & World, Inc., 1959), pp. 110–16. Compare Henry G. Manne, "Corporate Responsibility, Business Motivation and Reality," *Annals*, CCCXLIII (September 1962), 55–64.

[15]Emmette S. Redford, "Business as Government," in Roscoe C. Martin (ed.), *Public Administration and Democracy* (Syracuse, N.Y.: Syracuse University Press, 1965), p. 78.

[16]John Kenneth Galbraith, *The New Industrial State* (Boston: Houghton Mifflin Company, 1967), Chap. 10. See also William J. Baumol, *Business Behavior, Value and Growth* (New York: The Macmillan Company, Publishers, 1959); Neil W. Chamberlain, *Enterprise and Environment: The Firm in Time and Place* (New York: McGraw-Hill Book Company, 1968), pp. 55–56; Robin Marris, *The Economic Theory of 'Managerial' Capitalism* (New York: The Free Press, 1964); and Joseph W. McGuire, *Theories of Business Behavior* (Englewood Cliffs, N.J.: Prentice-Hall, Inc., 1964).

[17]R. Joseph Monsen, Jr., and Anthony Downs, "A Theory of Large Managerial Firms," *Journal of Political Economy*, LXXIII, No. 3 (June 1965), 221–36.

[18]Monsen and Downs, "A Theory . . . ," p. 230.   Apparent em-

pirical support for the Monsen and Downs theory is found in R. Joseph Monsen, John S. Chiu, and David E. Colley, "The Effect of Separation of Ownership and Control on the Performance of the Large Firm," *The Quarterly Journal of Economics*, LXXII, No. 36 (August 1968), 435–51.

[19]See, for example, Gene Bylinsky, "Hughes Aircraft: The High-Flying Might-Have-Been," *Fortune*, LXXVII, No. 4 (April 1968), 101; and William S. Rukeyser, "Litton Down to Earth," *Fortune*, LXXVII, No. 4 (April 1968), 139. See also Richard Austin Smith, *Corporations in Crisis* (Garden City, N.Y.: Doubleday & Company, Inc., 1963).

[20]Aaron Wildavsky, "The Political Economy of Efficiency: Cost-Benefit Analysis, Systems Analysis, and Program Budgeting" (Berkeley: Institute of Urban and Regional Development, Center for Planning & Development Research, University of California, Berkeley, September 1966), pp. 45–46. Mimeograph. A slightly revised version of Wildavsky's monograph is found in *Public Administration Review*, XXVI, No. 4 (December 1966), 292–310.

[21]Crawford H. Greenewalt, "A Political Role for Business," *California Management Review*, II, No. 1 (Fall 1959), 9.

[22]Michael D. Reagan, *The Managed Economy* (Fair Lawn, N.J.: Oxford University Press, Inc., 1963), p. 132.

[23]For an examination in theoretical terms of the political role of corporations, see Sheldon S. Wolin, *Politics and Vision* (Boston: Little, Brown and Company, 1960), pp. 414–34.

[24]Arthur Selwyn Miller, *The Supreme Court and American Capitalism* (New York: The Free Press, 1968), p. 54.

[25]See cases collected in Edwin M. Epstein, *Corporations, Contributions and Political Campaigns: Federal Regulation in Perspective* (Berkeley: Institute of Governmental Studies, University of California, Berkeley, 1968); pp. 194–95, fns. 279–81.

[26]*Eastern R.R. Presidents Conference* v. *Noerr Motor Freight, Inc.*, 365 U.S. 127, 139 (1961).

[27]2 U.S.C., §§ 261–270 (1946).

[28]29 U.S.C. § 164(b) (1947).

[29]See Stanley S. Surrey, "The Congress and the Tax Lobbyist—How Special Tax Provisions Get Enacted," *Harvard Law Review*, LXX, No. 7 (May 1957), 1145–82. For an account of the success of a single company in obtaining "private" tax benefits, see "Aluminum & Politics," *The Wall Street Journal*, April 26, 1967, p. 1, col. 6.

³⁰12 U.S.C. § 1828 (1966), *amending* 15 U.S.C. § 18 (1914) as amended.

³¹Legislation referred to in this paragraph can be cited as follows: National Traffic and Motor Vehicle Safety Act, 15 U.S.C. §§ 1381–1425 (1966); Fair Packaging and Labeling Act, 15 U.S.C. §§ 1451–1461 (1966); Air Quality Act of 1967, 42 U.S.C. §§ 1857–18571 (1967); Water Quality Act of 1965, 33 U.S.C. §§ 466–466j (1965); and the Wholesome Meat Act, 19 U.S.C. § 1306(B) (1967), and 21 U.S.C. §§ 96, 601–624, 641–645, 661, 671–680, 691 (1967).

³²Theodore Levitt, "Why Business Always Loses," *Harvard Business Review*, XLVI, No. 2 (March-April 1968), 81.

³³See Herbert E. Alexander, *Financing the 1964 Election* (Princeton, N.J.: Citizens' Research Foundation, 1966), p. 97; "Vanishing Vote," *Time*, November 25, 1966, p. 34; "Unions Fail to Deliver the Goods," *Business Week*, November 19, 1966, pp. 103, 106, 108. For an examination of organized labor's electoral failure in 1966, see J. Michael Eisner, "Implications for 1968: An Analysis of Labor's Recent Disaster at the Polls," *Business and Society*, VII, No. 2 (Spring 1967), 5–12.

³⁴V. O. Key, Jr., *Politics, Parties and Pressure Groups*, 5th ed. (New York: Thomas Y. Crowell Co., 1964), p. 142.

³⁵The Lewis Food Company was indicted for alleged violations of § 313 of the Federal Criminal Code (18 U.S.C. § 610 [1951]), arising out of several newspaper advertisements sponsored by the company in connection with the 1962 California congressional primaries. Ultimately, after two trials, the corporation was fined a nominal sum after it entered a plea of *nolo contendere* to the federal government's charges. See *United States* v. *Lewis Food Company, Inc.*, 366 F.2d 710 (9th Cir. 1966) *reversing* 236 F.Supp. 849 (S.D. Calif. 1964); and Epstein, *Corporations, Contributions . . .* , Chap. 4.

³⁶*Hearings* and *Report*, Parts I and II, *Investigation of Senator Thomas J. Dodd of Connecticut*, U.S. Congress, Senate, Select Committee on Standards and Conduct, 90th Cong., 1st Sess., S.Rept. 193 to accompany S.Res. 112, under the authority of S.Res. 338 (Washington, D.C.: U.S. Government Printing Office, 1967), pp. 20–22, 25, 26.

³⁷Peter Gall, "Battling Blade Man," *The Wall Street Journal*, June 24, 1966, p. 1, col. 6, quoted at p. 15, col. 1. See also Stanley H. Brown, "The Frawley Phenomenon," *Fortune*, LXXIII, No. 2 (February 1966), 136.

[38]See "Corporations: Is 'Right' Wrong?" *Newsweek,* March 18, 1968, p. 79.

[39]"Corporations . . ." (*Newsweek*).

[40]Raymond Moley, *The Political Responsibility of Businessmen* (New Brunswick, N.J.: Johnson and Johnson, 1958), p. 7.

[41]Lemuel R. Boulware, quoted in Andrew Hacker and Joel D. Aberbach, "Businessmen in Politics," *Law and Contemporary Problems,* XXVII, No. 2 (Spring 1962), 267.

[42]*Policy Declarations—1965/1966 Adopted by Members of the Chamber of Commerce of the United States of America* (Washington, D.C.: Chamber of Commerce of the United States of America, 1965), p. 79. See also "Why Politics Needs Business in '66," *Nation's Business,* LIV, No. 6 (June 1966), 42.

[43]George Meany, "Foreword" in *Labor Looks at Congress 1967: An AFL-CIO Legislative Report,* Publication No. 77-1 (Washington, D.C.: AFL-CIO Department of Legislation, January 1968), p. 1.

[44]"Unions Fail to Deliver the Goods," *Business Week,* November 19, 1966, pp. 103, 106, 108.

[45]Theodore Levitt, "Business Should Stay Out of Politics," *Business Horizons,* III, No. 2 (Summer 1960), 47.

[46]John Kenneth Galbraith, *The New Industrial State* (Houghton Mifflin Company, 1967), p. 296.

[47]For an analysis of alternative ways of structuring economic activity in modern industrial society, see Robert A. Dahl and Charles E. Lindblom, *Politics, Economics, and Welfare: Planning and Politico-Economic Systems Resolved into Basic Social Processes* (New York: Torchbooks, Harper & Row, Publishers, 1963), pp. 3–54.

[48]Andrew Shonfield, *Modern Capitalism* (Fair Lawn, N.J.: Oxford University Press, Inc., 1965), p. 301.

[49]"Why Politics Needs Business in '66," *Nation's Business,* June 1966, p. 76.

Chapter Seven

The Managerial Naysayers: Why Corporations Should Not Be in Politics

Just as the managerial proponents advance a number of reasons to explain the necessity and the propriety of corporate political involvement, the opponents of political participation by business firms also offer a variety of explanations to support their view. These critics base their opposition on economic, political, and philosophical considerations, at times combining the three grounds in offering their position. Among the various contentions made by the opponents of corporate political involvement, the five most important will be analyzed in detail and are summarized below:

    1. The business of business is business; therefore, political activity does not come within the purview of proper corporate action.

    2. Increased corporate involvement could lead to renewed political activity by organized labor with

the possible consequence of polarizing American political parties on a class basis.

3. Political involvement could ultimately lead to a loss of corporate autonomy in American society through the elimination of the distinction between "public" and "private." This result could take the form of either total public regulation or nationalization of corporations, with the intention of precluding any possibility of business domination of government.

4. Corporate participation in the political arena is akin to Gulliver frolicing among the Lilliputians. Since business firms possess a superabundance of power, they have an inordinate advantage over other social interests, which is detrimental to the political system.

5. Corporations lack political legitimacy, since democratic theory is based on political participation by human beings acting either individually or through associations. Political theory provides no rationale to explain the political activities of fictional corporate "persons" who are not accountable to any recognizable constituency.

The first three explanations, interestingly enough, are given primarily by managers and other supporters of the business system who are hostile to corporate political activity. Underlying these reasons are the fear of impairing the corporate system through political participation and the desire to preserve the freedom of economic action that corporations have traditionally enjoyed in American society. The remainder of this chapter will be devoted to a discussion of the three managerial reasons for opposing corporate political involvement.

The other two—excessive corporate power and a lack of political legitimacy—will be analyzed in subsequent chapters. Unlike the first three rationales, these arguments are made not by managers out of concern for possible dangers to the corporate system, but rather by representatives of other social interests and by scholars who fear possible adverse effects to or even destruction of American democracy as a result of corporate political involvement. Since the issues of excessive corporate power and legitimacy are basic to any understanding of the implications of this involvement for social pluralism in the United States, they warrant separate and extensive analysis. These two questions will be treated respectively in Chapters Eight and Nine. With this introduction, the analysis now centers on the three reasons advanced for managerial opposition to corporate involvement.

POLITICS IS NOT A PROPER CORPORATE ACTIVITY

One objection raised by critics of corporate political participation is that such participation will interfere with the business objectives of the firm. Proponents of this view apparently fear that political activity will catapult the corporation along the path of economic decline. The contention is made, for example, that

> involvement in politics can lead only to corporate inefficiency and possible ruin. The corporation that becomes deeply involved in party politics will necessarily dilute its basic profit-making function. The politically active corporation will have to become less seriously profit-minded. When that happens, it will cease to deliver the goods abundantly and efficiently.[1]

Such fears are chimerical. The author of the above statement seems to envision at least a substantial, if not a total, dedication of the corporate enterprise to the business of politics. As he apparently views the prospect, ordinary corporate activities, such as the production and distribution of goods and services, would either grind to a halt or, at very least, would stumble along the path of economic inefficiency. Underlying this position, moreover, is the unwarranted assumption that corporations are not already deeply involved in politics, including partisan politics. Enough has been said regarding this point to make further discussion redundant.

The misgivings expressed above are illusory for yet another reason. Even if existing legal restrictions against corporate political participation were eliminated, thereby enabling companies to engage in any political activities without fear of sanction, it is exceedingly doubtful that corporations would commit substantial additional company manpower or resources to political endeavors. (The most important legal constraints are (1) federal and state statutory prohibitions of certain types of corporate political contributions and expenditures, and (2) the possibility of shareholders' suits challenging the use of company funds for political purposes.) Several important reasons prompt this conclusion.

PRESENT LEVEL OF CORPORATE POLITICAL COMMITMENT IS SUFFICIENT

In the first place, many companies are already committed to the extent they consider necessary to accomplish their political objectives. As we have seen, corporate funds and personnel presently go into a wide variety of electoral and governmental activities. A substantial number of the larger firms now have governmental relations and public affairs departments and other groups of specialized personnel which are concerned with political matters of a very broad character. Thus, utilization of additional company resources for political purposes is basically unnecessary.

INTRACORPORATE COMPETITION LIMITS POLITICAL INVOLVEMENT

Second, competition within the corporation limits the amount of company resources that are devoted to political endeavors. Public affairs or governmental relations departments constitute merely one of many staff services available in the modern corporation. Consequently, political activities involve only a small number of individuals and receive only a minor budgetary allotment within any given enterprise. In their efforts to obtain organizational resources, the various staff and production departments compete with one another in attempts to increase their own allocations. Often the success of one unit occurs

at the expense of other company departments whose budget
requests are not met. The tendency toward empire-building,
which exists within the component parts of all large organizations, serves as a countervailing force against the expansionist
aspirations of any particular component part of the corporate
structure. The emergence of Galbraith's "technostructure"—a
body of technically proficient specialists with strong professional,
as opposed to organizational, identifications and loyalties—
increases this intracorporate competition. These technocrats
tend to be oriented toward specific problems and projects which
draw upon their technical expertise, rather than toward the
broader objectives of the corporation.[2] Moreover, as this chapter indicates, there is hostility by some managers to corporate
political involvement, and their opposition operates as a brake
upon such involvement. Finally, as we shall see in a subsequent
section, serious political differences may exist among the subsidiary divisions of a firm, thereby restricting the political activities of the company. Thus sufficient internal constraints exist
to prevent any allocation of corporate resources to political activity to an extent that would impair the fulfillment of the basic
economic functions of the firm.

CORPORATE POLITICS:
A SUPPORTIVE FUNCTION

Corporate officials and employees who are concerned with
political affairs are in a position analogous to that of other staff
personnel, such as legal counsel, industrial relations advisors,
economists, and systems analysts. Their function is basically
supportive—contributing to the profitability and growth of the
company as a producer and merchandiser of goods and services
and promoting the longevity and stability of the enterprise. As
suggested earlier, certain business managers may view corporate
political participation as an opportunity for implementing their
personal predilections, but more often they seek merely to create
a favorable climate within which to pursue their firm's basic
economic goals. Political activity is viewed simply as a normal

concomitant of doing business in a politically charged environment.[3]   Managers who have the responsibility for corporate political action are not likely to act in a precipitate fashion that might jeopardize the position of their companies—and ultimately their own careers.   Indeed, if anything, such individuals have tended "to go slow" in increasing either the scope or the magnitude of political activities.

POLITICS AND PROFITS

Another aspect of the argument that politics is not the business of the corporation relates to the goal of profit maximization. The contention is made that corporations have only one function —to maximize profits for the stockholders—and that any expenditures of company time, money, and personnel that do not directly further that goal are improper.   Corporate political activity is not considered by its critics to be a profit-maximizing endeavor.

This contention is not novel but has its counterpart in the opposition of some business managers to the tendency of many large firms to undertake public service activities of an assertedly socially responsible character.   Among these activities are slum rehabilitation; job training for minority-group members; financial contributions to educational, cultural, and religious institutions; installation of smoke- and water-pollution control equipment not required by law; or sponsorship of scholarship programs.[4]   Since corporate social responsibility has been the subject of innumerable books and articles in the past few years and has only limited relevance to an analysis of corporate political activity, a thorough discussion of the implications of this notion is unnecessary in the context of this book.[5]   It should be noted, however, that the managerial search for the holy grail of social responsibility represents an explicit recognition by businessmen that the classic economic model is no longer in accord with the reality of an economy in which huge multinational corporations dominate their markets and exceed many governmental units in resources and social impact.   This classic model incorrectly portrays the business firm as a strictly economic organization forced by a highly competitive environment to concentrate on the single-minded purpose of profit maximization.

While large managerial firms seek profits because profits are necessary for the stability and growth of the enterprise, they do not attempt to *maximize* their profits except, perhaps, in a very long-run sense; this "maximization" strains the generally understood meaning of the concept. Instead, corporations today are confronted with the task of balancing the claims made of them by many diverse social interests. The pursuit of social responsibility—shadowy though this concept may be—is, accordingly, an inescapable corporate goal based upon the desire of business managers to preserve their autonomy by demonstrating that corporations act in accordance with public expectations and interests and should not, therefore, be subjected to additional social controls.[6] By preserving corporate autonomy through socially responsible activity, the profit-making objectives of the firm are, thereby, facilitated.

As was suggested earlier, corporate political involvement serves a similar purpose. Corporations undertake political activities to maintain and to extend company autonomy through the creation of a hospitable environment. Indeed, the correlation between the utilization of corporate resources and the furtherance of organizational interests is frequently more discernible in the case of company political involvement than in instances of broader, more general, "socially responsible" pursuits. To the degree that corporate managers can identify their political interests, their political activities presumably correspond closely with these interests.[7]

•   •   •

Seen from the corporate viewpoint, therefore, political involvement is a proper company activity if it serves to enhance the long-run economic prospects of the organization. In fact, it can be argued that corporate managers are derelict in their duties if they do not seek to further the stability and profitability of the enterprise through legitimate political means. While the business of business is indeed business, company objectives often have political dimensions that can be furthered only by political means.

THE LABOR BUGABOO REVISITED

A second reason frequently advanced in opposition to corporate political participation, particularly on a partisan basis, is that company involvement might energize labor into increased political activity. According to this view, a likely consequence of heightened activity on the part of these antagonists would be the polarization of American politics along economic lines, with labor forming the nucleus of one party and business corporations the core of another.[8] Should such a dichotomy develop, it is argued, the weight of numbers would inevitably be on labor's side, thereby resulting in political defeat for business and perhaps, ultimately, in the imposition of restrictions upon corporate independence. At very least, it is suggested, business interests cannot possibly match the overwhelming human and financial resources of organized labor and must, therefore, be disadvantaged political competitors. Accordingly, concludes the argument, it is preferable for business firms to forego political action rather than experience inevitable defeat.

These fears are—both individually and collectively—unfounded. A restructuring of the two major American political parties is always possible, though not very probable; however, for several reasons the likelihood of a recasting of the party structure along a business-labor axis is virtually nonexistent.

ORGANIZED LABOR HAS LIMITED
POLITICAL POWER

A most important reason is that the reputed labor dreadnought does not exist. This is not to deny that organized labor, like many other interest groups, has political power. It possesses in reasonable abundance two necessary political assets—manpower and money. Furthermore, since the early 1930's the labor movement has had a close relationship with the Democratic Party which, on the national level, has been in power during most of this period. Labor's political strength has not, however, resulted in political dominance. Moreover, whatever potential for such dominance may, at one time, have existed has long since disappeared. Three broad developments particularly illustrate this decline in political power.

Declining union affiliation. First, organized labor affiliation has been declining in recent years, due in large measure to (1) a shrinkage in employment in the organized industries; (2) a change in certain industries from strongly unionized areas to the largely nonunion South; and (3) a shift in the composition of the labor force from blue-collar to white-collar workers. By the mid-1960's, approximately 16–2/3 million American workers, less than 30 per cent of civilian, nonagricultural employees, belonged to unions. The lessening support for unions among workers is reflected in the continuous decline both in the percentage of NLRB representation elections won by unions and in percentage of votes that the unions have received in such elections. While in the decade between 1936 and 1945, unions won more than 83 per cent of all representation elections and polled more than 81 per cent of the vote, in the decade between 1956 and 1965 the figures had declined to slightly more than 60 per cent and 61 per cent respectively.[9]

The prospects for union growth are not encouraging. Projections of manpower needs have indicated that employment growth will take place primarily in what have been predominantly nonunion areas—white-collar and highly skilled blue-collar occupations. Although white-collar workers have made up more than 14 per cent of total union membership in the 1960's, these unionized employees have been concentrated largely in public organizations rather than in business firms. Accordingly, the prospects for extensive unionization of white-collar workers in private industry seem particularly bleak.

Moreover, while it is possible that white-collar groups will seek and will develop some form of collective representation, this representation will probably differ from traditional blue-collar unions. As Everett M. Kassalow has suggested, "we now know . . . the special qualities of white-collar workers have not really disappeared; in most western countries white-collar workers are much less unionized than are manual workers, and for the most part they give no signs of becoming like manual workers in their social outlook."[10] This observation suggests that even if unions succeed in organizing large numbers of white-collar workers, these workers are likely to be even less politically dependable than blue-collar operatives have been.

Leadership-membership tensions. The second factor that derogates from the political strength of organized labor is the inability of union leadership to rely upon unswerving political support from union members. In the United States, union members have been noted for their political apathy generally and, specifically, for their failure to respond as a malleable cadre for organizational political activity. E. E. Schattschneider has estimated that, at most, half of the total membership of the AFL-CIO voted and that among those who did vote, union activities increased the Democratic bias of union voters by no more than 10 per cent.[11] If this analysis is accurate, among those union members who do vote, a large number base their political positions on personal predilection rather than on union affiliation.

Membership adherence to organizational political policy is, to a substantial degree, a function of the strength of the identification that the member has with the group. Thus, only where there is a strong worker commitment to union goals do labor organizations wield significant influence over their membership.[12] For example, the United Auto Workers (UAW) union, under Walter Reuther, has for many years had the reputation of being a democratic union, which has avoided excessive bureaucracy and centralization, and has probably had a greater degree of worker loyalty than most other unions. Not surprisingly, therefore, Kornhauser, Sheppard, and Mayer found in the mid-1950's that "Detroit area auto workers are . . . predominantly oriented in agreement with the [United Auto Workers] union; they approve of union political activities; they trust labor's voting recommendations and the great majority cast their ballots accordingly."[13]

Nevertheless, in the 1966 Michigan elections, incumbent

Republican Governor George Romney, a one-time president of American Motors, won reelection; and the senatorial candidate, former Governor G. Mennen Williams, lost despite vigorous UAW support. Moreover, both Romney and Republican senatorial winner Robert P. Griffin—one of the authors of the Landrum-Griffin Act which labor finds repugnant—polled well in overwhelmingly Democratic and heavily labor-oriented Detroit and surrounding suburbs. Interestingly, two years later, *The Wall Street Journal* reported that

> despite Mr. Reuther's diligence [to snuff out tendencies within the UAW that tend to subvert democratic processes or dilute members' rights] there is fairly widespread feeling within the UAW that with its 1.4 million members the union is suffering from the same problems of size that are vexing most other major institutions, from churches and universities to the AFL-CIO. Symptoms of the problems are laments about "internal communications" and how to reach the growing horde of new members, who have no loyalty to the past.[14]

While obviously no causal relationship can be drawn between reported union discontent in 1968 (even assuming that the same conditions were present in 1966) and the electoral defeats sustained by UAW-endorsed candidates in 1966, it is pertinent to note that (1) even those unions with the strongest reputations for member loyalty have been experiencing tensions between the leadership and the rank and file; and (2) membership adherence to the union's political views is always precarious. And what is true for the UAW, which has been characterized as "probably the union most fully committed to political action on the national level and most influential in the use of its political arm in relation to broad economic and social policies,"[15] is even more likely to be true for other unions.

For several years, both the trends noted above have been evident throughout organized labor. With the influx of younger members who have no recollections of either the difficulties which unions had in obtaining recognition from a hostile business community or the poverty associated with the Great Depression, the hold of the union leadership has weakened. In a few instances, long-time labor leaders (notably David McDonald of the Steel Workers and James Carey of the Electrical Workers) were defeated in bids for reelection. Another manifestation of this generational gap has been the increasing political independence of workers. In addition to the labor defeats in Michigan, candidates supported by the AFL-CIO's political arm, the Committee on Political Education (COPE), fared poorly in 1966—much worse, we have seen, than in the 1962 off-year elections. Indeed, a COPE publication reports that "there's no question about it, the results were dispiriting: More than 40 liberal House Members defeated, six liberal governors and two liberal senators swept aside."[16] Notable among the COPE-supported losers were Governor Edmund G. Brown of California and Senator Paul H. Douglas of Illinois.

COPE's 1968 performance was mixed. Although Vice-President Hubert H. Humphrey was defeated in his bid for the Presidency, it is likely that the narrow margin of his defeat is attributable, at least in part, to the strong support he received from organized labor in critical industrial states. On the other hand, only 57 per cent (201 out of 353) of COPE-endorsed Congressional candidates (186 of 326 Representatives, 15 of 27 Senators) and 35 per cent (6 out of 17) of the gubernatorial candidates whom it supported were elected.[17] Prominent losers were Senators Joseph S. Clark of Pennsylvania and A. S. Mike Monroney of Oklahoma.

Candidates with strong union backing have been defeated in the past. For example, the endorsement of presidential hopeful Wendell L. Willkie by United Mine Workers leader John L. Lewis failed to move many miners into the Republican ranks in 1940. Senator Robert A. Taft handily defeated union-backed candidate Joseph Ferguson in 1950, despite the designation of the Ohio Republican as the enemy of labor. Moreover, prospects for a substantial improvement in organized labor's future political performance in the electoral arena are not bright, as was well explained a few years ago:

Despite increasing political involvements of union leaders, particularly in campaigns, there are a substantial number of union members who vote contrary to the public endorsements of their leadership; who note with disapproval, as detracting from the vital business of contract and grievance negotiation, any display of political activity by union leaders; or who remain politically apathetic, leadership exhortation to the contrary notwithstanding. Moreover, within the union movement, a substantial number of union leaders still attempt to stay out of the partisan election campaigns, and refuse to allow their unions to become closely identified with any political party or its candidates.[18]

A 1965 study conducted among members of union locals in the Central Labor Council of Alameda County in California indicates that while slightly more than 50 per cent of the membership generally voted for candidates endorsed by the union, more than 8 per cent of those polled specified that they exercised independent political judgment by pointing out that their adherence to union views "depends on the candidate," even though this choice was not included in the sampling questionnaire. The survey also indicated that a large majority of union members felt that labor unions had either "just the right amount of power" (49.8 per cent), or "too much power" (26.4 per cent), while less than a quarter (23.8 per cent) were of the opinion that unions had "too little power."[19]

In late 1966, a COPE-conducted survey of AFL-CIO member attitudes was reportedly so unsettling to the leadership that the results of the survey were not officially released. However, accounts of the survey indicate that it confirmed a widening gap between union leadership and membership.[20] In light of the foregoing, it is highly unlikely that union members would be willing participants in a political movement that would further increase the power of their leaders.

The above discussion does not suggest that union leadership has been totally without influence on political activities of its membership. The point is, rather, that the alleged labor political hegemony does not exist and that the influence of the leadership varies greatly. Like other voters, union members have other affiliations, including ethnic, religious, and fraternal ties, which subject them to diverse social pressures. At times, workers feel these other pressures more intensely than those exerted by their union. V. O. Key, Jr., well summarized the influence of labor leaders when he stated:

> Whether a labor vote exists that can be delivered by labor leaders is in a way a nonsense question. The influence of labor leaders over their members probably differs enormously with time and circumstances and in each instance is so intermingled with other influences as to be beyond measurement. . . . Yet the influence of labor organization should not be dismissed as of no import because labor-endorsed candidates do not invariably win. Organization doubtless re-enforces the loyalties of the hard core of labor votes. At times labor leaders manage to get to the polls a larger vote than would be cast without their efforts. And on occasion, their exertions may account for victory.[21]

Limited financial resources. The third factor that limits labor's political power stems from the fact that although unions are important contributors to political candidates and groups (overwhelmingly on the Democratic side of the rostrum), most experts agree that organized labor does not possess the financial resources it is purported to have. Although, as we saw in Chapter Six, the Chamber of Commerce of the United States views labor political expenditures as a threat to American political democracy, the total of labor's political contributions has hardly been overwhelming.

In 1964, for example, 31 national labor committees made total political disbursements of only $3.7 million. Of this amount, nearly $1 million was expended by COPE in the form of contributions to candidates and parties. An additional $1 million was spent by COPE on voter registration campaigns, particularly in marginal Congressional districts. While these figures do not include expenditures by state and local labor groups, it is questionable whether such expenditures have significantly raised the proportion of labor moneys to total political funds expended.

By way of comparison, reported campaign contributions of
$10,000 or more were made by 130 individuals and these contri-
butions totalled more than $2.16 million in 1964, while approxi-
mately 10,000 persons who each contributed $500 or more gave
$13.5 million.[22] In terms of direct comparisons with known con-
tributions by corporate officials, Alexander Heard points out that
in 1956 about 17 million union members gave approximately $2
million while the same amount was donated by only 742 businessmen (all of whom were officials of the nation's 225 largest
business concerns) who were reported contributing $500 or more
apiece.[23]

As with business campaign contributions and expenditures,
it is impossible to ascertain the total amount spent on elections
by labor organizations; however, Heard noted in his study of
election financing that "the conclusion seems inescapable that
labor money in politics from all sources pays a much smaller
share of the nation's campaign-connected costs than union members constitute of the population of voting age.[24] Accordingly,
business fears of political inundation by unlimited labor funds
represents more rhetoric than reality.

ORGANIZED LABOR'S POLITICAL EGOCENTRICITY

Even if the union movement possessed all the political
power attributed to it, organized labor is not likely to become
the nucleus of a new party alignment. Labor has eschewed
partisan leadership in the past, and traditionally, its political concerns have been of narrow scope rather than ranging broadly
over a wide spectrum of social concerns.

Early in this century, the American Federation of Labor
(AF of L) under the leadership of Samuel Gompers firmly established the policy that it is inexpedient for labor to create a
separate party to accomplish its political objectives. Accordingly, organized labor has worked within the existing party structures and has rejected the labor party model of a number of

Western European countries. Indeed, from its beginnings, the AF of L pursued a political policy of "voluntarism," which consisted of political nonalliance, of reliance by workers on their own union organizations, and of labor economic self-help.[25] As has been suggested earlier, even though organized labor at the national level has been closely aligned with the Democratic Party, this relationship has had its rocky moments. Significantly, the AFL-CIO remains officially nonpartisan in order to retain political flexibility. On occasion, individual unions even support Republican candidates, although this has been uncommon.

Moreover, even if union leadership were to aspire to partisan political leadership within the Democratic Party, such a path is today filled with obstacles. The southern wing of the party (which still wields considerable power) has largely maintained its antiunion bias. Furthermore, given its policy of rapprochement with the business community, the national Democratic Party leadership would undoubtedly be chary of any efforts by labor to increase its influence.

Throughout their history, American unions, with their nonideological bent, have been more concerned with bread-and-butter gains than with political hegemony. Labor has not sought the responsibilities of national political leadership. Indeed, one labor expert has suggested that

> if one were to look for political leadership in the United States, the labor movement would be about the last place one would expect to find it. The eyes of the union, no less than management's, are directed to the contest in the corporation—to the struggle over a little more money, a little more job security.[26]

Labor's political activities have been basically egocentric and defensive; that is, they have been designed primarily to contribute to organizational stability and to counteract attempts by other social groups (primarily business) to undermine union interests. Although some of its legislative goals, including social security, Medicare, and consumer-protection legislation, have benefited the population generally, union political interests remain essentially parochial. Significantly, when union leadership

supports broader social welfare and civil rights legislation, it
often meets with considerable opposition from its membership.

The labor movement has been characterized not by a drive
to achieve basic alterations of the American socioeconomic system, but rather by efforts to obtain for the working classes—more
specifically, those belonging to unions—a larger share of the
bounty of the American capitalist order. It aims not at over-
throwing capitalism or at preventing the exercise of business
influence on public opinion and government, but at balancing
and offsetting what it judges to be one-sided pressures in these
areas.[27] The socialistic ideological foundations of many European working-class parties have never taken root in our political
system. Thus far, the labor union movement in the United
States has been conspicuous in its failure to propose any real
or grand alternatives to the present social organization. In this
sense, labor's approach has been a conservative one.

As a result of this egocentricity, organized labor has increasingly incurred the antipathy of certain groups that previously were supportive—minorities, intellectuals, unorganized
members of the work force—not to mention a portion of its own
rank and file. Moreover, in this country, labor unions have had
a legacy of suspicion and hostility, for several reasons. Based
on a policy of collective action, organized labor has acted contrary to the individual achievement ethic of American society.
Furthermore, its origins as a protest movement and its history
of sporadic violence have contributed to public disapproval.
Finally, occasional revelations of labor corruption and of infiltra-
tion of some unions by criminal elements have contributed to a
tarnished image for the union movement. Considered together,
these factors make it probable that in this country a labor party
would attract only a narrow and undependable constituency and
would hardly provide the basis for a restructuring of the political
order. Shortly after World War II, Arthur M. Schlesinger, Jr.,
commented on labor's political potential as follows:

> The rise of the politicalized labor leader introduces a new and
> possibly valuable element in American politics. . . . If labor
> accepts the rôle of partnership in government and subordinates

its sectional demands to the public welfare, it may become as politically significant as the British Labour Party.[28]

This potential has not been realized and the prospects for the future do not look any brighter.

THE LABOR MOVEMENT AND
MIDDLE-CLASS VALUES

A third tendency that makes a business-labor political axis unlikely is the class structure of American society, with its developing trend toward what may be designated upward homogenization. The socioeconomic climate has become less favorable for development of political parties based on class or occupational lines. This homogenization has been marked by the conversion from a predominantly blue-collar to a white-collar society, characterized by an increasing level of education and by employment in salaried positions within large organizations (particularly corporations). A study by the United States Bureau of Labor Statistics projects that by 1975, 48 per cent of the civilian labor force will be employed in white-collar occupations while only 34 per cent will be in blue-collar positions.[29] Although there is some evidence that white-collar workers from blue-collar families continue to identify with the "working class,"[30] this retention of working-class values has not manifested itself in increased success of union organizing efforts among lower level white-collar workers. Nor, as we have indicated, does the future hold out the prospect of greater union political success.

There is disagreement among sociologists concerning the degree to which there has been an "enbourgeoisment" of the most successful manual workers, with an attendant growth of a middle-class style of life and behavior patterns. However, there are apparently valid indications of some changes in working-class attitudes and behavior—particularly among the more highly skilled and more prosperous employees. The safest position that can be ventured is that "the working class is heterogeneous, in terms of both social background and class views."[31]   The class perspective of the worker is affected by such factors as the nature of the industry, the ratio of mental to physical activity that the worker engages in, the autonomy of the worker in performing his tasks, job security and benefits associated with the job, and the contact of the operative with white-collar employees.   Robert Blauner has noted, for example, that

> the social personality of the chemical worker tends towards that of the new middle class, the white-collar employee in bureaucratic industry. . . .   Generally lukewarm to unions and loyal to his employer, the blue-collar employee in the continuous-process industries may be a worker "organization-man" in the making.[32]

Suburban living appears to have some impact on the class consciousness of union members and a negative effect on their attitudes toward union political activity.   For example, while the move to the suburbs apparently does not make workers anti-union per se or more politically conservative, it seemingly results in diminished union activity and militancy.[33]   Significantly, organized labor has acknowledged the eroding effect of the move to the suburbs.   The results of a survey released by COPE in late 1967 indicate that by the mid-1960's nearly 50 per cent of all union members and approximately 75 per cent of the membership under the age of 30 lived in the suburbs.   The under-30 group constitutes about one-quarter of total union membership. Terming the suburbs the "New Frontier for union politics," a COPE publication suggests the combined effect of membership, youth, and suburban residence on labor political solidarity:

> Those under 30 know of Franklin Roosevelt and the issues of the Great Depression and its aftermath only through the history books.   They have grown up in an era of unprecedented prosperity.   The issues that stirred union members of 30, 20, or even 10 years ago have lost their bite with younger members. . . .   For many of the suburbanite unionists—young and old—strictly local, and even neighborhood, issues dominate their

interest. Property taxes and sewer lines have bumped jobless pay standards and minimum wage and other "gut" issues.

This does not mean the union member changes entirely the moment he crosses the city line into suburbia. It does mean, however, that he sees some things in a different light and becomes concerned with matters previously of little interest to him. He becomes more neighborhood and community conscious.[34]

The COPE publication reflects a trend among union members toward status politics as opposed to class politics. The former refers to "political movements whose appeal is to the not uncommon resentments of individuals or groups who desire to maintain or improve their social status," while the latter refers to "political division based on the discord between the traditional left and the right, i.e., between those who favor redistribution of income, and those favoring the preservation of the *status quo*."[35] On class issues, union members tend to retain a liberal or progressive perspective; but on noneconomic status issues, the tone of the membership of organized labor has been increasingly conservative, particularly as a consequence of concerted efforts by lower-status groups (primarily, of course, the black Americans) to emulate the successes achieved by organized labor in past generations.

Indeed, traditional socioeconomic categories—namely business versus labor—are becoming less and less meaningful in providing a basis for a class-cleavage theory of political activity. In the offing may be a new political formulation, in which racial factors will play a significant role. Several factors militate for this development: (1) economic class and race are closely correlated in present-day American society with the blacks occupying the bottom positions of the stratification structure; (2) a substantial number of working-class whites appear to view the Civil Rights movement as a direct threat to their social and economic status, particularly the black demand for positions in what historically have been white occupations; and (3) the increasing emphasis by black groups on militant, collective, direct social, economic, and political action—Black Power—to accomplish their objectives. For many white workers, race is undoubtedly a factor that could become a more important determinant of political identification and affiliation than is union membership. In California, for example, the so-called backlash among working-class and middle-class whites against black demands has been viewed as one of the causes of the conservative swing in recent state-wide voting, which resulted in the election of political conservatives such as Senator George Murphy and Governor Ronald Reagan, as well as the passage of a constitutional referendum abrogating a state open-housing statute. The extent of this nascent development is not, however, clear at this time. In 1964, when Californians passed by a ratio of two to one Proposition 14, which repealed a recently enacted open-housing act, the measure received heavy support among working-class and middle-class whites.[36] However, in 1968, Governor George C. Wallace failed, outside of parts of the South, to attract at the polls the so-called "backlash" vote among blue- and white-collar Caucasian workers despite his efforts to woo this constituency.

One other factor connected with social class in American society warrants mention. The belief in equalitarianism, which has been a basic component of the American democratic ideology, has prevented union members from maintaining a parochially working-class perspective, since the possibility (albeit not the probability) of mobility into a higher class exists. This equalitarianism causes the worker to identify, at least in some measure, with Americans on higher social levels and to avoid the intensity of class-based politics present in some other countries. While finding that there is "no evidence of either a decline of class voting or any substantial change in the pattern of class voting among major United States regions or religious groups," Robert Alford concludes that class-oriented voting in the United States is considerably less than in Great Britain or Australia and exceeds only that found in Canada. Significantly, of the four variables (education, income, subjective social class, and trade-union membership) which he analyzes to determine the correlation between social class and voting—occupation is held constant—trade-union membership is statistically the least significant.[37]

The several factors analyzed above suggest that the current class structure of American society is not conducive to a restructuring of our political parties on a (corporate) business-labor basis. If anything, there is reason to believe that union affiliation will be an even less important determinant of political identification than in the past.

ORGANIZED LABOR IS NOT A POLITICAL MONOLITH

A fourth shortcoming of the thesis predicated on a business-labor dichotomy of political parties is that it is premised on an overly monolithic conception of business-union antipathy. Indeed, John Kenneth Galbraith suggests that

> The industrial system has now largely encompassed the labor movement. It has dissolved some of its most important functions; it has greatly narrowed its area of action; and it has bent its residual operations very largely to its own needs. Since World War II, the acceptance of the union by the industrial firm and the emergence thereafter of an era of comparatively peaceful industrial relations have been hailed as the final triumph of trade unionism. On closer examination it is seen to reveal many of the features of Jonah's triumph over the whale.[38]

While Galbraith's thesis of the virtual demise of the labor movement is overstated, it does make a valuable point. Organized labor within the United States has consciously pursued its goals within a capitalistic system. Given its acceptance of the existing socioeconomic order, labor shares a wide collaborative interface with business. This is true both on the level of our national economy and within particular industries. Joint union-industry efforts in periods of national emergency are well documented. Moreover, leading labor and business leaders frequently serve together on governmental and communal committees, thereby increasing contact and lessening hostility. In certain situations (connected, for example, with tariff policy, industry subsidies, foreign aid, and government contracts), the interests of particular corporations and of certain unions may be very closely aligned, and the opposition may be business firms or labor organizations in other industries or in other countries. For example, the Teamsters have consistently demonstrated a closer degree of cooperation with the trucking industry in its efforts to obtain contracts for the handling of government goods on new routes than with the railroad unions, which sided with the rail carriers in their opposition to such efforts. Similarly, the maritime unions and the shippers have collaborated to obtain increased federal subsidies against the opposition of other labor groups, while the steel producers and the steel workers have cooperated in efforts to restrict imports of foreign steel.

Moreover, dissension exists within the union movement. For a number of years, the important Teamsters Union and the West Coast Longshoremen's Union have been outside the AFL-CIO fold. Whatever the reasons for their expulsion (alleged union corruption for the Teamsters and Communist leadership for the Longshoremen), the fact remains that their absence from the AFL-CIO has lessened its strength. In 1968 the United Auto Workers, with over 1 million members, separated from the parent union as a result of a long period of hostility between UAW president Walter Reuther and AFL-CIO leader George Meany. Almost immediately after this schism, the UAW and the Teamsters formed an Alliance for Labor Action to coordinate and to promote organizing activities and social-action programs. Although no federation between the two unions was planned, formal affiliation may occur, with other unions solicited to join the Alliance. In any event, it is probable that the Alliance will differ with the AFL-CIO in many of its policies relating to social and political action, thereby further weakening the purported solidarity of the labor movement.

Even within AFL-CIO ranks, there are competition and hostility among the constituent international unions and their leaders. Jurisdictional conflicts hamper unions in their efforts to organize particular industries, and intraindustry union rivalries may affect other aspects of labor relations. In the electrical industry, for example, the deep split between the International

Union of Electrical Workers (IUEW) and the International Brotherhood of Electrical Workers (IBEW) has impeded labor's effectiveness in dealing with such industrial giants as General Electric and Westinghouse. This example illustrates the frequent unwillingness of unions to cooperate even to protect vital economic interests and the existence of strong ideological splits within the union movement itself. These intralabor tensions dissipate union energies and resources and weaken the effectiveness of organized labor as a political force.

If there were no interindustry competition and no interunion dissension, labor would still not be a unified political force. A substantial part of the union movement has had a conservative political orientation—demonstrating either political apathy, an overwhelming concern with parochial union problems, or a careful avoidance of partisan commitments. Moreover, organized labor is hardly monolithic in its political organization and affiliation.

> The American labor movement is a highly complex social phenomenon with myriads of dissimilar features at lower levels. These diversities are multiplied in the alliances and organizational arrangements improvised for political purposes within organized labor and between labor organizations and other political groups.[39]

For these several reasons, we can justifiably conclude that organized labor is not unified politically and probably will not be so unified in the foreseeable future. Accordingly, apart from the other three impediments discussed in this section, internal organizational difficulties would prevent the union movement from becoming the nucleus of a labor-centered political party.

THE NATURE OF THE AMERICAN PARTY SYSTEM

The nature of the party system within the United States constitutes a final reason why a restructuring of American politics on a business-labor basis is most unlikely. Both major parties have been required to accommodate diverse social interests within their membership.

Because political resources have been widely (although unequally) distributed within the American political system, the success of each social interest is dependent on its ability to make alliances with other groups. This situation has also existed within our political parties, which, in essence, constitute alliances of diverse social interests. American politics has, historically, been coalition politics.[40]

The importance of two-party hegemony in the United States is not to be underestimated. It is Clinton Rossiter's view that "the most momentous fact about the pattern of American politics is that we live under a persistent, obdurate, one might almost say *tyrannical* two-party system."[41] Third-party movements have failed to retain their separate identities, but have experienced considerable success in that the Democratic and Republican Parties have absorbed their platforms and have effectuated many of their policy goals. Third parties constitute deviations from the two-party norm of American politics, and their primary significance stems from their influence on the major parties. Conservative and liberal factions are present in both major parties, with the congressional wing of both the Democratic and Republican Parties tending more to the political right than the presidential wing of each with regard to social and economic issues. Also, while there are real ideological differences between the parties and their leaderships, the Democrats and Republicans have demonstrated of late a fair measure of similarity in their party platforms and legislative proposals. This disjunctive similarity between the parties has been termed "dualism in a moving consensus."[42]

As a consequence, throughout the years, business has not been able to totally dominate the Republican Party nor labor the Democratic Party. Each has had to compete against hostile social interests within "its" party, and each has, on occasion, operated within the opposition party. For example, corporations and their managers are not totally estranged from either the Republican or the Democratic party. Some firms maintain close relations with both parties on national, state, and local levels. Other companies indicate a preference for one party nationally and the other party regionally, participating actively in Democratic Party affairs in their southern divisions while identifying with the national Republican Party. Similarly, some unions support Republican candidates locally while backing Democrats in national politics. Each party desires to receive the support of business groups and attempts, within the limits of political feasibility, to make its policies compatible with what it perceives to be the position of significant corporate interests; and both parties welcome labor support and funds when they can obtain them. The result is a "blurring of the outer edges of each party's area of loyalty and service . . . [and a] deep overlapping of the beliefs and programs and even voters of the parties."[43] This blurring has contributed to the stability of the American political order. As John H. Fenton points out,

> In some ways, the entrance of interest groups into active membership in political parties facilitates the development of a closer consensual bond in society. So long as interest groups stand outside parties, they feel free to make the most extreme and self-seeking demands on the parties and government. However, once inside the parties, they are forced to think in broader terms. More precisely, when interest group leaders are members of political parties, they must actively participate in the aggregative and synthesizing functions of the parties. This invariably affects the policies of the interest groups and reduces the policy differences between the interest groups and the parties.[44]

Accordingly, while the Republican Party has traditionally been the party of business and the Democratic Party the party of labor, these labels do not indicate the important facts that (1) neither industry nor the unions has hegemony within the party usually associated with it and, thus, each has been obligated to work with both parties, and (2) the internal structures of both parties are pluralistic, accommodating a variety of social interests. These facts have significant implications for future political development within the United States. Assuming for the moment total group cohesiveness, we can predict failure for any attempt by either business or labor to capture a party which would pursue its political objectives to the exclusion of those of other social interests. Similarly, any effort by corporations or labor unions to establish an autonomous party would meet the fate of other third-party groups. There is no reasonable expectation under the informal rules of American politics that a business party or a labor party could make a respectable showing in two successive elections. "Indeed, if a new third party were to make such a showing in just one election, the major party closest to it would move awkwardly but effectively to absorb it."[45] The practical result would be a return to the partisan system which exists at present.

Therefore, the wisest course for both organized labor and industry is to operate within the existing party structure and to seek to accomplish their political objectives as in the past.

•   •   •

Corporate political involvement will not result in a restructuring of party lines on a labor-corporate axis as long as the aggregate involvement does not grossly interfere with the economic and social aspirations of the mass of American workers or take the form of extortionate demands upon a wide variety of social interests, including labor. Accordingly, a party system in which organized labor and business corporations would meet as inevitable and unremitting antagonists is not probable in the American context. In this section, I have suggested five reasons why American politics is unlikely to polarize on class lines: (1) labor's political power is much more limited than its opponents realize, in terms of number of union members, of loyalty of the membership, and of financial resources; (2) organized labor has historically eschewed national political leadership for parochial goals; moreover, it does not enjoy the confidence of many other social interests; (3) the American class structure is not conducive to a labor-based party, given the prominence of middle-class values and the increasing importance of status rather than class politics; (4) labor is not a political monolith, either in terms of its reputed hostility to business or its intraunion solidarity; and (5) the nature of the present American party structure is such that the two major parties have been able to absorb many disparate social interests. All in all, these factors indicate scant justification for business fears of upsetting the "hornet's nest" of organized labor through corporate political involvement, with resultant harm to the American business system.

LOSS OF CORPORATE AUTONOMY

Managers offer a final major argument against corporate political involvement—an argument that is likewise voiced by supporters of the American corporate system rather than by its opponents. The primary concern of this last group of naysayers is that continued and intensified political activities by business firms will result in the eventual destruction of the American economic system as it now exists or in its takeover by the federal government. This outcome, they claim, will result from pressures applied by other social interests to prevent corporations from achieving complete supremacy in the political arena. As with the other reasons that are asserted in opposition to corporate political activities, the above argument conjures up a picture of horrors that we are not likely to witness. There are a number of factors pointing toward this conclusion.

ABSENCE OF A CORPORATE
POLITICAL MONOLITH

In the first place, like labor unions, corporations do not constitute a monolithic political bloc, but are diverse in terms of interests, philosophies, and political goals. To assume the contrary is to indulge in an overly mechanistic view of political affiliation. Intercorporate political conflict manifests itself on many levels. Competition may be partisan in character. For many years, for example, the big two of the auto industry— General Motors and Ford—have often been pitted against each other in a factional struggle within the Republican Party in Michigan.[46]   Or, as we have seen, corporations compete increasingly on an interparty basis both locally and nationally.

Corporate political differences may exist on both an intra-industry and on an interindustry basis.   Turning to intraindustry differences, the quest for government contracts and licenses perforce brings normal business competition into the political context.   Boeing's gain in obtaining the contract to develop the supersonic transport is Lockheed's loss.   The grant of a license to one claimant to operate a TV channel is contrary to the interest of the unsuccessful suitor.   The award of an air route to a carrier means disadvantages for its competitors.   Furthermore, intraindustry competition may exist between large firms and smaller companies—witness the disagreement over fair-trade legislation.[47]   Similarly, examples of interindustry political competition abound.   We have already noted the legislative battle between the truckers and the railroads.   For years, savings and loan associations and commercial banks have been engaged in political warfare over attempts by the savings and loan organizations to increase their share of the nation's banking business.   Oil and gas producers compete with coal extractors for government contracts, subsidies, and tax advantages.   Governmental preference toward maritime firms may adversely affect the interests of the airlines.   These inherent conflicts among business firms contribute to the diversity of the political objectives that they pursue.

Diverse political interests and orientations may exist *within* individual corporations.   Large firms—particularly conglomerate enterprises which came into fashion during the 1960's—engage in many different economic activities, frequently spanning a number of industries.   On occasion, subsidiary divisions of a company may be direct economic competitors, having unrelated or even antithetical political interests.   For example, the ship-building division of a conglomerate firm may be well served by particular federal military policies or industry subsidies that are contrary to the welfare of a sister subsidiary in the aerospace business.   Bauer, Pool, and Dexter document the conflicts that can exist even within well-established nonconglomerate companies. In explaining the diverse positions taken by Du Pont's management on the issue of the renewal of the Reciprocal Trade Act in 1953, they point out:

> There is very real difficulty in discovering what DuPont's true interest is because the company has so many irons in the fire . . . DuPont had ten separate operating divisions. For many purposes, they acted as separate companies. . . . A DuPont economist in Wilmington said: "Don't ever talk of DuPont as being in *an* industry; it is in a lot of industries. . . . The sales manager for finishes, selling a fair amount of paint abroad, might want to support all this reciprocal trade, whereas the rayon-yarn people, who are very alarmed about foreign imports, would be on the other side. This whole problem is pretty academic to the people in nylon; they just would not care. . . . There is no over-all company policy."[48]

As a result of these intracorporate conflicts, a company is prevented from taking a unified stand on certain important issues, thereby lessening its political impact.

David T. Bazelon has suggested still other plausible bases for intercorporate political competition. In his opinion, a natural division is developing in business political affiliation between large and small corporations, between old money and new, and between national and regional enterprises, yet further vitiating the concept of business as a political monolith.[49] The precise borders of this division may not be as sharply delineated as Bazelon indicates. However, the merit of this thesis was demonstrated by the 1964 Presidential campaign, in which President Johnson received important support from the heads of large national firms but had very little assistance from the leaders of smaller companies, who tended to favor Senator Goldwater.

Additionally, corporate managers can be found along the entire spectrum of political persuasion ranging from the conservatism of Patrick J. Frawley to the liberalism of Sol M. Linowitz, the former board chairman of the Xerox Corporation. Within each of the parties, moreover, corporate leaders can be found among the liberal and the conservative factions. The politics of Republican Howard J. Pew of Sun Oil differ from those of Republican David Rockefeller of Chase Manhattan. Similarly, the political views of Democrat Charles B. Thornton of Litton Industries differ from those of Democrat Marshall Field, the Chicago department store chief. This political diversity among top business leaders is a further impediment to the formation of a corporate political bloc.

Through the years there has been both (1) "a network of common interest [which] pulls the business community together on major issues when its security is threatened,"[50] and (2) a marked preference among corporations and corporate executives for a single party (the Republican); however, as we have seen, business interests are frequently in political opposition to each other. Accordingly, there is little likelihood of an attempted corporate political takeover that would result in widespread public agitation for the imposition of stringent governmental control of corporate activities.

POLITICS IS A LIMITED CORPORATE ENDEAVOR

Second, as was mentioned earlier, political activity commands but a small percentage of the human and material assets of an enterprise and occupies a position of relatively low priority in evaluations of corporate organizational objectives. Political activity is an instrumental, rather than an end, value of corporations and is thus not permitted by corporate managers to derogate from the long-term interests of the firm, which, indeed, it is supposed to enhance. As Joseph A. Schumpeter pointed out:

> The attitudes of capitalist groups toward the policy of their nations are predominantly adaptive rather than causative, today more than ever. Also, they hinge to an astonishing degree on short-run considerations equally remote from any deeply laid plans and from any definite "objective" class interests.[51]

Corporate political involvement is, accordingly, narrow in orientation, as opposed to being programmatic in character. Managers are generally concerned with the specific needs of their companies rather than with basic issues. Organizational requirements rather than social ideology are the catalysts for business political action. Just as it is unlikely that organized labor will attempt to assert national political leadership, it is equally improbable that any such effort would arise from the corporate sector.

THE VIGILANCE AND POWER OF
OTHER SOCIAL INTERESTS

Yet another factor militating against the theory that corporate political activity poses a grave danger to the autonomy of the enterprise is the vigilance and power of other social interests in American society. Competing interest groups would be quick to oppose, from the very inception, any efforts by business corporations to achieve hegemony in the political arena. If political history is a guide for future events, it is highly unlikely that the stage would be reached where total public regulation of corporations or the destruction of the corporate system would be the only alternatives to corporate domination of political processes. Power, as a political resource, is sufficiently diffused in America to permit other social groups to take necessary prophylactic measures to prevent corporate political control.

Since the question of the comparative political power of business corporations and of other social interests constitutes much of the subject matter of the next chapter, further discussion of this point will be reserved until then. Suffice it to say that the current power relationships among major social interests indicate that the outlook for corporate political control—assuming for the moment that this is a goal of the business community—is bleak. In his examination of the power structure in the United States today, Arnold M. Rose indicated the reasons for this conclusion, noting

> that [the] power structure of the United States is highly complex and diversified (rather than unitary and monolithic), that

the political system is more or less democratic (with the glaring exception of the Negro's position until the 1960's), that in political processes the political elite is ascendant over and not subordinate to the economic elite, and that the political elite influences or controls the economic elite at least as much as the economic elite controls the political elite.[52]

There is little prospect that this analysis of the American political picture will be invalidated in the foreseeable future. In any event, whatever changes may occur will not be the result of the political aspirations and activities of business corporations.

NO CORPORATE DESIRE FOR
POLITICAL HEGEMONY

A fourth reason for the complete unlikelihood of the demise of the corporate system as a consequence of business political activities is the fact that there has been virtually no evidence in the statements and activities of business managers that such a corporate political takeover is either contemplated or desired. The role of a limited but effective participant in the creation of a political environment sympathetic to corporate goals and interests is the extent of involvement that most business leaders appear to consider appropriate for themselves and their enterprises.

Indeed, there is respectable opinion among political scientists that, at least on the local level, the problem posed by the political activities of business firms has been underparticipation rather than overparticipation. In concentrating their attentions on their professional careers within their companies, managers give but little attention to local politics. By way of illustration, as was noted in Chapter Five, corporate efforts to involve their employees in politics have met with limited success. This lack of success is a result of a "real and important . . . conflict between the corporation as an institutionalized center of [employee] loyalties and the local territorial community."[53] However, as will be developed in Chapter Eight, this picture of corporate abstinence from local political involvement is not accepted with unanimity by students of community power.

Much of the hostility felt by those who fear business political involvement has its origins in the post-Civil War era of the nineteenth century, when there was substantial domination of the political sphere by corporate interests. As we have seen, however, since that time, and particularly since the Depression era, business interests have lost whatever monopoly of control over political decision making they may have had. The analogies drawn to corporate political activity during the late nineteenth century are not applicable today as a result of a restructuring of the American political order. Several factors have been important to this restructuring, including (1) the growth of government at all levels; (2) urbanization; (3) international commitments; (4) technological development; (5) the emergence of new social-interest groups as effective political forces, and (6) the growth of other large-scale organizations including universities and foundations, not to mention unions. Moreover, corporations have continually been politically active during the past half century without overwhelming our governmental order. There is no evidence that business managers are today any less committed to the democratic "rules of the game" than are other citizens. Indeed, if commitment to these "rules" is a function of the frequency and effectiveness of political participation, they are probably more committed to them than are many other Americans. There is little reason to believe that corporate leaders seek a return to a time when "politics was largely a Punch and Judy show . . . [in which] . . . business ran politics, and politics was a branch of business."[54]

DEEP-SEATED ACCEPTANCE OF CORPORATE CAPITALISM IN THE UNITED STATES

A final reason that the fears of the opponents of corporate political activism are unnecessary is the deep-seated popular acceptance of corporate capitalism in the United States. As Andrew Shonfield remarked in his book, *Modern Capitalism*,

The United States is indeed one of the few places left in the

> world where "capitalism" is generally thought to be an OK
> word. . . . Among the Americans there is a general commit-
> ment to the view, shared by both political parties, of the natural
> predominance of private enterprise in the economic sphere and
> of the subordinate role of public initiative in any situation other
> than a manifest national emergency.[55]

It must be remembered that in this country, "private enterprise"
is dominated by large business corporations. A study published
in 1951 by the Institute for Social Research of the University of
Michigan suggests a basic public satisfaction with large corporations in this country. The authors report that 76 per cent of
the 1227 persons polled were of the opinion that the good things
about big business outweighed the bad things, while only 10 per
cent viewed the negative features as prevailing.[56]

These findings were confirmed by a study conducted by
pollster Louis Harris for *Newsweek* and the National Industrial
Conference Board in 1966. The study indicated that 96 per cent
of the 2000 individuals 18 years or over who were polled held the
opinion that "free enterprise has made this country great," while
91 per cent were of the view that "business in America has
changed for the better since the depression days," and 76 per
cent believed that "most businessmen are genuinely interested
in [the] well-being of the country." Although a sample of 800
college seniors expressed less confidence in business than did
their elders—particularly in terms of the public-spiritedness of
the private sector—they still overwhelmingly supported a private
business system. Of the students polled, 93 per cent rejected
the idea of government ownership of business. However, 74
per cent favored the present degree of government regulation[57]
as compared with 54 per cent of adults.

The reasonable inference to be drawn from these studies is
that the corporate system rests on very firm popular acceptance.
It is unlikely that corporate political activities will shake this
foundation. Barring the total failure of the present socioeconomic order to satisfy the social and economic expectations of
American society, there is little reason to believe that there will

be any public call for a replacement or stronger regulation of our system of corporate capitalism.

•   •   •

Despite the fears expressed by some managers, corporate political activity does not threaten the autonomy of business corporations. I have suggested five reasons for this conclusion: (1) corporations do not constitute a monolithic political bloc necessitating massive public resistance; (2) politics receives limited resources and attention from business firms; (3) other social interests would counteract at an early stage any putative corporate attempt of a political takeover; (4) there is no evidence that contemporary corporate leaders seek to dominate the political order, thereby arousing widespread public opposition; and (5) the corporate system enjoys wide acceptance among the American public, making total public control highly unlikely. As Clyde Kluckhohn has well stated, "This [America] has been a business civilization."[58] This underlying fact stands as a real buffer against any fundamental impairment of corporate autonomy.

SUMMATION

This chapter has been devoted to an analysis of the three major reasons offered by managerial opponents to corporate political activities to explain why business corporations have no place in the political arena. To recapitulate the contentions: (1) political activity will interfere with the underlying economic functions of the firm by misallocating corporate resources, by derogating from profit making, and by impeding the efficient production and distribution of goods; (2) corporate political involvement runs the risk of activating that already restive giant, organized labor, into intensified political activity, which could result in a polarization of American politics along a business-labor axis in which business would inevitably come out the loser;

and (3) continued corporate political activity carries the risk that other social interests will call for either public ownership or at least close public control of business in order to prevent corporate political domination, thereby destroying the autonomy historically enjoyed by business.

The common denominator of the three reasons is that political activity threatens the American business system rather than enhances its position. Those who make the arguments seek to preserve the socioeconomic status quo. For reasons discussed in this chapter, each of the three explanations of why corporations should be apolitical appears to be marred by erroneous assumptions and by misconceptions regarding both the present state of corporate political involvement and the potential threat posed by other social interests. The American corporate system as it exists today is likely to be with us until events much more significant than corporate political activities result in a fundamental alteration of our socioeconomic order.[59]

There are reasons for questioning whether corporations should be political participants. These reasons, however, are not those offered by the managerial critics; they revolve around the much more fundamental issues of the extensiveness of corporate political power, and of corporate political legitimacy. Ultimately, any resolution of the question of whether corporate political involvement is consistent with a democratic political order must be based on an analysis of power and legitimacy. Let us now turn our attention to an examination of the nature and extent of corporate political power.

NOTES

[1]Theodore Levitt, "Business Should Stay Out of Politics," *Business Horizons*, III, No. 2 (Summer 1960), 50.

[2]For a more extensive discussion of the nature of the "Techno-Structure," see John Kenneth Galbraith, *The New Industrial State* (Boston: Houghton Mifflin Company, 1967), pp. 60–71.

³Aaron Wildavsky, *Dixon-Yates: A Study in Power Politics* (New Haven, Conn.: Yale University Press, 1962), p. 3. See also Robert Engler, *The Politics of Oil* (Chicago: Phoenix Books, The University of Chicago Press, 1967), p. 366.

⁴The arguments against an expanded view of corporate social responsibility are found in Clarence C. Walton, *Corporate Social Responsibilities* (Belmont, Calif.: Wadsworth Publishing Company, Inc., 1967), pp. 54–82.

⁵Representative discussions of the "Social Responsibility Issue" are found in Walton, *Corporate Social Responsibilities*; Edward S. Mason (ed.), *The Corporation in Modern Society* (Cambridge, Mass.: Harvard University Press, 1961); Earl F. Cheit (ed.), *The Business Establishment* (New York: John Wiley & Sons, Inc., 1964); James W. Kuhn and Ivar Berg (eds.), *Values in a Business Society: Issues and Analyses* (New York: Harcourt, Brace & World, Inc., 1968); William T. Greenwood (ed.), *Issues in Business and Society* (Boston: Houghton Mifflin Company, 1964); Andrew Hacker (ed.), *The Corporation Take-Over* (New York: Harper & Row, Publishers, 1964); Edwin B. Flippo (ed.), *Evolving Concepts in Management: Proceedings of the 24th Annual Meeting* (University Park, Pa.: Academy of Management, 1965); and "The Ethics of Business Enterprise," *Annals of the American Academy of Political and Social Science,* CCCXLIII (September 1962).

⁶Earl F. Cheit, "Why Managers Cultivate Social Responsibility," *California Management Review,* VII, No. 1 (Fall 1964), 16.

⁷The question has been raised, however, whether businessmen always perceive and pursue their political interests. See Raymond A. Bauer, Ithiel de Sola Pool, and Lewis Anthony Dexter, *American Business and Public Policy* (New York: Atherton Press, 1963), Chaps. 9, 35; and Francis X. Sutton, Seymour E. Harris, Carl Kaysen, and James Tobin, *The American Business Creed* (New York: Schocken Books, 1962), Chaps. 1, 17.

⁸Michael D. Reagan, "The Seven Fallacies of Business in Politics," *Harvard Business Review,* XXXVIII, No. 2 (March-April 1960), 68.

⁹The statistics cited in this paragraph are drawn from *America's Industrial and Occupational Manpower Requirements, 1964–75* (Washington, D.C.: U.S. Bureau of Labor Statistics, 1966), p. 3; Table 3-A, "Membership of National and International Unions, 1930–64, in Absolute Figures and as Percentages of Total Labor Force and

of Nonagricultural Employment"; Table 3–1, "Results of NLRB Representation Elections, 1936–65"; and Table 3–2, "Membership Reported by National and International Unions, by Geographic Area and Affiliation, 1964" found in E. Wight Bakke, Clark Kerr, and Charles W. Anrod (eds.), *Unions, Management and the Public*, 3d ed. (New York: Harcourt, Brace & World, Inc., 1967), pp. 738–41. See also Solomon Barkin, "The Decline of the Labor Movement," in Andrew Hacker (ed.), *The Corporation Take-Over* (New York: Harper & Row, Publishers, 1964), pp. 223–45; and A. H. Raskin, "The Obsolescent Unions," *Commentary*, XXXVI (July 1963), 18–25. Compare Irving Bernstein, "The Growth of American Unions, 1945–1960," in Walter Fogel and Archie Kleingartner (eds.), *Contemporary Labor Issues* (Belmont, Calif.: Wadsworth Publishing Company, Inc., 1966), pp. 229–43.

[10]Everett M. Kassalow, "The Prospects for White-Collar Union Growth," *Industrial Relations*, V, No. 1 (October 1965), 37.

[11]E. E. Schattschneider, *The Semi-Sovereign People* (New York: Holt, Rinehart & Winston, Inc., 1960), pp. 50–51. Compare Arthur Kornhauser, Harold L. Sheppard, and Albert J. Mayer, *When Labor Votes* (New York: University Books, 1956), wherein it is estimated that approximately two-thirds of the members of the United Auto Workers voted in the 1956 Presidential election and of those who voted, one-quarter did not vote in accordance with the union's recommendation, pp. 31, 99; and Fred I. Greenstein, *The American Party System and the American People* (Englewood Cliffs, N.J., Prentice-Hall, Inc., 1963) for statistics indicating that 77 per cent of union members voted in the 1960 Presidential election, pp. 24–25.

[12]Angus Campbell, *et al.*, *The American Voter*, abridged ed. (New York: John Wiley & Sons, Inc., 1964), pp. 164–80.

[13]Kornhauser, Sheppard, and Mayer, *When Labor Votes*, p. 281.

[14]Laurence G. O'Donnell ". . . and Bum Rap for Reuther," *The Wall Street Journal*, May 10, 1968, p. 16, col. 4.

[15]Kornhauser, Sheppard, and Mayer, *When Labor Votes*, p. 14.

[16]" '66 Looking Back, '68 Looking Ahead," in *Memo from COPE*, No. 8–67 (Washington, D.C.: Committee on Political Education, AFL-CIO, April 17, 1967), p. 1.

[17]"COPE-Backed Candidates Win Majority of Races," *AFL-CIO News*, November 9, 1968, p. 12, cols. 2 and 3.

[18]Nicholas A. Masters, "The Organized Labor Bureaucracy as

a Base of Support for the Democratic Party," *Law and Contemporary Problems*, XXVII, No. 2 (Spring 1962), 252.

[19]Central Labor Council of Alameda County and the Center for Labor Research and Education, Institute of Industrial Relations, University of California, Berkeley, *Report on Union Member Attitude Survey* (Berkeley: Center for Labor Research and Education, Institute of Industrial Relations, University of California, Berkeley, 1965), pp. 23–24.

[20]For a journalistic account of the survey, see James P. Gannon, "Divided Unions," *The Wall Street Journal*, July 6, 1967, p. 1, col. 6. Other reports of rank and file discontent are given in A. H. Raskin, "Rumbles from the Rank and File," *Challenge*, March-April 1967, pp. 28–30, 46; and Murray J. Gart, "Labor's Rebellious Rank and File," *Fortune*, LXXIV, No. 6 (November 1966), 151.

[21]V. O. Key, Jr., *Politics, Parties, and Pressure Groups*, 5th ed. (New York: Thomas Y. Crowell Co., 1964), pp. 67–68.

[22]Herbert E. Alexander, *Financing the 1964 Election* (Princeton, N.J.: Citizens' Research Foundation, 1966), pp. 63, 84–88, 96–97.

[23]Alexander Heard, *The Costs of Democracy* (Chapel Hill, N.C.: University of North Carolina Press, 1960), pp. 169–211, esp. pp. 196, 208.

[24]Heard, *The Costs of Democracy*, p. 208.

[25]Michael Rogin, "Voluntarism: The Political Functions of an Antipolitical Doctrine," *Industrial and Labor Relations Review*, XV, No. 4 (July 1962), 521–35.

[26]Neil W. Chamberlain, "The Corporation and the Trade Union," in Mason (ed.), *The Corporation in . . .* , pp. 124–25.

[27]Kornhauser, Sheppard, and Mayer, *When Labor Votes*, p. 16.

[28]Arthur M. Schlesinger, Jr., *The Vital Center* (Boston: Sentry Editions, Houghton Mifflin Company, 1962), pp. 187–88.

[29]*America's Industrial and Occupational . . .* (Bureau of Labor Statistics), p. 3. The remaining civilian work force will be in services and miscellaneous occupations.

[30]Richard F. Hamilton, "The Marginal Middle Class: A Reconsideration," *American Sociological Review*, XXXI, No. 2 (April 1966), 192–99. Compare Seymour Martin Lipset and Reinhard Bendix, *Social Mobility in Industrial Society* (Berkeley, Calif.: University of California Press, 1963), p. 15; and C. Wright Mills, *White Collar* (Fair Lawn, N.J.: Galaxy Books, Oxford University Press, Inc., 1956), pp. 239–58.

[31]John C. Leggett, Sources and Consequences of Working-Class Consciousness," in Arthur B. Shostak and William Gomberg (eds.), *Blue Collar World* (Englewood Cliffs, N.J.: Prentice-Hall, Inc., 1964), p. 247. For discussions of working-class identification, see, for example, Kurt Mayer, *Class and Society*, rev. ed. (New York: Random House, Inc., 1955), pp. 40–42; Bennett M. Berger, *Working-Class Suburb* (Berkeley, Calif.: University of California Press, 1968), pp. 80–90; Richard F. Hamilton, The Behavior and Values of Skilled Workers," in Shostak and Gomberg (eds.), *Blue Collar World*, pp. 42–57; Gerald Handel and Lee Rainwater, "Persistence and Change in Working-Class Life Style," in Shostak and Gomberg (eds.), *Blue Collar World*, pp. 36–41; S. M. Miller and Frank Riessman, "The Working Class Subculture: A New View," *Social Problems*, IX (Summer 1961), 86–97; and S. M. Miller and Frank Riessman, "Are Workers Middle Class?" *Dissent*, VIII, No. 4 (Autumn 1961), 507–12, 516.

[32]Robert Blauner, *Alienation and Freedom* (Chicago: Phoenix Books, The University of Chicago Press, 1964), p. 181.

[33]William Spinrad, "Blue-Collar Workers as City and Suburban Residents—Effects on Union Membership," in Shostak and Gomberg (eds.), *Blue Collar World*, pp. 215–25. See also Berger, *Working-Class Suburb*, pp. 28–39.

[34]Reprinted from *New Frontier: Politics in the Suburbs*, COPE Publication No. 177C (Washington, D.C.: AFL-CIO Committee on Political Education, n.d.), p. 5.

[35]For further discussion of the distinction between class and status politics, see the book from which these quotes have been taken—Seymour Martin Lipset, "The Sources of the 'Radical Right,' " in Daniel Bell (ed.), *The Radical Right* (Garden City, N.Y.: Anchor Books, Doubleday & Company, Inc., 1964), pp. 308–9. See also Richard Hofstadter, "The Pseudo-Conservative Revolt," in Bell (ed.), *The Radical Right*, pp. 84–85; "Pseudo-Conservatism Revisited: A Postscript," in Bell (ed.), *The Radical Right*, pp. 98–99; and T. B. Bottomore, *Classes in Modern Society* (New York: Pantheon Books, a Division of Random House, Inc., 1966), pp. 103–11.

[36]See Raymond E. Wolfinger and Fred I. Greenstein, "The Repeal of Fair Housing in California: An Analysis of Referendum Voting," *The American Political Review*, LXII, No. 3 (September 1968), 753–69.

[37]Robert Alford, *Party and Society* (Chicago: Rand McNally & Company, 1963), pp. 102, 106, and 248.

[38]John Kenneth Galbraith, *The New Industrial State* (Houghton Mifflin Company), p. 281.

[39]Heard, *The Costs of Democracy*, p. 176.

[40]Nelson W. Polsby, *Congress and the Presidency* (Englewood Cliffs, N.J.: Prentice-Hall, Inc., 1964), p. 9; and Greenstein, *The American Party System* . . . , pp. 100–101.

[41]Clinton Rossiter, *Parties and Politics in America* (New York: Signet Books, The New American Library of World Literature, Inc., 1960), pp. 12–13.

[42]Key, *Politics, Parties, and* . . . , p. 222.

[43]Rossiter, *Parties and Politics* . . . , p. 20.

[44]John H. Fenton, *People and Parties in Politics* (Glenview, Ill.: Scott, Foresman & Company, Educational Publisher, 1966), pp. 63–64.

[45]Rossiter, *Parties and Politics* . . . , p. 167.

[46]John P. White and John R. Owens, *Parties, Group Interests and Campaign Finance: Michigan '56* (Princeton, N.J.: Citizens' Research Foundation, 1960), p. 8.

[47]See Joseph Cornwall Palamountain, Jr., *The Politics of Distribution* (Cambridge, Mass.: Harvard University Press, 1955).

[48]Bauer, Pool, and Dexter, *American Business and* . . . , p. 270.

[49]David T. Bazelon, "Big Business and the Democrats," *Commentary*, XXXIX, No. 5 (May 1965), 39–46. A few years ago, John H. Bunzel pointed out that there exist significant differences in political ideology between small businessmen and corporate managers. See John H. Bunzel, "The General Ideology of American Small Business," *Political Science Quarterly*, LXX, No. 1 (March 1955), 87–102.

[50]Key, *Politics, Parties, and* . . . , p. 72.

[51]Joseph A. Schumpeter, *Capitalism, Socialism and Democracy* (New York: Harper Torchbooks, Harper & Row, Publishers, 1962), p. 55.

[52]Reprinted from Arnold M. Rose, *The Power Structure* (London: Oxford University Press, 1967), p. 492.

[53]Norton E. Long, "The Corporation, Its Satellites and the Local Community," in Mason (ed.), *The Corporation in* . . . , p. 217. A similar thesis is developed by Andrew Hacker, "Politics and the Corporation," in Hacker (ed.), *The Corporation Take-Over*, pp. 246–69.

[54]Samuel Eliot Morison and Henry Steele Commager, *The*

Growth of the American Republic (Fair Lawn, N.J.: Oxford University Press, Inc., 1950), II, p. 217.

[55]Andrew Shonfield, *Modern Capitalism* (London: Oxford University Press, 1965), p. 298.

[56]Burton R. Fisher and Stephen B. Withey, *Big Business as the People See It* (Ann Arbor, Mich.: The Survey Research Center Institute for Social Research, University of Michigan, 1951), p. 20.

[57]The statistics cited in this paragraph are found in the *Newsweek*-National Industrial Conference Board Study, "The Public Mandate for Business," reported in Louis Harris, "What the Public and College Seniors Think About Business," in *Public Affairs in National Focus*, Public Affairs Conference Report, No. 5 (New York: National Industrial Conference Board, Inc., 1966), pp. 20–36, esp. 20–22, 31–33. For additional student opinion about the role of business, see Louis Harris and Associates, *Money and Its Management* (An Attitude Study Among College Students Conducted by Louis Harris & Associates), sponsored by *Newsweek* Magazine in conjunction with the National Industrial Conference Board, released September 1967.

[58]Clyde Kluckhohn, *Mirror for Man* (New York: McGraw-Hill Book Company, 1949), p. 229.

[59]For a suggestion as to the factors that might lend to a basic restructuring of capitalism, see Robert L. Heilbroner's provocative essay, *The Limits of American Capitalism* (New York: Harper Torchbooks, Harper & Row, Publishers, 1966).

Chapter Eight

Corporate Political Power: A Threat to Democracy?

Apprehension prompted by the purported super-abundance of corporate political power underlies much of the opposition to corporate political involvement by critics from outside of the business community. To borrow Andrew Hacker's colorful language—"when General Electric, American Telephone and Telegraph, and Standard Oil of New Jersey enter the pluralist arena we have elephants dancing among the chickens."[1] Although Hacker's metaphor is overstated and neglects to mention that other pachyderms are involved in the frolic, the fact remains that the corporate presence on the political scene raises important questions concerning the possession and exercise of power in a democracy.

The political power of economic organizations is a fundamental issue in this country. Indeed, it is the view of E. E. Schattschneider that

> American democracy was an early attempt to split the political
> power from the economic power. This is the great American
> experiment. . . . The function of democracy has been to pro-
> vide the public with a second power system, an alternative
> power system, which can be used to counterbalance the eco-
> nomic power.[2]

However, the suggestion of the possibility of a clear-cut dichotomy of political power and economic power is misleading. Although disagreeing about the causality and consequence of the
relationship between the political and the economic, such diverse
students of society as Beard, Madison, Marx, Parsons, Weber,
and Webster have pointed out the inextricable relationship between polity and economy, between political power and economic power.[3] Significantly, students of the process of industrialization have demonstrated the necessity and inevitability of
some quantum of fusion of economic and political power in
nations before significant economic development can occur. As
we have seen, moreover, this same tendency for fusion has been
observed in mature, industrialized countries as a consequence of
technological change and of social and economic interdependence. In the United States, for example, corporations have
assumed important positions as part of the apparatus of government.

   The real issue, therefore, is not one of separation of political
and economic power, but rather "the subordination of economic
power to a political conception of the public interest."[4] Toward
the end of achieving compatibility between our economic order
and our political system, the centers of economic power should
be as diffused and as balanced as possible, and must operate
within a broad *Weltanschauung* consistent with the character of
a democracy.

A FEAR OF CORPORATE
POLITICAL POWER

   The primary concern of critics of business political power
is that the modern corporation—characterized by the divorce of

control from ownership and lacking, accordingly, clearly defined guidelines of managerial accountability—places in the hands of politically irresponsible managers "a force able to compete on equal terms with the modern state."⁵ The fear exists that large corporations, acting either in concert or through intermediaries such as trade associations or national business organizations, will be in a position to overwhelm other social interests competing in the political process and, thereby, to achieve dominance over the formal and informal institutions of American government. In the words of Walton Hamilton, "Business enterprise, sparked by the march of technology, is beating forever against the political frontier. . . . The spirit of business enterprise is like the wind, it goeth where it listeth."⁶

The specter of a potentially uncontrollable group of corporations making the political decisions for the rest of society looms so large in the minds of some social commentators that the question has been posed whether the large corporation is the lesser commonwealth or, in fact, the greater. At very best, we are told, there will exist (if there does not already) a "pluralism of elites," with giant corporations among the very few competing elements.

The remainder of this chapter will be devoted to an analysis of these apprehensions. In my opinion, the fears expressed above are exaggerated. To state this is not, however, to suggest that business corporations collectively do not have political power or that the extensiveness of such power should not be a matter of concern. To indulge in either of these assumptions is foolish and dangerous. As we shall see, business firms and their managers do possess and do utilize the essential resources of power.

The critical problem, however, is not the mere possession of power. Rather, the crux of the matter is how this power is utilized and what impact it has on the political viability of other social interests. In making the analytically useful distinction between "power to do" and "power over," Edward S. Mason has correctly noted that "unfortunately, in any group or society there is little power to do without some power over."⁷ For a democratic political system, it is essential that the latter dimension of power not be elevated to an end value sought and exercised for its own sake, but rather that power exist and be utilized for the accomplishment of legitimate social goals. The critical factor is the consequences of power, rather than power per se. Bayless Manning has framed the issue thusly: "It is not power we fear, but the power to effectuate particular policies to which we object. The question is—what are they and who is in a position to carry them out. . . . The question is not Power; it is policy."[8]

THE NATURE OF POWER

Like all basic concepts, *power* is difficult to define. Various definitions can be found in the literature of political science, sociology, and economics.[9] However, for purposes of the analysis which follows, the essential attribute of power is the capacity to determine or influence some aspect of the behavior of others, either individually or collectively. The hallmark of power is effectiveness. In and of itself, power is value-free. It is neither inherently good nor intrinsically bad, but is simply a resource which manifests itself in fluid relationships between and among individuals and groups in society. As was suggested in the previous section, in a democracy the basic social values associated with the possession and exercise of power by any social interest are that (1) a high degree of fluidity be maintained in the relationships among the diverse groups in society—that there be no monopoly over social power—and (2) power not be utilized in a manner that is inimical to this fluidity.

Power does not exist in a vacuum. Rather it is, in two senses, relational. In the first place, any social actor possesses power only in relation to another social actor—two or more protagonists are necessary before it is appropriate to speak of their comparative power positions. Second, there is no fixed quantity or lump of power in a society. Power is not analogous to a pie which can be cut into an indeterminate number of slices of varying sizes, all of which together, however, must total the whole. On the contrary, all power is comparative. A may possess *more* power *than* B and *less than* C. The fact that one social actor possesses power does not mean that another actor lacks power.

Rather they possess degrees of power which vary with time and circumstance. Accordingly, A may be more powerful than B in situation 1, but less powerful than B in situation 2.

Power must also be distinguished from power potential. Although a social actor may possess both *a base of power* (resources or assets) and the *means of power* (the specific actions by which one can use these resources to influence the behavior of another), the mere existence of these power possibilities is not, per se, power.[10] By way of illustration, S. E. Finer suggests that business possesses five principal political advantages or resources: (1) organization, (2) riches, (3) access (to those in authority), (4) patronage (the dependency of others upon businessmen's private decisions), and (5) surrogateship (the performance of public tasks). He goes on to point out, however, that

> Our list merely records abstract possibilities. It does not record capital's *effective* capacity to act. What may or can conceivably happen is not the same as something likely to happen. And in this way if we identify bare possibilities with effective capacity, we in effect assume the very thing we are trying to prove—that the power of government is ineffective to curtail or abrogate the political potentialities of private capital.[11]

The critical factor is not the mere existence of potential resources —the assets listed above by Finer and those which will be discussed later in this chapter—but the efficacy of actual utilization.

While Nelson W. Polsby is correct in suggesting that the concept of potential political power is fraught with both theoretical and empirical difficulties, it is not without value.[12] If over the course of time (1) a political actor does not utilize his base of power through his means of power, which together constitute his potential power ability, and (2) other social actors are aware of this fact and, consequently, no longer feel constrained or influenced in their behavior by this actor, his actual ability to influence behavior—power—is less than his potential ability. The presence of this psychological constraint or influence factor distinguishes *power* from *potential power*.

If we are to understand the nature of the power relation, in addition to

1. The base of power,
2. The means of power, and
3. The distinction between power and potential power, several other factors must be taken into account. John C. Harsanyi has suggested the following elements:

> 4. The scope of power (the set of specific actions one can get another to perform),
> 5. The amount of power (the net increase in the probability of one performing some specific action as a result of a utilization of the means of power by one against another),
> 6. The extension of power (that is, power over whom?),
> 7. The costs of power (the opportunity costs of using power), and
> 8. The strength of power (the opportunity costs of the one on whom power is being exerted to resist this power).[13]

The total of these ingredients determines the nature of a social actor's political power in a given context.

Before terminating this discussion and launching into a detailed analysis of the political power of corporations, one comment specifically apropos of business organizations is necessary by way of both conclusion to this section and introduction to the next. Corporate political power does not exist per se. Rather, there exists in certain places, at certain times, and under certain circumstances, the ability on the part of corporations to influence the behavior of other political actors in certain ways and to a certain extent. Rather than an all-or-nothing phenomenon, corporate power is a matter of degree.

CORPORATE POLITICAL RESOURCES

As we have seen, the *possession* of power resources—the first determinant of power—does not by itself constitute power. The *means* of utilizing these resources is the second crucial determinant of political power. Since in Chapter Five we examined the means of corporate power through an analysis of the nature and extensiveness of political activities by business firms, the present section will be devoted to a study of the power resources possessed by corporations.

_____Corporations possess political assets of considerable magnitude—assets which, on the whole, are utilized with a reasonable degree of effectiveness. Some of these resources have already been suggested by Finer: organization, riches, access, patronage, and surrogateship. In addition, corporations have several other resources, including the influence of business firms over mass media, the backlog of political success accumulated by corporations over the years, and the high status and reputation of business and of business managers in American society. Let us now consider each of these resources.

ORGANIZATION

Business corporations are large-scale organizations. As such, they are characterized by

> (1) divisions of labor, power, and communication responsibilities, divisions which are . . . deliberately planned to enhance the realization of specific goals; (2) the presence of one or more power centers which control the concerted efforts of the organization and direct them towards its goals . . . ; (3) substitution of personnel . . . .[14]

As we saw during our discussion of corporate political behavior, these organizational attributes are valuable for the conduct of their political activities.

In the first place, business corporations can draw upon and coordinate a wide variety of talents valuable for politics. Consider the number of corporate departments that perform politically useful functions. Governmental relations or public affairs, public relations, legal counsel, Washington office, and government contracting are obvious examples of corporate units devoting some or all of their time to tasks that are relevant to the political concerns of the firm. Moreover, in a broader context, research and development, procurement, production engineering, and marketing units concern themselves with matters of political import when they deal with agencies of government. In addition to these departmental resources, corporations can draw upon the technical expertise of their employees, which, for large diversified companies, covers a wide spectrum of skills and knowledge. Hence, from their own resources, firms often have the necessary manpower to assist in the resolution of the political problems that confront them.

A related matter is the gamut of nonhuman resources possessed by large corporations. Frequently, these include the latest available communications, transportation, and electronic informational equipment, which are of invaluable assistance to the diverse corporate personnel concerned with political matters. These material resources enable business firms, to an extent possible for few other social interests, to pursue political goals with the support of modern technology.

Organization is an important asset in yet another respect—large corporations have branches in many geographical locations, both nationally and internationally. Despite the extent of company decentralization and the degree of policy initiative exercised by subunits, basic corporate policies are formulated and coordinated at a focal point within the organization, thence implemented by subsidiary divisions. Accordingly, corporations can pursue political objectives over broad geographical areas while, at the same time, coordinating their activities from a central location. As was suggested in the preceding paragraph, the development of modern transportation equipment and communications media facilitates this coordination effort.

Another aspect of organization is the wide variety of human contacts that corporations have. Employees, shareholders, suppliers, customers, and the general public all have varying degrees of exposure to the corporation as a consequence of their business relationships. While this contact does not necessarily translate into political support for the firms in terms of votes or legislative backing—indeed, contact may result in political hostility—it gives the enterprise a *corporate* political identity, which is of value. In our examination of corporate political education programs, we noted how corporations use these human contacts to attempt to create a favorable political environment. Similarly, corporate public relations affords another type of contact that is designed to promote the interests of the firm. To put it in another way, organization assists corporations in developing an image or an identity, which is of political utility.

Lastly, organization enables corporations to coordinate their political activities and objectives with other social interests. Trade-association involvement provides an example of such coordination. Similarly, on issues of mutual political interest, corporations cooperate with other business firms or social groups with which they maintain relationships.

Before leaving this discussion of organization as a corporate political resource three points warrant mention. As with the other political resources possessed by corporations, other social interests also have, in varying degrees, the advantage of organization. Indeed, the very reason for forming such groups as labor unions, farm groups, professional associations, and veterans' interests is to benefit from organization and the strength of numbers. Second, the effectiveness with which corporations utilize this resource differs. Intracorporate competition or disharmony concerning company goals is dysfunctional to optimal utilization of organization for political purposes. Finally, as all students of business operations are aware, the quality of organization differs among corporations and directly affects the utility of this resource as a political asset. In sum, the nature and the value of organization as a corporate political resource vary considerably.

RICHES

Corporate wealth as a political asset is closely related to the resource of organization.

Mobilized and concentrated in this way [through organization], business can dispose, immediately, of large sums of money. As a group it tends to be considerably wealthier than other interest groups; it can produce the money much more quickly than they can, and can spend it for a longer period.[15]

The wealth possessed by large corporations enables them to obtain the human and technological resources that are the cornerstones of effective organization. Wealth also enables business firms to fund the numerous governmental and electoral activities that are essential to promoting company political interests. It is expensive to finance such ventures as maintaining employees who concentrate full time on political matters; contributing (indirectly, of course) to political parties and candidates; engaging in administrative, legislative and executive lobbying; conducting litigation; and purchasing media time and space.

While corporations do not exercise a monopoly on wealth in the United States, the largest firms have a financial advantage over most other social interests. Some of the largest firms hold assets that run into the multi-billion-dollar range. The 1968 "*Fortune* Directory" indicates that nine United States corporations had assets in excess of $10 billion. American Telephone and Telegraph led the list with assets of more than $37.6 billion. Standard Oil of New Jersey (nearly $15.2 billion) and General Motors (nearly $13.3 billion) were the leading industrial corporations in terms of assets. All told, 194 publicly held firms (including 73 industrials) listed by *Fortune* had assets in excess of $1 billion. Within the corporate community, the largest firms enjoy a distinct financial advantage. In 1962, the 100 largest industrial corporations held more than 46 per cent of the assets of all industrial corporations; they also made nearly 58 per cent of the after-tax profits reported for all corporate industrials. Of the 420,000 manufacturing units in the United States in 1962 (of which 180,000 were corporations and the remainder proprietorships and partnerships), the total assets of the 20 largest firms were approximately the same as those of the 419,000 smallest. Income statistics provide additional perspective regarding the magnitude of corporate wealth. Save for the federal government, which was first, and the state of California, which was tenth, corporations occupied eight of the first ten positions in terms of the size of annual revenue in 1958. Of the first 55 places, only 9 were filled by governmental entities.[16]

Obviously, because there are so many internal demands on company moneys, only a very small—one might even say minuscule—percentage of corporate assets or revenues is used for political purposes. However, for the large firms, the financial resources are at hand to accomplish company objectives without the necessity of having to search for funds from outside sources. The concentration of substantial wealth in the hands of a relatively small number of firms provides these companies with the potential (even if unexercised) for behavior of political significance, which governmental decision makers must take into account in formulating policy. While other social interests often possess ample wealth for political purposes, our large corporations are even wealthier. Together with organization, wealth constitutes the basic political resource possessed by corporations. It is a necessary but not a sufficient precondition of corporate political power.

ACCESS

A third important corporate political resource is access—the chance to get a hearing and the opportunity to make one's case at crucial times and places. Close connections between governmental decision makers and corporations result from a number of factors. As was noted in Chapter Four, in an interdependent economy in which business organizations are charged with the task of performing important public functions, corporate managers are thrown into continual contact with governmental officials and are involved in the formulation of public policy. This dimension of access will be examined in detail in conjunction with the political resource which Finer has termed surrogateship.

Another aspect of access has already been considered in connection with our analysis of corporate political activities. For example, political contributions afford corporations access to governmental decision makers, since public officials do not wish to offend past contributors. While contributions by no means guarantee favorable results, they do assure corporations of a forum in which to present their case. In the words of Senator John L. McClellan of Arkansas:

> I don't think anybody that gave me a contribution ever felt he was buying my vote or anything like that, but he certainly felt he had an entree to me to discuss things with me and I was under obligation at least to give him an audience when he desired it to hear his views.[17]

The fact that governmental agencies are often required by law to consult with groups that are affected by their regulations provides an automatic route of access. Access is thus a concomitant of continuous political activity, whether such activity is voluntary or obligatory.

Access also results from the size, importance, and reputation of corporations. A high-level representative of General Electric, Du Pont, or Alcoa can readily get to see an important governmental official, largely on the basis of his organizational affiliation. Witness, for example, the apparent ease with which Roger M. Blough, chairman of the board of United States Steel, obtained "an abruptly arranged appointment" in 1962 with the President of the United States, John F. Kennedy, at which he informed the President of the increase in steel prices by the corporation.[18] Business corporations constitute important social interests which public officers must take into account in making their decisions. As pointed out earlier, the needs and the welfare of an important corporate constituent are automatically of concern to a legislator, notwithstanding the fact that the corporation may have opposed his election. Indeed, public officials and political leaders frequently seek the support of important business figures—just as they seek that of leaders of many other social interests—and are, therefore, accessible to them. Organizational prestige is, accordingly, an important ingredient of access.

Corporations also consciously cultivate access. For example, a few years ago a series of dinners was arranged between business leaders and top officials in the federal administrative agencies and executive departments by Dan H. Fenn, Jr., vice-chairman of the United States Tariff Commission, and officials of the Manufacturing Chemists' Association. The dinners, which were attended by groups of about 20 men equally divided between business executives and government officials, served the following function:

> The purpose on the part of the businessmen was not to persuade any government official that he ought to change his policy on any specific subject, and not on the part of the government people to persuade any businessman that he ought to support any particular government policy. The purpose was instead really to bring the people together under relaxed conditions for general discussions which might range widely, and which would be designed primarily to enable them to become better acquainted and to foster mutual respect.[19]

The net result of the dinners was to enhance access.

Corporate political access and the access of individual business leaders to governmental decision makers are intimately associated. The personal influence of corporate managers, both within the formal institutions of government and on an informal, personal level with leading governmental officials, constitutes a significant political asset. On the formal, institutional level, this influence arises from two sources. In the first place, the chief executives of the largest corporations frequently don (or have bestowed upon them) the mantle of "leader of industry" or of "industrial statesman" and are accorded the status of semiofficial spokesmen for the business community. Second, as we have seen, business leaders have considerable influence as a consequence of their capacity as the managers of the most important economic enterprises in the country, whose cooperation and assistance is critical to the national interest. In adopting new policies and implementing existing ones, governmental officials seek wherever possible to achieve the acquiescence, if not the active support, of influential businessmen. Such efforts take place on the commission and departmental levels where top governmental officers speak to leading corporate executives to "get readings" on the acceptability of particular governmental actions. At the highest level of our government, American Presidents have, in recent years, frequently sought to bolster their positions on critical matters by obtaining the support of the Business Council. As we shall see later in this chapter, there is considerable disagreement among scholars who study community power about the nature and the degree of influence of business executives in their localities; however, there is evidence that, on occasion, political officials do "clear" policies with economic notables and in some instances formally co-opt them into the decision-making structure.[20]

Mention was made earlier of another means by which business leaders have an impact upon governmental institutions and activities—actual service in official capacities. The names of cabinet members Robert S. McNamara (Ford Motor), C. Douglas Dillon (Dillon, Reed & Co.), Charles E. Wilson (General Motors), George M. Humphrey (Hanna Mining), and Thomas S. Gates, Jr. (Morgan Guaranty) readily come to mind as corporate leaders who have occupied positions at the highest levels of federal officialdom in recent years. Similarly, corporate heads serve on top-level Presidential public-service commissions. For example, a few months after the disorders during the summer of 1967, Henry Ford II was chosen by President Johnson to head the National Alliance of Businessmen, a presidentially appointed group of business leaders charged with assisting the federal government in upgrading the socioeconomic position of black Americans. One would be hard put to assemble a comparable list of labor leaders who have held positions in government of comparable importance. On less lofty planes, businessmen serve in various capacities with administrative agencies and executive departments. Business leaders participate as WOC's (without compensation) or as paid consultants on a myriad of advisory panels, boards, councils, and commissions concerned with both broad policy decisions and with the minutiae of policy implementation affecting their industries. While corporate executives run the gamut of political and economic persuasions, a common element binding them together is their familiarity and sympathy with the problems of large-scale business organizations, as well as a general orientation toward and acceptance of business values. The fact that many of these officials are still actively engaged in corporate activities or intend to return to business firms after their tour of governmental service also reinforces their pro-business propensities.

A related fact is that a corporate executive who formerly was a government official is frequently called upon to speak with individuals with whom he was associated while in the public employ. The high value placed by companies upon these contacts is illustrated by the frequency with which leading governmental figures are hired by large corporations, the presence of former government attorneys in corporate legal departments, and the eagerness of aerospace and defense contractors to hire ranking military officers. Indeed, the last-mentioned practice became so prevalent that in 1964 the Department of Defense issued regulations that required retiring regular officers to abstain from selling to defense agencies on behalf of a contractor for a period of three years after retirement. The converse of the situation of the former governmental official working in private industry is that of the erstwhile corporate executive doing a tour of duty with the government. Here too, the accessibility of former business associates is enhanced by the prior associations. This is not a result of malfeasance or corruption but rather a consequence of the natural inclination to be available to one's friends.

Turning now to informal political access, two factors warrant mention. The first pertains to social class. Most sociologists agree that social class in contemporary American society is primarily a function of occupation. In terms of income, prestige, and power, the corporate executive places high on any ranking of occupations. Since high social status is in large measure a result of important functional position within the society, business leaders qualify as members of social elites. As such, business leaders are thrown into social contact with other notables, including leaders in politics and government. This social contact serves to enhance the access that the firm, via its executives, has to governmental decision makers.

The second source of informal influence is related. Although finding that, in terms of socioeconomic origins, civilian federal executives are "more representative" of the occupational structure of the United States than are leaders of big business, a study of federal officials concluded that "the similarities between the executives of big business and those who occupy the top ranks of the federal government are more evident than the differences."[21] In discussing the backgrounds of corporation presidents and United States senators, Andrew Hacker notes that, in terms of regional origins, level of education, national origins, and pre-career mobility, "the pictures are pretty much the same."[22] Moreover, as was mentioned earlier, a significant number of senators possess substantial wealth—in 1968, at least a fifth of the members of the Senate were classified as millionaires.[23] Accordingly, economic and political elites possess, in terms of socioeconomic background, important similarities, which facilitate contact and contribute to understanding between the two groups.

It must not be concluded, however, that there is identity of interest or of outlook between corporate heads and political leaders. Unlike Great Britain's "old-boy" ties—based on attendance at prestigious public schools and Oxbridge—the "Alma Mater mystique" is relatively insignificant in the United States. Because of such factors as the large geographical size of the United States, the impact of physical and social mobility upon the class structure, the diversity of social and educational institutions servicing elites, and the ideological equalitarianism which is deeply imbedded in American culture, a homogeneous ruling class has not emerged.[24] Indeed, Hacker concludes that a basic provincialism in the outlooks of senators as opposed to the more urbane and national perspectives of the business executives results in "a real lack of understanding and a failure of communication between the two elites."[25] Although Hacker's thesis appears overstated since the Senate, more so than the House, has been sympathetic to business interests, he does point out that there exists significant diversity between these two elites. Yet another factor contributing to the disparity in outlook between governmental officials—particularly in administrative or executive departments—and corporate executives is the professionalization process which each group undergoes. This process emphasizes different norms and goals for business activity than for governmental service.[26]

While the above discussion of the formal and informal sources of access to governmental decision makers that corporate interests possess may conjure up a picture of political leaders and governmental officials jumping about in response to the every urging of business managers, such is hardly the case. Greater accessibility does not assure businessmen of success in their political contacts. While friendship and commonality in socioeconomic background are important, "you can't go far on friendship alone" in the political sphere.[27]   The primary advantage of access to any political participant is the increased opportunity to state his position to the relevant public official. The access enjoyed by corporations and their managers should not be regarded as insidious. It is an inevitable characteristic of human relations that individuals deal more easily and more sympathetically with those whom they know or with whom they feel an affinity than with strangers or persons to whom they cannot relate. Other social interests possess this valuable resource and use it with great effectiveness.

PATRONAGE —

The concept of patronage in this context denotes the dependency of other social groups upon the activities of the corporation. This dependency manifests itself in numerous ways. Employees are dependent upon the firm for their livelihoods. Job mobility is often possible and, to the extent that it is, lessens worker dependency; but lower-level employees whose skills are widely available in the labor market are largely denied the advantages of mobility. Moreover, in certain locations, companies possess a geographical monopoly as a source of employment. Dependency, therefore, is a function of the existence of practical employment alternatives. A firm is provided with leverage over its workers by the potency of a possible threat to close a plant in a particular area unless certain conditions considered by management to be undesirable are changed. While in times of rising unemployment such threats may be particularly forceful, even under normal conditions workers are dependent upon job incomes to enable them to meet the financial obligations that they have assumed.

In those industries that are organized, unions have substantially lessened the degree of worker dependency, but have not eliminated it. Although such practices as company intimidation and blacklisting of workers have been largely eliminated and unions are often able to provide counter pressures against corporations in terms of organization and financial resources, employees are still ultimately dependent upon the firms for their jobs. There exists, therefore, the necessity in the long run for corporations and their employees to reach an accommodation.

While the above discussion has focused upon the dependency of blue-collar workers on the corporation, white-collar workers, particularly at lower levels, are similarly dependent. Moreover, they usually do not have the advantages of union support. The net result of this dependency is to give employees some sense of identity with corporate objectives and interests. Although this sense of identity may be weak, it still results in the employee taking into account the company's position—in instances where the firm has taken a strong stand on a matter of public policy, the firm's needs may affect his employment situation. Similarly, local businessmen, who are essentially dependent on the operations of a company for their livelihoods, have a stake in its well-being. Since these reliant enterprises are directly affected by strikes, layoffs, or declining business of the corporation, there is good reason for their owners to attempt to foster an environment that is favorable for the dominant enterprise.

Corporate patronage assumes yet another form. A satellite or patron-client relationship may also develop with governmental units such as states and municipalities because of the overriding economic importance of the corporation to the area in which it is located. The classic legal model of the corporation having its genesis as a result of a concession of power from the state and remaining a creature of the state, dependent upon governmental grace for its survival, is hardly appropriate to the realities of the large international business firm operating under general incorporation laws. For example, Bauer, Pool, and Dexter have found that in Delaware, Du Pont has been circumspect in exerting political pressure—at least in the area of foreign economic policy—yet the fact remains that it is critical for the state of Delaware to provide congenial social, political, and economic environment for its single most important economic asset.[28] In other words, not infrequently, a governmental entity exists in a greater state of dependency upon the business firm than contrariwise. Although the era of the company town is largely past history, instances still can be cited of firms occupying critical positions in their communities—Phillips Petroleum in Bartlesville, Oklahoma; Boeing in Seattle, Washington; Crown Zellerbach in Bogalusa, Louisiana; Bethlehem Steel in Bethlehem, Pennsylvania; United States Steel in Gary, Indiana; and Kodak in Rochester, New York. For example, *The Wall Street Journal* reports that "Phillips Petroleum casts its long shadow on just about every aspect of Bartlesville's community life"—including the town's economy, cultural affairs, civic projects and social activities, and politics—and quotes a local businessman to the effect that "when Phillips twitches, . . . Bartlesville jumps."[29]

The threat of a company to leave a locality or, conversely, the promise to consider relocation in a community, can be of great significance in determining policy decisions made by governmental bodies, since there is a desire to create a favorable business environment. One need only read the business-publications advertisements sponsored by municipalities, counties, and states to have evidence of this desire. South Carolina advertises "We'll train your workers *free*"; Tennessee proclaims "We grow plants and they live better here"; Erie County, New York, indicates to businessmen that "the Niagara frontier is hot all year long . . . for you"; Sunnyvale, California, claims that it "offers outstanding advantages to two types of companies"; and Philadelphia, Pennsylvania urges "Move your plant to Port instead of your cargo. It's cheaper." A full-page *The Wall Street Journal* advertisement in the form of a letter from the governor of Ohio demonstrates the importance which governmental entities place upon providing a favorable business environment. It states, "In Ohio we believe that the greatest contribution that anyone can make to the people of the state is to create an economic climate and attitude toward industry that will, in the end, provide more and better jobs. That is why 'Profit is Not a Dirty Word in Ohio.' "[30]

Another source of dependence arises from the fact that, increasingly, business corporations serve as the administrative arm of government. For example, large firms in their capacity as prime contractors on government contracts are delegated the discretion of determining which among a number of potential participants will be subcontractors on particular projects. When one considers the volume of contracts between corporations and the Defense Department—in fiscal 1967 military procurement contracts with United States business firms exceeded $40 billion —the importance of this power of delegation can be appreciated. Numerous smaller entities are greatly dependent upon the award of subcontracts, and it is reasonable to assume that the degree of their dependence is related to the extent of influence which a large prime contractor can exercise upon them. Although there is no evidence on this point, firms that are politically antagonistic to a major contractor might find themselves in an unfavorable position in attempting to gain subcontracts. In any event, the delegation to large firms of the right to subcontract presents an opportunity to influence, even informally, other businessmen, since the interests of the latter tend to become more and more closely identified with those possessing the power of decision making.

In a more general sense, economic interdependence among businessmen may have political consequences. As V. O. Key, Jr., has pointed out:

> Quite apart from the conformity induced by the fear of the frowns of one's fellows, pecuniary relations within the business system may discourage dissent. The concentration of business in large corporate organizations establishes a large number of dependency relations . . . which may be used to purchase acquiescence or to penalize deviation. Let a vulnerable manufacturer espouse unbusinesslike views, and he may discover that he has

become an undesirable credit risk and that his customers are seeking other sources of supply. The intricate network of relationships within business creates mechanisms for punishment as well as reward.[31]

Once again, these dependency relationships would likely cause satellite business firms to identify with the political needs of the dominant enterprises.

In summation of this point, patronage as a political resource is most valuable where the alternatives available to the dependent social interest are quite limited. More often, dependence results in a sense of identity of interest with the dominant firm rather than in formal coercion by it. As with other corporate resources, the importance of patronage should not be overestimated. Dependency relationships are rarely so complete as to give even the most dominant firm unbridled control. For example, despite the dominant position held by the copper companies in the communities where they are situated—usually they are the only employer for miles around—they were subject to a strike in 1967–1968 which lasted more than half a year. In this instance, the national solidarity of the copper workers through their union was able to counteract the local dominance of the producers.[32] Corporations that have large investments in plant and equipment or are tied to a particular geographical area because of its strategic location or the presence of important natural resources must be concerned with maintaining the good will of the community. They cannot simply pick up and leave if displeased by the business climate. The dependency relationship is weakened by the fact that, in an era of a nation-wide economy, customers and suppliers usually have commercial alternatives. Patronage, moreover, does not necessarily result in an abuse of power. Indeed, the very size of a firm may constitute an inherent limitation to such abuse.

In general, it may be said that, the larger a firm is, the more concern its chief officers must have for the interaction of their own behavior and that of the economic, social, and political environment in which they operate. For one thing, their own

actions may have predictable second-order consequences back
on themselves via the economy as a whole. Also, once a business reaches a certain size, it acquires a good deal of social
visibility. Because it can have an effect on the economy or on
the society as a whole, public agencies keep an eye on it. This
does not necessarily mean that every head of a large organization develops a social conscience. But he must at least acquire
a sensitivity to the reactions of those people who do have social
consciences and to the reactions of politicians who may capitalize on the social consciousness of others.[33]

Accordingly, patronage, important though it may be, is subject
to constraints.

SURROGATESHIP

Another important political resource possessed by corporations is surrogateship.

The fact that the businessman's work, although conducted as his
private enterprise is nevertheless something which affects all
members of the community (it is in fact a very highly decen-
tralized form of public administration) permits us to express its
relationship to government as that of a surrogate, a deputy.[34]

Surrogateship is a fundamental ingredient of an interdependent
capitalistic order and assumes a number of forms.

First of all, there is the economic power resulting from the
significant absolute and relative positions that large firms occupy
in national, regional, and local markets. As we saw during our
discussion of the concentraton of corporate assets and revenues,
our largest firms equal and frequently exceed governmental entities in terms of wealth. Moreover, as we have noted, in the
American socioeconomic order, the fundamental responsibility
for performing the economic tasks of the nation remains with

business corporations. The net result is that economic power lies primarily in private hands. While there is no direct correlation between economic power and political power, the fact remains that important firms influence the formulation and implementation of public policy in areas relevant to their operations, since the government cannot afford to espouse policies that are in opposition to the basic needs of the largest corporations. While the degree of influence undoubtedly varies with the time and the issue, it is probably true that "public policy necessarily tends to be oriented, especially over the long run, in a direction which is fundamentally in line with the interests of the great corporate enterprises."[35]

The important role of business firms in fulfilling governmental functions, which has already been mentioned in a number of contexts, is another dimension of surrogateship. Among other functions, corporations operate our basic communications and transportation facilities; develop and construct the nation's military defense and aerospace systems; supply most of the goods and services required by governmental bodies; operate governmental facilities; and engage in regional planning, urban rehabilitation and manpower-training activities on behalf of public agencies. On the local level, corporations satisfy many of the fundamental requirements of the community.

As a consequence of this public dependence upon private industry for the fulfillment of basic economic tasks and the fact that corporations often assume governmental functions, business firms have two important sources of leverage upon governmental decision makers. First, they can threaten, or deliberately take, action that slows down activities government wishes to encourage or speeds up processes government is attempting to discourage. Second, they can threaten a political strike—nonperformance of their valuable economic tasks—unless political authorities either take certain actions which they demand or refrain from taking certain actions of which they disapprove.

As examples of the first type of leverage, a firm may refuse to locate a plant in a pocket of unemployment unless the governmental body that is attempting to encourage industrial relocation in the area makes certain concessions or provides particular advantages; or a corporation may invest abroad at a time when the government is attempting to redress an unfavorable balance of payments situation and may thereby thwart governmental policy.

The use of the political strike, which is analogous to the threat of a small child to go home unless his companion "plays right," is even more common. Business firms frequently threaten to locate elsewhere if state or local taxes are not adjusted in a desired manner. Such a threat occurred in Minnesota, where the iron-mining industry warned "in a threatening manner" of dire economic consequences to the state economy unless the legislature passed the "taconite amendment," which would freeze taxes on taconite production at the then current low rate for 25 years.[36] Similarly, the New York Stock Exchange threatened a few years ago to leave New York City if the state passed a stock transfer tax. Although in neither of the instances cited did the industry leave despite its failure to receive the favored tax treatment, it should not be thought that the political strike is strictly a ruse. In 1968, the state of New York did pass legislation reducing the levy imposed by the 1966 stock transfer tax.[37] Moreover, during the decade following World War II, a large segment of the New England textile industry moved to the South in response both to the state governments' pressures for taxes and to organized labor's demands on an industry which was experiencing serious economic difficulties. "The important point is that it is the threat that counts, not the exercise of the threat. As long as people think that business might move, their behavior will, at least in part, be effectively controlled by business."[38]

Another dimension of the political strike, illustrated by the 1962 steel controversy, is the threat by business to "lose confidence" in government if it takes undesirable actions. From the time he assumed office, President John F. Kennedy had attempted to assure the business community of the friendliness of his administration. When confronted with the announced price increase by United States Steel, he was aware that negative governmental action would be considered antibusiness by businessmen and would impair his attempts at rapprochement. Indeed, some observers contend that the stock market decline of 1962 could be attributed, at least in part, to a show of "no confidence" by the business community following the administration's actions forcing the steel companies to rescind the price increase. The steel dispute was a "political contest . . . in that major problems of public policy were involved, in that government became embroiled, and that . . . [the] . . . contest became a problem of power."[39]

It would seem that Democratic administrations desiring close ties to the business community are more susceptible to the pressures of the political strike than are Republican leaders. Since the Democratic Party has traditionally had a reputation of being antibusiness, a Democratic President must assiduously woo business support and demonstrate his good faith. As *Fortune* reported in an article entitled, "What Business Wants from Lyndon Johnson,"

> Washington's ear is cocked toward the business community as it has not been in decades. President Johnson has called for a business-government "partnership" and has actively sought the friendship and advice of the nation's corporate chiefs. He also wants desperately to maintain an atmosphere of business confidence. For these reasons, therefore, the hopes and fears of the nation's corporate leaders have taken on new importance. Pieced together, they add up to the business leadership's economic policy for the next four years—or, put more bluntly, its terms for getting along with the President.[40]

Interestingly, however, although President Johnson attempted to maintain close ties to business during his administration, he did not hesitate in late 1965 to use techniques against the aluminum and copper industries similar to those which President Kennedy used with the steel industry. Although to a lesser extent than was his predecessor, he was subjected to a barrage of criticism from businessmen who threatened their loss of confidence. While this form of political strike has not been successful under crisis conditions, its importance should not be underestimated in an economy that is dependent on close government-business cooperation.

CORPORATE INFLUENCE OVER MASS MEDIA

The influence of large corporations upon the mass media is a political resource of prime value. "The political tone of the media is far from reflecting even approximately the distribution of attitudes and opinions in the society as a whole."[41] Corporate influence derives primarily from four sources: (1) the advertising dollar, (2) the ownership of some media outlets by industrial firms, (3) the fact that the media comprise sizable corporate enterprises with political interests of their own and a natural inclination to be sympathetic to a business point of view, and (4) the continuous exposure of the public—via the mass media—to efforts by business firms (a) to project a positive image of the importance of corporate enterprise to the American way of life and (b) to create a store of public empathy and support of business, which can be valuable in times of political crisis.

Let us look first at the use of the advertising dollar to purchase media time and space. In 1967, the top 125 national advertisers expended nearly $3.3 billion, of which more than two-thirds was allocated to radio and television advertising, and the remainder to the daily and periodical press.[42] Although direct censorship of media content is not commonplace, advertisers can exert influence, through their supervision of program packaging, over the media time that they have purchased. Similarly, a firm's willingness or refusal to sponsor programs in the public-affairs category is a form of media control. An indirect source of influence arises from the fact that, since the media are dependent on business advertising, they are often reluctant to publish or transmit criticism of corporate practices. On the opposite side, the costs associated with the use of mass media often prohibit other social groups from utilizing these facilities to the same extent as business firms.

Turning to the second point—media ownership by corporations—the 1967 Federal Communications Commission hearings on the proposed merger between the American Broadcasting Company (ABC) and International Telephone and Telegraph Company (ITT) raised in bold relief the question of media freedom from business influence. Accusations were made by members of the press during the time of the hearings that ABC was attempting to control the reporting of news about the merger. Had the merger between ABC and ITT been completed, it would not, however, have presented a novel situation with regard to the relationship between a manufacturing company and a communications firm. The National Broadcasting Company is a wholly owned subsidiary of the Radio Corporation of America, and General Tire and Rubber Company owns a string of radio and television stations. Until 1959, Anaconda Copper owned eight daily newspapers in Montana.[43] Other examples of media ownership by industrial firms can be found on the local level. Although there is no evidence of direct exploitation of such ownership interests so far as the general substance of programming is concerned, it is still highly improbable that a subsidiary would publicize views that are incompatible with the interests of its parent.

A third point is that many media organizations are themselves big business, with political interests aligned with those of other large corporations. Thus, media executives identify and associate with their counterparts in other industries. This orientation can be and sometimes is reflected in editorial policy, in the content of programs and articles, and in the differential treatment accorded business as opposed to labor and governmental organizations. It is also manifested in the pattern of political endorsements by the media at election time. There is evidence that editorial support is reflected in news coverage. Robert E. Lane reports that, regarding the political bias of the press, "analysis of a substantial body of material reveals consistent but moderate bias in the news columns favoring the candidate given support in the editorial pages."[44]

A plausible explanation of the conservatism of the publications media is that nowadays the conservative bias of the American newspapers is usually attributed to more subtle factors, related to the nature of the industry. A major daily newspaper is a large business enterprise, having most of the characteristics of all large business enterprises. It usually has a corporate form, a large and expensive plant, and a management separated from its ownership. . . . That large newspapers tend to be conservative in their economic and political views may be, in part, the natural conservatism of big and middle-sized business in America.[45]

A critical question posed by the pro-business orientation of the media is the extent to which other social and political groups obtain access to the publication and communications media for expression of their views. Some readily obtain media support; others cannot hope to make their views known.

In the context of this discussion, incorporated media possess a direct political resource in their ability to take editorial positions on issues and candidates and to selectively edit program content. Newspapers and magazines have made editorial endorsements for many years. A recent study indicates that, in 1960, 939 daily newspapers endorsed a presidential candidate. Of this number, 731 (78 per cent) backed Republican Richard M. Nixon and 208 (22 per cent) endorsed Democrat John F. Kennedy. In 1964, 789 dailies made endorsements; 349 (45 per cent) supported Republican Barry Goldwater and 440 (55 per cent) supported Democrat Lyndon B. Johnson. As of January 15, 1962, there were 1,761 dailies in circulation. Interestingly, although individual radio and television stations have been free since 1949 to take positions on issues and candidates, it was not until 1960 that an American radio station endorsed a Presidential candidate. In that year, 62 stations (almost all radio) editorialized for or against candidates, and 148 did so in 1962 Congressional races.[46] Although evidence regarding the direct influence of the media upon voter opinion is limited, a number of studies suggest that the media function more effectively as agents of reinforcement than as agents of change.[47]

Lastly, the continual public exposure that large firms enjoy through the media emphasizes the importance of the corporation to American life and contributes to the store of corporate good will, which is a definite political asset in time of company need. A number of years ago, for example, the Atlantic and Pacific Tea Company (A & P) used the media to lead a successful fight against a proposed California "chain-store tax." Assisted by an advertising firm, A & P won consumer support by stressing its low prices and efficiencies and had great success in its appeal to agricultural groups.[48] The public, long advised that "Progress" is General Electric's "Most Important Product," or that Du Pont is providing "Better Things for Better Living Through Chemistry," is thereby more inclined to view the company as somehow associated with the public good, rather than merely as a business organization. As mentioned earlier, AT&T was among the earliest and most successful practitioners of the art of corporate public relations and still maintains one of the most extensive and highly rationalized public relations networks in the country. Combined with its large number of stockholders, this continual and favorable public exposure has contributed to the creation, over the years, of a political environment that has been favorable to "Ma Bell."

The over-all impact of corporate expenditures on the mass media is difficult to assess. For one thing, the media are "to a very large degree, apolitical—if not antipolitical,"[49] since relatively small amounts of space and time are devoted to political subjects. Moreover, in some instances, the expenditure of large the creation over the years of a political environment that has is completely wasted. Yet, in the opinion of one expert,

> the chances are that the cumulative impact over the years is imposing. The great political triumph of large-scale enterprise has been the manufacture of a public opinion favorably disposed toward, or at least tolerant of, gigantic corporations.[50]

If nothing else, the mass media have historically been the primary agents for disseminating the fundamental tenet of American business ideology — that a capitalist economic order is the necessary precondition of a democratic political system. By their continuous stress upon the equation

$$\text{CAPITALISM} = \text{DEMOCRACY}$$

the media have placed those groups that propose changes in the American economic order in an unfavorable light, since any deviation from a traditional free enterprise system is, by definition, considered to be antidemocratic.[51] Consequently—although the ideological bias of the media, particularly network television and nationally circulated publications, has become less pronounced in recent years—established economic interests have held an important advantage over their critics as a result of the support given them by the media.

A BACKLOG OF POLITICAL SUCCESS

Another political asset of significance to some corporations is the backlog of favorable results that they have enjoyed over the years in their relationships with legislative bodies and with administrative agencies and executive departments. While past success does not inevitably breed future success, it does serve to (1) provide a favorable climate within which to pursue political objectives, (2) bolster the confidence of corporate officials engaging in political activities, (3) give experience regarding the most efficacious means of accomplishing political goals, and (4) make other social interests more cautious in their opposition to corporate objectives. For example, it is easier both psychologically and practically for oil and gas producers to fight a proposed elimination of the depletion allowance, given the past success that they have had with Congress when this matter has previously arisen. By like token, industries that have been recipients of federal subsidies in prior years find it much easier to request assistance than do groups that have never received such aid.

Administrative agencies have been primary areas of past corporate political success. As we have already seen, there is strong evidence that regulatory commissions have life cycles during which their enforcement activities range from the aggressive, crusading vigor of youth to the debility and decline of old age. Consequently, in certain industries, client control has been a prime characteristic of the regulatory process. That is, particular companies and industry groups have carved out spheres of influence within the very governmental agencies charged with their supervision, achieving thereby a high degree of autonomy in terms of effective governmental control. Marver H. Bernstein, a leading analyst of administrative commissions, has noted that

> the hostile environment in which regulation operates is pervasive. It provides the frame of reference for the regulatory process and makes the process conditional upon the acceptance of regulation by the affected groups. It forces a commission to come to terms with the regulated groups as a condition of its survival.[52]

An even more pessimistic critique of administrative regulation is offered by Walter Adams and Horace M. Gray. In their opinion, "legalized private monopoly under public regulation is a snare and a delusion, productive of little good and much evil. In no single instance has it fulfilled the roseate expectations of its original advocates."[53]

Examples of governmental agencies that have been characterized in the past by client control are the Departments of Commerce and the Interior, the Federal Power Commission (FPC), the Federal Communications Commission (FCC), the Food and Drug Administration (FDA), the Interstate Commerce Commission (ICC), and the Civil Aeronautics Board (CAB). Indeed, the last two mentioned agencies had their geneses in legislative designs to protect the regulated industry and, particularly in the case of the CAB, to promote it. The relationship between corporations and administrative agencies can, in a very loose sense, be analogized to the system of "closed politics" which, as Sir C. P. Snow notes, frequently exists between governmental decision makers and their scientific advisors.[54] Scientific decisions are "closed," or virtually immune from outside scrutiny, since once a decision has been made by a governmental body after deliberation with its advisors, there often exists no effective appeal by dissenters to a larger assembly of outside opinion. Similarly, in the case of regulatory agencies, decisions frequently have been a result of consultation between the agency and the client group, with other social interests playing a limited and often ineffective role.

Of all the many aspects of corporate political activity, this success that business firms have enjoyed with administrative agencies has caused the greatest concern among observers of American politics. For example, Grant McConnell has expressed the view that "in this capture of public authority in particular areas lies the most important problem," since the consequence of such a capture is "the formulation of separate narrow constituencies for particular parts of government."[55] Were public agencies to become so thoroughly subverted by corporations that there was complete identity between business policy and governmental policy, thereby effectively eliminating access to points of public decision making, the interests of other relevant constituencies in American society would be adversely affected. Notwithstanding the instances of client control cited above, this total subversion has not occurred, if for no other reason than that other governmental agencies have frequently served as counterbalancing influences. Witness, for example, the antagonism between the Justice Department and the Comptroller of the Currency over bank mergers. However, it is this area of business political activity more than any other that most bears close watching for any potential manifestation of exorbitant corporate political power.

This close relationship between regulator and client group is, of course, not unique to corporations and administrative agencies. Organized labor has enjoyed great success within the National Labor Relations Board. Social welfare and public health agencies have client status within the Department of Health, Education and Welfare. In each instance, these groups have a political asset comparable to the backlog of success relevant to their activities that some corporations enjoy with governmental bodies.

A history of political success does not mean that success is inevitable. A case in point is the struggle of the drug manufacturers with the Food and Drug Administration over the testing and labeling of drugs. Similarly, firms in regulated industries continually bemoan the fact that their rate structures are much lower than is justified by their costs. Thus, the point is only that past political success carries with it a greater likelihood of success in the future than does a prior history of political failure. Success contributes to the creation of a favorable climate in which to conduct political activity.

THE STATUS OF BUSINESS AND BUSINESS MANAGERS IN AMERICAN SOCIETY

Lastly, as a result of their position as social and economic notables, corporate managers are frequently opinion makers within their communities. In keeping with the business emphasis of our society, economic leaders in America possess higher social status than is enjoyed by their counterparts in Europe. In the United States, "in the social hierarchy of occupations, the politician rates lower than he should and the businessman higher. Great deference is paid to the corporation executive, whose job is the symbol of success and who reputedly has mastered the art of managing men and making money."[56] This high status has its political consequences. As suggested previously, it contributes to the access that corporations have to governmental decision makers. Moreover, the reputation enjoyed by businessmen has an impact upon the general public. Many persons feel that business leaders are practical and efficient and that therefore the policies they espouse are also practical and efficient; consequently, on certain issues, particularly of an economic nature (for example, monetary and fiscal policy and taxation), leading business executives have found that their public pronouncements carry weight with the electorate. Indeed, in 1967 and 1968, the Johnson administration sought to bolster its attempt to obtain from a reluctant Congress passage of a 10 per cent surcharge on the federal income tax by soliciting the public support of business leaders who were of the opinion that the tax proposal was necessary for national "fiscal responsibility." The administration hoped that business acceptance of the tax increase would make the surcharge proposal more palatable to the general public and hence to an election-minded Congress.

Policy pronouncements by business leaders are probably even more influential on the local level, where there are fewer competing influences, than in national politics. For example, a few years ago, officials of Olin Mathieson were instrumental in helping to defeat a school bond issue in Hannibal, Ohio, where the firm had a plant. In newspaper advertisements and statements by company officials, Olin argued that over its 22-year period the $3.5-million bond issue would cost in excess of $6 million. The voters rejected the proposal by nearly 4 to 1 and subsequently passed a $1.9 million pay-as-you-go program that was supported by the corporation. It should be noted that Olin, which accounted for 90 per cent of the real estate taxes paid in Hannibal, was the primary beneficiary of the defeat of the bond issue.[57]

The effectiveness of business leaders in influencing public opinion varies substantially with the issue. Corporate managers generally have greater success in obtaining support for their views on taxation than on right-to-work legislation or on fiscal policies rather than on social welfare legislation. Their success is largely a function of both the expertise they bring to bear on the issue and the lack of blatant self-interest. Moreover, the more moderate the views advocated by a businessman, the more probable a broad public acceptance of them. Extreme positions usually attract but limited support. Indeed, among some segments of the society, any position taken by a business leader more often than not meets automatic opposition. It should also be remembered that the high status and reputation of corporate heads is also enjoyed by prominent individuals associated with other social interests—public officials, educational leaders, professional men, and ethnic notables.

We have concentrated on the status and reputation of business leaders; the related point, that business per se is highly regarded in American society, has been discussed in a number of contexts throughout this book and need not be amplified here. Suffice it to say, the corporate assets of public acceptance, reputation, and good will constitute an important political resource.

•　　•　　•

In this section, eight important political resources possessed by corporations were analyzed: organization; riches; access to political decision makers; patronage that is a consequence of the dependence of other social interests upon business firms; surrogateship, resulting from the fact that in our socioeconomic order many important social tasks have been delegated to corporations; influence over mass media; the backlog of political success; and the high status and reputation enjoyed by business and business managers in American society. While not exhaustive, the above listing of political assets possessed by corporations indicates the most significant resources available to business firms in the political arena. This discussion of political assets does not imply that a corporate cabal has been engaging in a nefarious and successful effort to undermine the foundations of American democracy, but rather indicates—contrary to the assertions frequently made by business managers—that corporations possess certain valuable bases of political power. At this point, however, any attempt to evaluate the extent and impact of this power on our political process would be premature. Preliminarily, we must examine those limitations upon corporate political power that are present in American society.

LIMITATIONS UPON CORPORATE POLITICAL POWER

Notwithstanding the impressive political resources possessed by corporations, business firms do not constitute a threat to political democracy in the United States because of several factors. These limitations, which go to the heart of any analysis of corporate political power, are considered in this section.

POLITICAL RESOURCES ARE NOT EQUIVALENT TO POLITICAL POWER

The first point is that, as suggested earlier, political resources are not synonymous with political power. Resources constitute merely one of the ingredients of power and must be used efficaciously—thereby affecting the behavior of other political actors—before they are converted into power. The effective capability to act varies substantially among business firms. Some corporations that possess a wide spectrum of political resources have demonstrated an inability to utilize them effectively. For example, since the end of World War II, in the deployment of their substantial political resources, aerospace firms have demonstrated greater political efficacy than have steel companies. Indeed, the effective capability of a single firm may vary over time or in response to particular issues. By way of illustration, for a time during the early 1960's the political capability of General Electric was reduced, following the revelation of its extensive violation of the antitrust laws. Similarly, the effective capability of the automobile manufacturers to oppose auto safety legislation was reduced in 1966, after their efforts to intimidate critic Ralph Nader became publicly known.

Psychological factors may affect the effective capability of a firm. David Riesman has pointed out that "power, indeed, is founded, in large measure, on interpersonal expectations and attitudes. If businessmen feel weak and dependent, they do in actuality become weaker and more dependent, no matter what material resources may be ascribed to them."[58] Accordingly, if the important political resources of a corporation are considered by its management to be inferior to the assets of a political competitor, the corporate leaders may be restrained from action, thereby reducing the firm's actual power. Similarly, the fact that, as suggested in Chapter Five, a greater number of executives perceive that business political activity is more "ineffective" than "effective" operates as a constraint upon corporate political endeavors.[59]

A related point is that the political resources of a given corporation are not constant. The quality of organization—in terms of personnel, management practices, coordination, and decision making—differs over the life of a company. The financial resources available for political purposes depend upon the other pressing intracorporate claims on these resources. Access may vary in accordance with the party in power, the public official in office, or the background and contacts of top management. Corporate good will is a variable asset. The net result is that, in both a quantitative and a qualitative sense, corporate political resources fluctuate over time.

Moreover, although we have been speaking of corporate political resources, the fact remains that business firms possess these assets to varying degrees. Some firms have greater wealth than others. Company A may have a greater legacy of political success than Company B; the organizational effectiveness of Corporation C is markedly superior to that of Corporation D; and so on.

POLITICAL RESOURCES OF OTHER SOCIAL INTERESTS

A second point is that corporations do not have a monopoly over political resources. Other social interests possess equivalent political assets. Labor unions possess organization and riches. Educational and professional interest groups have access, and social status and reputation. Farm groups have a history of political success. Moreover, certain resources possessed by other social groups—such as a large number of voters, unimpeachable legitimacy as political participants, and deep-seated organizational loyalty—are unavailable to corporations. One of the interesting dimensions of the Black Power movement among American blacks is the attempt to mobilize the primary political asset available to blacks—strength of numbers—for political purposes. Because the focus in this chapter has been upon *corporate* political resources, specific attention has not been given to the power bases of other social actors. If we were to similarly analyze the power resources of other interest groups, the tally sheet would be quite impressive. Since all power is relational, the fact that political assets are distributed throughout society is of great importance in limiting the effectiveness of any single social participant.

Thus, the various social interests exist in a perpetual state of tension. Each attempts to maintain or to advance its own political position against the efforts of other social interests to retain or to enhance their positions. Other interest groups can be counted upon, therefore, to utilize their own bases of power to counteract any untoward corporate advances. Labor, while weakened, is hardly moribund. Unions are quick to denounce and to oppose manifestations of corporate political strength. Political resources are possessed by small business groups, agricultural associations, conservation organizations, professional societies, ethnic and racial organizations, and consumer groups. Observers as diverse as Harold Brayman, former director of public relations of Du Pont, and John Kenneth Galbraith have pointed out that intellectuals and technocrats—both within and outside of the universities—are an increasingly important political force, possessing two significant bases of power—expertise and access.[60]   Since, by and large, this group tends to view corporate political power with suspicion, an additional important constraint upon this power is developing.

As was suggested earlier, the very necessity for both major political parties to accommodate the claims made by the variety of interests present in American society militates against domination of the party structure by corporations. Our political elites, particularly on the national level, are exceedingly jealous of their power, independence, and prerogatives, and thus they constitute a check against excessive corporate political power.   Furthermore, the many bureaucratic interests that exist at all levels of government can and do act as countervailing forces.   Because of these restraints within the institutions of government,

> officials of big corporations also come to realize that their relationships with government are continuous and that, if they press too hard for victory on one particular problem, even if they win, it may jeopardize their chances of success on some future and more important problem.[61]

This condition of group tension, which has developed as a result of the competing influences discussed above, has been called varyingly countervailing power, polyarchy, and interest group liberalism.⁶² Its effect is to limit the scope and the magnitude of corporate power relative to the political system.

OPPOSITION OF THE GENERAL PUBLIC: EMPHASIS ON SOCIAL PLURALISM

A related constraint upon corporate political power is the widespread public commitment to a pluralistic political order. For corporations to achieve sufficient political power to threaten democratic processes would require a largely apolitical, unaffiliated, and submissive populace that neither identified with nor formed competing social-interest groups and, accordingly, could not be energized into political action in order to forestall such a threat. The notion of a political man who is the thoroughly enlightened, rational, and concerned citizen of town-meeting fame has long since been cast upon the scrap heap of political mythology. However, the American electorate has, over the years, been sufficiently supportive of the democratic "rules of the game" to stifle extreme elements of both the left and the right, which have been perceived as threats to the pluralistic character of the American political order.⁶³

Efforts by the corporate community to exert power to an extent inconsistent with these "rules" would engender opposition. While business enjoys high status within American society, "the legitimacy of businessmen and their values is not accepted in all areas of community life and by all people."⁶⁴ Since the legitimacy of corporate political activity has traditionally been viewed with suspicion by various social interests, any deviation from widely accepted political practices would almost certainly arouse influential segments of the public and invoke political reprisal by agencies of government. Indeed, fears of an antagonistic public have been important in restraining corporate political activity. For example, Bauer, Pool, and Dexter report that

> GM's reluctance to speak up for its views on foreign trade was
> at least in part a reflection of the marked sensitivity which certain giant corporations in America have developed over their
> public image. Large firms which have been the object of anti-

trust action or have been generally viewed as throwing their weight around may indeed sometimes use their economic strength to influence public policy or to take advantage of their business competitors. But, if they sometimes do so in fact, such industrial giants must take all the more pains to avoid the appearance of so doing. And, as many of them have learned by harsh experience, the best way to maintain the image of probity is to maintain its practice, too.[65]

As we have seen, moreover, corporate political activity viewed by the public as extreme may result in direct financial loss to a business firm. Witness, for example, the decline in sales of the Eversharp Company, which has been attributed in large measure to public resentment of the support given by the firm and its chief executive officer, Patrick J. Frawley, to conservative political causes.

Some evidence indicates that, as a consequence of the growth of a more articulate and educated public, we are experiencing in this country an increase in ideological sophistication and an acceptance of liberal democratic values. Consequently, the future holds out the prospect of a "more numerous class of political influentials, committed to liberal democracy and aware of the rights and obligations which attend that commitment."[66] If such a prognostication is accurate and if commitment and awareness are reflected in an increase in the quality of political participation, in the future there should be less to fear by way of unchecked political power by corporations—or other interest groups—than there was in the past.

CONSTRAINTS WITHIN THE BUSINESS SYSTEM

A final set of constraints on excessive corporate political power exists within the business system itself. These internal limitations are every bit as important as the three other factors that have been discussed in this section.

The first constraint is intercorporate political competition. As we have seen, "conflict of interest and opinion among businessmen is as evident as cohesion."[67] Corporations utilize their political resources against each other as frequently as they do against other social interests. Indeed, internecine conflict among business organizations constitutes much of the substance of corporate political activity. The net result is a degree of political pluralism within the corporate community that has prevented the emergence of a monolithic business political force. Moreover, even were collective corporate action desired, there are certain inherent operational difficulties, in addition to the aspect of competition. William Spinrad suggests several in the context of local politics:

> Communication may not be as easy as assumed, especially through their far-flung organizations. The process of formal decision-making on an issue is not always readily available, and potentially divisive decisions, within business organizations or in the community, are avoided. Public relations may be more important than power wielding for its own sake.[68]

Operation of these factors has tended to constrain intercorporate political collaboration. A related point is that intracorporate conflict limits corporate political power. We have seen that competition exists within large, diversified organizations regarding both company goals and the allocation of organizational resources. As Bauer, Pool, and Dexter point out, since various divisions within Du Pont stood to benefit quite differently from the passage of reciprocal trade legislation, the company never took a unified stance on this issue. Consequently, Du Pont's political effectiveness with regard to the tariff fight was reduced.[69]

A third internal factor limiting the possibility of corporate domination of the political order is the absence of any demonstrable desire on the part of corporate leaders to achieve business political hegemony over either other social interests or the formal institutions of government. Corporate managers have been content to work within the pluralistic political order for the parochial interests of their firms. In this context, it should be recalled that corporate political activity has been instrumentally oriented—to enhance the economic environment of the firm —rather than directed toward the accomplishment of any grandiose scheme for social power. As a group, corporate managers have eschewed general political leadership and have concerned themselves with limited politics for limited purposes. Business leaders historically have heeded the admonition of Eugene V. Rostow that "the economic job of directors and management is quite difficult enough to absorb the full time of first-rate minds."[70] Consequently, political activity is generally viewed by business leaders as a necessary means to corporate well-being rather than as an end pursued for its own sake. Indeed, excessive political activity on the part of a corporate manager is looked upon somewhat askance by his professional colleagues.

While a sizable majority of executives polled by the *Harvard Business Review* in 1968 thought, as a general proposition, that the political involvement of business should be more extensive than at present, when queried about specific political activities in which business should engage, respondents were much more reluctant to recommend additional corporate participation. Significantly, moreover, in the 1968 survey the percentage of executives (68 per cent) who thought that business should increase its involvement was smaller than the percentage in the 1964 poll (72 per cent) or the percentage in a 1959 *HBR* study (89 per cent).[71] Accordingly, an intensification of managerial political activity to an extent which endangers political democracy is remote.

Political power seems to have accrued to corporations more from the manifold social, economic, and political developments that have taken place during the past half century as a result of the emergence of an organizational society than from any deliberate design by business managers to acquire power. Like other members of the populace, moreover, the acceptance by corporate leaders of the rules of the game is sufficient to preclude the possibility of a takeover of political institutions even if their organizations possessed the requisite power. Thus far, the American political order has been able to accommodate the demands of a large variety of social interests without limitations being either attempted or effectuated by the corporate com-

munity. There is little reason to believe that the relative openness of the political system will change in the years to come as
a consequence of corporate involvement.

•   •   •

In this section we have dealt with several major limitations
upon corporate political power. In the first place, since political
resources are not synonymous with political power, the effective
capability of corporations to act is a critical determinant of
power. Second, other social interests also possess important
political resources with which they counteract corporate power
—in essence, a pluralism of power exists in American society.
A third restraining factor is the opposition of the general public
to any business political behavior that transcends the "rules of
the game." Finally, there are several constraints within the
business system, including intercorporate antagonisms and the
lack of motivation on the part of corporate managers to pursue
political activity beyond the limited needs of the firm. As a
consequence of these limitations, despite the impressive array
of political assets, corporate political power does not constitute
a threat to democracy in the United States. As Adolf A. Berle,
Jr., has pointed out,

> Yet the fact was, and is, that centralization of industrial eco-
> nomic power to a point where it could dominate the political
> state has been avoided in the American political system. It is
> not at present a major threat. . . . There is no high factor of
> unity when several hundred corporations in different lines of
> endeavors are involved. There is still less when a substantial
> degree of competition prevails among them. Dominance by
> them over the political state in major matters is not a present
> possibility.[72]

No mention has been made in this section of the various
legal restrictions on business political activities—notably, the
federal prohibition of corporate campaign contributions and ex-

penditures and the requirement that corporate lobbyists register
with Congress. These statutory constraints have been omitted
from this discussion because they have been singularly unsuccessful in limiting corporate power. As we have seen, corporations have carried on their electoral and governmental activities
virtually as effectively as if the prohibitions did not exist. At
very best, these limitations have caused corporations to be a
little more careful in their political involvement than they would
otherwise have been.[73] Accordingly, it is inappropriate to include these legal prohibitions in a discussion of actual constraints
on corporate power.

A CORPORATE POWER ELITE?

No discussion of corporate political power would be complete without specific treatment of the role of business leaders
as wielders of political power—a subject that has been of abiding
interest to social scientists. We have already referred to formal
participation by business executives in partisan politics and in
their capacities as governmental advisors and to the equally
important informal political role of the corporate manager, which
derives solely from his economic and social position rather than
from any official political position that he might occupy. Sociologists have emphasized that, in American society, class (wealth),
status (prestige), and power (influence or control) are determined largely by occupation, which in turn is a function of organizational affiliation. The question that has been posed, therefore, is whether business executives—sitting at the apex of the
economic structure—constitute a dominant political elite.
Both sociologists and political scientists have demonstrated
considerable energy and ingenuity in attempting to ascertain
the influence of businessmen in (1) determining the candidates
and policies of political parties and (2) in making or controlling
governmental decisions. Much of the analytical research on the
subject has been in the form of community-power studies, which
have focused upon local political life. The conclusions of these
studies have been dramatically inconclusive.[74]

ELITE THEORY CONSIDERED

Sociological studies on the local level by Floyd Hunter, Robert S. and Helen Merrell Lynd, W. Lloyd Warner, August Hollingshead, and Roland J. Pellegrin and Charles H. Coates, and by C. Wright Mills and G. William Domhoff on the national scale have resulted in a body of literature emphasizing the power of economic elites, whose members are viewed as the critical decision makers in the political arena.[75]   For example, in his study of Atlanta, Georgia, Hunter concluded that a small group of powerful men, operating behind the scenes, informally determined community policy. "The test for admission to this circle of decision-makers is almost wholly a man's position in the business community" in Atlanta.[76]   According to Hunter, the top economic leaders made the basic community decisions, which were then implemented by the "under-structure," composed of the economic subordinates of the elite, small businessmen and political and social-service professionals.   "The men in the under-structure of power become the doers and are activated by the policy-makers—the initiators."[77]

On the national level, C. Wright Mills concluded that a power elite consisting of high military chieftains, corporate heads, and, to a lesser extent, political leaders, makes the critical public decisions in America.   "Inside military circles and inside political circles and 'on the sidelines' in the economic area, these circles and cliques of corporation executives are in on most all major decisions regardless of topic."[78]   Ironically, Republican President (and former general) Dwight D. Eisenhower has borne witness to Mills' thesis.   In his "Farewell Radio and Television Address to the American People," he warned the nation that it must "guard against the acquisition of unwarranted influence, whether sought or unsought, by the military-industrial complex" consisting of the conjunction of "an immense military establishment and a large arms industry . . . new in the American experience."[79]

Similarly, G. William Domhoff expressed the view that the business elite constitutes a national ruling class.   In response to his rhetorical question, "Who Rules America?," Domhoff concludes that, the income, wealth, and institutional leadership of . . . the "American business aristocracy" are more than sufficient to earn it the designation "governing class." . . . This "ruling class" is based upon the national corporate economy and the institutions that economy nourishes. It manifests itself through . . . the power elite.[80]

By way of summary, at the heart of elitist theory relative to both local and national politics "is a clear presumption of the average citizen's inadequacies."[81]   Power is viewed as resting in the hands of the few who make decisions for the many and about the many.   These few consist primarily of business leaders.

THE PLURALIST ALTERNATIVE

Research by political scientists has not generally supported the findings in a number of sociological studies concerning the existence of an economic (particularly a corporate) power elite that is the dominant political decision maker on either the community or the national level.   Instead, political scientists have tended toward a pluralist interpretation of the distribution and use of political power.[82]   Robert A. Dahl described this pluralistic model as follows:

The theory and practice of American pluralism tend to assume . . . that the existence of multiple centers of power, none of which is wholly sovereign, will help (may indeed be necessary) to tame power, to secure the consent of all, and to settle conflicts peacefully.[83]

In his study of New Haven, Dahl found a situation of "dispersed inequalities" in the distribution of political resources, in which no single elite held the key to control over all decisions of communal importance.[84]   Edward C. Banfield has commented on the conspicuous failure of economic notables to exercise political power in Chicago.[85]   Wallace S. Sayre and Herbert Kaufman pointed out in their study of New York City that (1) decisions of the municipal government emanated from a variety of sources; (2) conflicts and clashes were settled, not at a single point, but at many levels; (3) no single group could guarantee either the success of any proposal it supported or the defeat of every idea it opposed; (4) every separate decision center consisted of a cluster of interested contestants, with a core group formally invested with authority to make the decision and a constellation of related satellite groups seeking to influence the core group; and (5) every decision of importance was consequently the product of mutual accommodation.[86]

Perhaps the best summary of the hypotheses underlying pluralist theory is found in Nelson W. Polsby's *Community Power and Political Theory*:

> One of the most common patterns of behavior to be observed in American community life is that participation in the making of decisions is concentrated in the hands of a few. But this does not mean that American communities are ruled by a single all-purpose elite, after the fashion suggested by stratification [elite] theory. At least three significant modifications to the finding of limited participation in decision-making must be made. First, different small groups normally make decisions on different community problems, and likewise, the personnel of decision-making groups often change, even over the short-run. Secondly, the decisions made by small groups are almost always considered routine or otherwise insignificant by most other members of the community. Thirdly, when small groups undertake innovation or decision-making in cases salient or likely to become salient to others in the community they must achieve special kinds of legitimacy or risk the likelihood of failure.[87]

After reviewing most of the available literature of elite theory (including the work of Hunter, Warner, the Lynds, Hollingshead, Delbert Miller, E. Digby Baltzell and Robert O. Schulze), Polsby concludes that "no properly documented instances of communities where hierarchy [elite rule] predominates have come to light."[88]

ELITISM AND PLURALISM:
A MODUS VIVENDI?

The differences in the conclusions of sociologists and political scientists regarding community power are largely attributable to the research perspectives that each group brings to bear in studying the problem.[89]   Sociologists have focused their attention on *individuals* and on *classes of individuals* and have attempted to ascertain which persons in the community occupy high economic and social position and are *reputed* to be political decision makers.   Position and reputation are seen as the keys to the question of who governs.   They have found pyramidal power structures in which, more often than not, persons holding economic power are the key wielders of influence and control.[90]

On the other hand, political scientists have tended to focus on *issues*—such as urban renewal, the grant of a subsidy, the passage of a piece of legislation—and have concentrated on the actual decision-making process.   This approach "eschews both position and reputation as effective means of ascertaining the power structure or generalizing about power, and stresses the actual determination of community decisions and the persons involved in making them."[91]   As we have seen, the pluralists find that power is fragmented among a variety of persons who specialize in issue areas of particular interest to them.

While the discussion, thus far, has concentrated on the opposing views of the sociology and political science fraternities, it should be noted that disagreements exist within both disciplines concerning the political power of business leaders in the local community and on the national level.   As long ago as the early 1950's, sociologist David Riesman concluded that nationally there existed, rather than a "ruling class of businessmen," a series of "veto groups, . . . each of which has struggled for and finally attained a power to stop things conceivably inimical to its interests and, within far narrower limits, to start things."[92]   The principal effectiveness of these veto groups stems from their ability "to neutralize those who might attack them."[93]

Robert O. Schulze, another sociologist, concluded in his study of Ypsilanti, Michigan, that "the recent economic dominants—

and especially those representing the growing number of large, absentee-owned corporations—appear indeed to have dissociated themselves from active involvement in . . . [Ypsilanti's] power structure."[94] Schulze found that, while in the old days locally owned economic dominants participated actively in the political-civic life of the community, today "the overt direction of the political and civic life of . . . [Ypsilanti] has passed almost wholly into the hands of a group of middle-class business and professional men, almost none of whom occupies a position of economic dominance in the community."[95]

A recent sociological study by Arnold M. Rose of the perceptions of political power and influence among selected groups in Minnesota is of particular interest. Using a technique of research akin to the "reputational approach" to community power (which examines the reputation which persons within a community have for possessing and exercising power) associated with Floyd Hunter and other elite theorists, Rose found that his results failed to support virtually all of the leading hypotheses of Hunter and C. Wright Mills concerning the existence of a power elite. He reports:

> The picture that emerges from this study is of a highly diversified, highly specialized and fractionated, image of power and influence structure in Minnesota. . . . There is little support for a theory that an economic elite, openly or secretly, has the reputation of controlling people's opinions and decisions (except that this opinion is found, to a slight extent, among business leaders themselves). If any group has ascendancy in our respondents' minds, it is the top political office-holders of both political parties.[96]

Similarly, William V. D'Antonio and William H. Form found after their study of two southwestern border cities that their evidence failed to document the existence of a solitary, unified influence system. They state, "In a dynamic metropolitan American community, there is little probability that a single coordinated power elite controls all the decisions in the community."[97]

On the other hand, political scientist Henry S. Kariel has concluded that this country has experienced the "decline of American pluralism."[98]   Kariel assumes a posture not unlike that of Mills—and interestingly, John Kenneth Galbraith in his *New Industrial State*—that national political power is not exercised solely by political office holders, but is shared with the leaders of the major pluralistic power centers of the nation, particularly business corporations.   He attributes the decline of pluralism to two factors: (1) the principles of federalism and separation of powers make for governmental disorganization and stalemate; and (2) the growth of the private power of "corporate citizens" as a result of the integrating tendencies of technology and the fragmented nature of public power.   Accordingly, Kariel concludes,

> However sensitive to the aspirations of the groups that they govern, however inefficient their rule in practice, and however responsive to a government-endorsed national interest when it is virtually unanimous, they [the corporate giants] wield power in a stupendously large sector of our economic order. . . . Insofar as corporate oligarchies effectively control industrial systems, and insofar as the systems manage to bring under their influence vast areas of the public, it is corporate oligarchies that control public life.[99]

Kariel's view finds support in the writings of two other political scientists, Michael D. Reagan and Alpheus T. Mason.[100]

While the pluralists have had the better of their argument with the elitists, increasingly there is an awareness by scholars that neither approach is sufficient to analyze the character of community power and that power structure is dependent upon a large number of factors and can assume a variety of forms. Among the relevant factors are size of the community; party structure (one party, two parties, or nonpartisan); nature, number, ownership and size of business interests (types of industries represented, extent of local and absentee ownership); regional location; relationship among business groups; presence of other highly organized social interests; and the socioeconomic composition of the population.[101] With regard to the various power-structure forms, it has been suggested that communities can be ranked along an elitist-pluralist continuum with numerous gradations between the poles of one-man rule and a situation where there is such a high degree of fragmentation of power that the power structure can best be described as amorphous.[102] Accordingly, it is more sophisticated to view the question of community power in terms of a variety of power-models existing in a wide assortment of communities possessing differing characteristics than to think in terms of polarities.

CORPORATIONS AND COMMUNITY POWER: AN APPRAISAL

The various community-power studies indicate, on balance, that business leaders, as a distinct elite group, at one time exerted substantial political influence in communities in which business ownership and management were in the hands of individuals who were locally raised and based. Indeed, those firms that still manifest great concern with and influence over community politics today tend to be locally owned and managed businesses in older, smaller towns and cities. Conversely, the larger and more industrialized the community, the more likely is the existence of a pluralistic political structure.[103] Today, corporate leaders—particularly in the case of the managers of absentee-owned corporations—have largely withdrawn from local political affairs. The close relationship, discussed earlier, between Phillips Petroleum and Bartlesville, Oklahoma, is today far less typical than that between the United States Steel Corporation and Birmingham, Alabama, as far as corporate community political involvement is concerned. Indeed, during the height of the civil rights demonstrations of 1963, United States Steel was severely criticized for its hands-off policy concerning racial integration in Birmingham, where it is the single largest employer; charges of absenteeism and corporate civic indifference were leveled against the company.[104] There appears to be one principal exception to this general proposition of the political withdrawal of absentee-owned firms. Corporations that are highly immobile—

engaging in either extractive activity (for example, mining) or dependent upon the locale for distributive purposes because of the high costs of transporting raw materials and finished goods —and hence sensitive to inescapable local conditions must necessarily involve themselves in local politics.[105]

Corporate withdrawal on the local level is attributable to several factors: (1) the transiency of company management, which therefore lacks roots in the social and political fabric of the community; (2) the commitment to organizational as opposed to community goals; and (3) the fact that, for large national corporations, the most important political arenas typically have been of a wider dimension than the community. Concerning this latter point, Robert O. Schulze has commented, "It seems tenable that it was the very sensitivity of the large corporations to socio-political determinations at the regional and national levels which militated against their involvement in these matters at the level of the local community."[106]

Where corporate leaders involve themselves in local politics, they have generally concentrated their efforts on influencing policy decisions that are closely related to their perceived business interests—urban renewal in New Haven and a convention-exhibition hall in Chicago—rather than attempting to influence more general political decisions.[107]   Indeed, Robert A. Dahl concluded from his research on New Haven that the direct influence of business leaders on local political nominations is "virtually nil."[108]   Similarly, Edward C. Banfield observed in his Chicago study that the "leading Chicago businessmen" do not capitalize on their almost unlimited power potential.[109]

Before concluding this discussion on local community power, two admonitions are necessary. First, most of the available studies predate the business-in-politics movement of the late 1950's and early 1960's. It will be recalled that the primary purpose of this movement was to involve corporate employees in local politics. Second, these studies do not take into account the recent corporate emphasis on social responsibility, which has involved many companies in extensive relationships with local government. However, given (1) the lack of effectiveness of the business-in-politics movement, and (2) the relatively apolitical manifestations of these new corporate responsibilities, the general pattern of community power that has emerged from our examination does not appear to have been altered greatly by recent developments. In summation, the available evidence tends to support the conclusion that

> most American communities reveal a relatively pluralistic power structure. On some community-relevant questions, power may be widely dispersed. On the most salient questions, many groups may have an effect on what is decided, but the directing leadership comes from some combination of particular business groups, local government, and, in recent developments, professionals and experts. Communities differ and communities change in the power relations among these elements. A suggestive hypothesis holds that the tendency has been towards their coordination into a uniquely composite decision-making collectivity.[110]

What has been said about local community power holds true in the sphere of national politics. There is little evidence of the existence of a power elite as described by C. Wright Mills, consisting of the highest leadership of the large corporations, the government, and the military. Even so critical a student of the role of private power in American democracy as Grant McConnell concludes that "the 'power elite' today rather obviously suffers from internal disarray. It lacks the organization and unity necessary to give it the capacities which are feared from it."[111]

As has been pointed out, among the leadership of our largest corporations can be found a wide variety of viewpoints and, more importantly, conflicting interests regarding specific issues of public policy. Consequently, these economic elites do not act cohesively with each other on many issues. "They do not 'rule' in the sense of commanding the entire nation. Quite the contrary, they tend to pursue a policy of noninvolvement in the large issues of statesmanship, save where such issues touch their own particular concerns."[112] The net result is that the power structure of this country is highly complex and diversified

—essentially pluralistic—rather than characterized by the political domination of corporate elites. Indeed, even Floyd Hunter indicates that notwithstanding their positions of importance, corporate leaders "do not and cannot exercise personal, decisive public power."[113] While interest groups do influence important parts of our federal government, these groups are narrowly based and largely autonomous of each other. Corporations, moreover, constitute merely one class of interest group—a highly atomistic class, at that. Estimates of the power of these corporate constituencies also vary substantially. Whereas Robert Engler found that the major oil companies constitute a potent political force in pursuing their interests, Bauer, Pool, and Dexter concluded that, with regard to tariff policy in the 1950's, the business community was beset with strife and accomplished little by way of tariff reductions.[114] Corporations appear to have greater national political power when pursuing narrow interests than when engaging in broader policy issues.

SUMMATION

In this chapter, we initially discussed the fears expressed by critics of business political involvement that corporate power is a danger to political democracy; then, after a general analysis of the nature and sources of power, we turned to the important corporate political resources: organization, wealth, access, dependence of other social interests, the delegation to corporations of critical social tasks, influence over mass media, past political success, and the status and reputation of business managers. Corporations possess these resources in widely varying degrees. The mere possession of political resources does not, in and of itself, constitute political power. There are several limitations upon the exercise of corporate political power, among them: numerous constraints upon the effective capacity to utilize power resources, the political power of other social interests, public commitment to a pluralistic society, and internal constraints within the business system.

In the final section, we analyzed the elitist-pluralist argument which has raged among social scientists studying community power. This discussion focused specific attention on whether economic elites control the political decision-making processes at the local and national levels and concluded that, while neither the elitist nor the pluralist models accurately describe the power structure of local communities, the weight of the evidence tends toward the latter. However, there are wide variations among communities with regard to the influence of business leaders. It is generally true that (1) the older and smaller the community, (2) the more dependent business firms are upon the locale, and (3) the greater the self-identification of the economic dominants with the community, the greater the political influence of the business leadership. Conversely, on local levels, absentee-owned national corporations have tended to eschew political leadership and to concentrate their attention on socially responsible civic causes. Nationally, the pluralist model appears to be accurate, with corporate interests—just as other social groups—concentrating their political energies on those areas of government that immediately affect their operations and pursuing a policy of noninvolvement in other areas. There is little evidence of a power elite or of a governing class dominated by the heads of our largest corporations.

Without question, business corporations possess political power, if *power* is defined as the ability to determine or influence the behavior of others; however, so also do other interests in American society. As we have seen, all power is relational, and the extent to which corporations are more powerful or less powerful than other social interests varies with time, place, circumstances, and the character of political goals and opponents. As Robert A. Dahl has suggested, it is a basic fact of political life that neither control over political resources nor political influence is distributed evenly in political systems.[115] This holds equally true with regard to the distribution of political power among corporations.

Accordingly, no definitive statements regarding the extensiveness of corporate political power in America are possible, except to note that such power does not monopolize the social order and does not constitute a threat to political democracy.

In this context, it is pertinent to reiterate that, very frequently, corporations use their political power to maximize their interests vis-à-vis other corporations. Political competition follows in the wake of economic competition. Therefore, it is necessary to maintain a realistic perspective regarding the ubiquity and exclusivity of corporate power in the social order.

To enhance our presently limited knowledge of the impact of corporate political power, much additional empirical research on the subject is necessary. Specific cases provide the acid test. Such research is not, however, without its difficulties. As was noted a number of years ago in a statement quite apropos the political power of American corporations,

> There is an elusiveness about power that endows it with an almost ghostly quality. It seems to be all around us, yet this is "sensed" with some sixth means of reception rather than with the five ordinary senses. We "know" what it is, yet we encounter endless difficulties in trying to define it. We can "tell" whether one person or group is more powerful than another, yet we cannot measure power. It is as abstract as time yet as real as a firing squad.[116]

NOTES

[1]Andrew Hacker, "Introduction: Corporate America," in Andrew Hacker (ed.), *The Corporation Take-Over* (New York: Harper & Row, Publishers, 1964), pp. 7–8.

[2]E. E. Schattschneider, *The Semi-Sovereign People* (New York: Holt, Rinehart & Winston, Inc., 1960), pp. 120–21.

[3]See James Madison, "The Federalist, No. 10," in Alexander Hamilton, James Madison, and John Jay, *The Federalist Papers* (New York: New American Library of World Literature, Inc., 1961), pp. 77–84; Karl Marx, *Critique of Political Economy* (New York: International Library, 1904); Charles A. Beard, *An Economic Interpretation*

of the Constitution of the United States (New York: The Macmillan Company, 1913); and *The Economic Basis of Politics* (New York: The Macmillan Company, 1912); H. H. Gerth and C. Wright Mills, *From Max Weber: Essays in Sociology* (Fair Lawn, N.J.: Oxford University Press, Inc., 1958), Chaps. 4, 14; Talcott Parsons, "On the Concept of Political Power," in Reinhard Bendix and Seymour Martin Lipset (eds.), *Class, Status and Power*, 2d ed. (New York: The Free Press, 1966), pp. 240–65; and Daniel Webster "Speech in the Massachusetts Convention, 1820–21," in Alpheus Thomas Mason (ed.), *Free Government in the Making*, 3d ed. (Fair Lawn, N.J.: Oxford University Press, Inc., 1965), pp. 411–16.

⁴Leslie Lipson, *The Democratic Civilization* (Fair Lawn, N.J.: Oxford University Press, Inc., 1964), p. 571.

⁵Alpheus T. Mason, "Business Organized as Power: The New Imperium in Imperio," *American Political Science Review*, XLIV, No. 2 (June 1950), 324.

⁶Walton Hamilton, *The Politics of Industry* (New York: Vintage Books, Random House, Inc., 1957), pp. 100, 109.

⁷Edward S. Mason, "Introduction," in Edward S. Mason (ed.), *The Corporation in Modern Society* (Cambridge, Mass.: Harvard University Press, 1961), p. 7.

⁸Bayless Manning, "Corporate Power and Individual Freedom: Some General Analysis and Particular Reservations," *Northwestern University Law Review*, LV, No. 1 (March-April 1960), 46.

⁹The concept of power has absorbed the attention of scholars and political practitioners throughout the ages and has given rise to a voluminous literature. For contemporary analyses of power, see Bertrand De Jouvenel, *On Power* (Boston: Beacon Press, 1962); R. M. MacIver, *The Web of Government* (New York: The Free Press, 1965), Chap. 5; Harold D. Lasswell, *Power and Personality* (New York: The Viking Press, 1962); Harold D. Lasswell and Abraham Kaplan, *Power and Society* (New Haven, Conn.: Yale University Press, 1950); Robert A. Dahl, *Modern Political Analysis* (Englewood Cliffs, N.J.: Prentice-Hall, Inc., 1964), Chapt. 5; Floyd Hunter, *Community Power Structure* (Garden City, N.Y.: Anchor Books, Doubleday & Company, Inc., 1963); David Riesman, *The Lonely Crowd*, abridged ed. (New Haven, Conn.: Yale University Press, 1961), Chap. 10; Robert A. Nisbet, *Community and Power* (Fair Lawn, N.J.: Oxford University Press, Inc., 1962), and *The Sociological Tradition* (New York: Basic Books, Inc., Publishers, 1966), pp. 107–73; Hannah

Arendt, *On Revolution* (New York: The Viking Press, 1965), Chap.
4; John Kenneth Galbraith, *American Capitalism*, rev. ed. (Boston:
Houghton Mifflin Company, 1956), Chap. 9, and *The New Industrial
State* (Boston: Houghton Mifflin Company, 1967), pp. 46–71; William A.
Gamson, *Power and Discontent* (Homewood, Ill.: The Dorsey
Press, 1968); C. Wright Mills, *The Power Elite* (Fair Lawn, N.J.:
Oxford University Press, Inc., 1959); Adolf A. Berle, Jr., *Power Without
Property* (New York: Harvest Books, Harcourt, Brace & World,
Inc., 1959), Chap. 3; Arnold M. Rose, *The Power Structure* (Fair
Lawn, N.J.: Oxford University Press, Inc., 1967); Joseph Tussman,
Obligation and the Body Politic (Fair Lawn, N.J.: Oxford University
Press, Inc., 1960), Chap. 1; Max Weber, *The Theory of Social and
Economic Organization*, A. M. Henderson and Talcott Parsons (trans.)
and Talcott Parsons (ed.) (New York: The Free Press, 1964), pp.
152–57 and Part III; Robert A. Dahl, "The Concept of Power," *Behavioral
Science*, II, No. 3 (July 1957), 201–15; Parsons, "On the
Concept of Political Power," in Bendix and Lipset (eds.), *Class,
Status and Power*, pp. 240–65; Nelson W. Polsby, *Community Power
and Political Theory* (New Haven, Conn.: Yale University Press,
1963), and "The Sociology of Community Power: A Reassessment,"
Social Forces, XXXVII, No. 3 (March 1959), 232–36; Herbert
Kaufman and Victor Jones, "The Mystery of Power," *Public Administration
Review*, XIV, No. 3 (Summer 1954), 205–12; John C.
Harsanyi, "Measurement of Social Power, Opportunity Costs, and
the Theory of Two-Person Bargaining Games," *Behavioral Science*,
VII, No. 1 (January 1962), 67–80; Dow Votaw, "What Do We
Believe About Power?" *California Management Review*, VIII, No. 4
(Summer 1966), 71–88; Peter Bachrach and Morton S. Baratz, "Two
Faces of Power," *The American Political Science Review*, LVI, No. 4
(December 1962), 947–52; and Richard M. Merelman, "On the Neo-Elitist
Critique of Community Power," *American Political Science
Review*, LXII, No. 2 (June 1968), 451–60.

[10]For a fuller discussion of the *base* and the *means* of power,
see Harsanyi, "Measurement of Social Power . . . ," p. 67.

[11]S. E. Finer, "The Political Power of Private Capital," Part I,
Sociological Review, III, No. 2 (December 1955), 287.

[12]Polsby, *Community Power and . . .* , p. 60.

[13]Harsanyi, "Measurement of Social Power . . . ," pp. 67–80.

[14]Amitai Etzioni, *Modern Organizations* (Englewood Cliffs,
N.J.: Prentice-Hall, Inc., 1964), p. 3.

[15]Finer, "The Political Power . . . ," p. 282.

[16]The statistics in this paragraph are drawn from the following sources: *Economic Concentration: Hearings . . . Pursuant to S. Res. 262*, Part 1, U.S. Congress, Senate, Subcommittee on Antitrust and Monopoly of the Committee of the Judiciary, 88th Cong., 2d Sess. (Washington, D.C.: U.S. Government Printing Office, 1964), pp. 113–15; "The *Fortune* Directory," *Fortune*, LXXVII, No. 7 (June 15, 1968), 186–220; Dow Votaw, *Modern Corporations* (Englewood Cliffs, N.J.: Prentice-Hall, Inc., 1965), pp. 3–4. For studies of economic concentration in the United States, see Joe S. Bain, *Industrial Organization*, 2d ed. (New York: John Wiley & Sons, Inc., 1968); A. D. H. Kaplan, *Big Enterprise in a Competitive System*, rev. ed. (Washington, D.C.: The Brookings Institution, 1964); Norman R. Collins and Lee E. Preston, "The Size Structure of the Largest Industrial Firms, 1909–1958," *The American Economics Review*, LI, No. 5 (December 1961), 986–1011; Richard Caves, *American Industry: Structure, Conduct, Performance*, 2d ed. (Englewood Cliffs, N.J.: Prentice-Hall, Inc., 1967); and Walter Adams, ed., *The Structure of American Industry: Some Case Studies* (New York: The Macmillan Company, 1961).

[17]*Hearings . . . Pursuant to S. Res. 219 of the 84th Congress*, U.S. Congress, Senate, Special Committee to Investigate Political Activities, Lobbying and Campaign Contributions, 84th Cong., 2d Sess. (Washington, D.C.: U.S. Government Printing Office, 1957), p. 1046.

[18]Grant McConnell, *Steel and the Presidency—1962* (New York: W. W. Norton & Company, Inc., 1963), p. 3.

[19]Reprinted from Harold Brayman, *Corporate Management in a World of Politics* (New York: McGraw-Hill Book Company, 1967), p. 72.

[20]See, for example, Robert A. Dahl, *Who Governs?* (New Haven, Conn.: Yale University Press, 1961), Chap. 6; Robert Presthus, *Men at the Top* (Fair Lawn, N.J.: Oxford University Press, Inc., 1964), Chaps. 7, 8, 12; and Edward C. Banfield, *Political Influence* (New York: The Free Press, 1965), Chaps. 4, 5.

[21]W. Lloyd Warner, *et al.*, *The American Federal Executive* (New Haven, Conn.: Yale University Press, 1963), pp. 37–38.

[22]Andrew Hacker, "The Elected and the Anointed: Two American Elites," *American Political Science Review*, LV, No. 3 (September 1961), 545.

[23]"20% of Senators Are Millionaires," *The New York Times,* April 7, 1968, p. 68, cols. 2 and 3.

[24]For a penetrating analysis of the American upper-class, see E. Digby Baltzell, *The Protestant Establishment* (New York: Vintage Books, Random House, Inc., 1964). Compare: G. William Domhoff, *Who Rules America?* (Englewood Cliffs, N.J.: Prentice-Hall, Inc., 1967).

[25]Hacker, "The Elected and . . . ," p. 547.

[26]Robert E. Lane, *The Regulation of Businessmen, Social Conditions of Government Economic Control* (New Haven, Conn.: Yale University Press, 1954), pp. 72–88.

[27]Donald R. Matthews, *U.S. Senators and Their World* (New York: Vintage Books, Random House, Inc., 1960), p. 191.

[28]Raymond A. Bauer, Ithiel de Sola Pool, and Louis Anthony Dexter, *American Business and Public Policy* (New York: Atherton Press, 1964), Chap. 16.

[29]James C. Tanner, "One-Company Town," *The Wall Street Journal,* August 4, 1966, p. 1, col. 1.

[30]The advertisements quoted in this paragraph are found respectively in *Business Week,* May 18, 1968, p. 106 (South Carolina); *Business Week,* March 23, 1968, p. 85 (Tennessee); *Fortune,* LXXVII (May 1968), 44 (Buffalo and Erie County, New York); *Business Week,* March 23, 1968, p. 116D (Sunnyvale, California); *The Wall Street Journal,* May 13, 1968, p. 7, cols. 4–6 (Philadelphia, Pennsylvania); and *The Wall Street Journal,* September 19, 1967, p. 9 (Ohio).

[31]V. O. Key, Jr., *Politics, Parties, and Pressure Groups,* 5th ed. (New York: Thomas Y. Crowell Co., 1964), p. 91.

[32]See A. H. Raskin, "A Kind of Economic Holy War," *The New York Times Magazine,* February 18, 1968, p. 25.

[33]Reprinted from Raymond A. Bauer, Ithiel de Sola Pool, and Lewis Anthony Dexter, *American Business and Public Policy* (New York: Atherton Press, 1964), p. 487. Copyright © 1963, Massachusetts Institute of Technology. All rights reserved.

[34]Finer, *The Political Power . . . ,* p. 285.

[35]Morton S. Baratz, "Corporate Grants and the Power Structure," *Western Political Quarterly,* IX, No. 3 (June 1956), 413.

[36]From Arnold M. Rose, *The Power Structure* (London: Oxford University Press, 1967), p. 102. Rose's analysis of the political

strike has influenced my subsequent discussion of this corporate political tactic.

[37]"Big Board Edges Toward New Site in New York City," *The Wall Street Journal*, May 28, 1968, p. 2, col. 2.

[38]Reprinted from Arnold M. Rose, *The Power Structure* (London: Oxford University Press, 1967), p. 102.

[39]McConnell, *Steel and . . .*, p. 63.

[40]Edmund K. Faltermayer, "What Business Wants from Lyndon Johnson," *Fortune*, LXXI, No. 2 (February 1965), 122.

[41]Carl Kaysen, "The Corporation: How Much Power? What Scope?" in Mason (ed.), *The Corporation in . . .*, p. 100.

[42]"Top 125 National Advertisers Put Record $4.54 Billion in Promotion," *Advertising Age*, XXXIX, No. 35 (August 26, 1968), 1, 80–81.

[43]R. T. Ruetten, "Anaconda Journalism: The End of an Era," *Journalism Quarterly*, XXXVII (1960), 3–12.

[44]Robert E. Lane, *Political Life* (New York: The Free Press, 1965), p. 279.

[45]Bernard C. Hennessy, *Public Opinion* (Belmont, Calif.: Wadsworth Publishing Company, Inc., 1965), p. 301.

[46]The statistics in this paragraph are drawn from Hennessy, *Public Opinion*, pp. 289, 303, 306. See also Herbert E. Alexander, "Broadcasting and Politics" in M. Kent Jennings and L. Harmon Zeigler (eds.), *The Electoral Process* (Englewood Cliffs, N.J.: Prentice-Hall, Inc., 1966), pp. 81–104.

[47]See, for example, Joseph T. Klapper, *The Effects of Mass Communication* (New York: The Free Press, 1960), p. 15; Elihu Katz and Paul F. Lazarsfeld, *Personal Influence* (New York: The Free Press, 1964), pp. 15–30, 271–95, 316–20; and Lane, *Political Life*, pp. 275–98.

[48]Joseph Cornwall Palamountain, Jr., *The Politics of Distribution* (Cambridge, Mass.: Harvard University Press, 1955), p. 173.

[49]Hennessy, *Public Opinion*, p. 273.

[50]Key, *Politics, Parties, and . . .*, p. 96.

[51]Francis X. Sutton, *et al.*, *The American Business Creed* (New York: Schocken Books, 1962), Chap. 2; and Marver H. Bernstein, "Political Ideas of Selected American Business Journals," *Public Opinion Quarterly*, XVII, No. 2 (Summer 1953), 258–67.

[52]Marver H. Bernstein, *Regulating Business by Independent*

Commission (Princeton, N.J.: Princeton University Press, 1955), pp. 100–101.

[53]Walter Adams and Horace M. Gray, *Monopoly in America* (New York: The Macmillan Company, Publishers, 1955), p. 71.

[54]C. P. Snow, *Science and Government* (Cambridge, Mass.: Harvard University Press, 1961), p. 56.

[55]Grant McConnell, *Private Power & American Democracy* (New York: Alfred A. Knopf, Inc., 1966), p. 254.

[56]Lipson, *The Democratic Civilization*, p. 267. For studies of the social status of various occupational groupings, see generally Albert J. Reiss, Jr., *Occupations and Social Status* (New York: The Free Press, 1961); and studies collected in Sigmund Nosow and William H. Form, *Man, Work, and Society* (New York: Basic Books, Inc., Publishers, 1962), Chap. 8; Theodore Caplow, *The Sociology of Work* (New York: McGraw-Hill Book Company, 1964), Chap. 2; Alex Inkeles and Peter H. Rossi, "National Comparisons of Occupational Prestige," *American Journal of Sociology*, LXI, No. 4 (January 1956), 329–39; Robert W. Hodge, Donald J. Treiman, and Peter H. Rossi, "A Comparative Study of Occupational Prestige," in Bendix and Lipset (eds.), *Class, Status and Power*, pp. 309–21; Robert W. Hodge, Paul M. Siegel, and Peter H. Rossi, "Occupational Prestige in the United States, 1925–1963," in Bendix and Lipset (eds.), *Class, Status and Power*, pp. 322–34; and David Granick, *The European Executive* (Garden City, N.Y.: Anchor Books, Doubleday & Company, Inc., 1964).

[57]See David J. Galligan, *Politics and the Businessman* (New York; Pitman Publishing Corporation, 1964), pp. 107–10.

[58]Reprinted from David Riesman, Nathan Glazer, and Reuel Denney, *The Lonely Crowd* (New Haven and London: Yale University Press, 1961), p. 219.

[59]Stephen A. Greyser, "Business and Politics, 1968 (Special Report)," *Harvard Business Review*, XLVI, No. 6 (November-December 1968), 4–6, 8, 10.

[60]Brayman, *Corporate Management in . . .* , p. 22; and Galbraith, *The New Industrial State*, pp. 379–87.

[61]Reprinted from Raymond A. Bauer, Ithiel de Sola Pool, and Lewis Anthony Dexter, *American Business and Public Policy* (New York: Atherton Press, 1964), p. 269. Copyright © 1963, Massachusetts Institute of Technology. All rights reserved.

[62]These terms are used respectively by Galbraith, *American Capitalism*, pp. 108–34; Robert A. Dahl, *A Preface to Democratic Theory* (Chicago: The University of Chicago Press, 1963), pp. 63–89; and Theodore Lowi, "The Public Philosophy: Interest-Group Liberalism," *American Political Science Review*, XLI, No. 1 (March 1967), 5–24.

[63]For a discussion of the adherence to the rules of the game, see generally Herbert McClosky,"Consensus and Ideology in American Politics," *American Political Science Review*, LVIII, No. 2 (June 1964), 361–82; and Dahl, *Who Governs?*, pp. 256–67.

[64]William Spinrad, "Power in Local Communities," *Social Problems*, XII, No. 3 (Winter 1965), 335–56, reprinted in Bendix and Lipset (eds.), *Class, Status, and Power*, p. 229.

[65]Reprinted from Raymond A. Bauer, Ithiel de Sola Pool, and Lewis Anthony Dexter, *American Business and Public Policy* (New York: Atherton Press, 1964), p. 258. Copyright © 1963, Massachusetts Institute of Technology. All rights reserved.

[66]McClosky, "Consensus and Ideology . . . ," p. 379.

[67]Spinrad, "Power in Local Communities," p. 229.

[68]Spinrad, "Power in Local Communities," p. 229.

[69]Bauer, Pool, and Dexter, *American Business and . . .* , pp. 265–76.

[70]Eugene V. Rostow in Mason (ed.), *The Corporation in . . .* , p. 69.

[71]Greyser, "Business and Politics, 1968," p. 10; Stephen A. Greyser, "Business and Politics, 1964 (Problems in Review)," *Harvard Business Review*, XLII, No. 5 (September-October 1964), 28, and Dan H. Fenn, Jr., "Business and Politics (Problems in Review)," *Harvard Business Review*, XXXVII, No. 3 (May-June 1959), 10.

[72]Adolf A. Berle, *The American Economic Republic* (New York: Harcourt, Brace & World, Inc., 1963), p. 13.

[73]For a discussion of the ineffectiveness of federal legislation of corporate campaign contributions and expenditures, see Edwin M. Epstein, *Corporations, Contributions and Political Campaigns: Federal Regulation in Perspective* (Berkeley: Institute of Governmental Studies, University of California, 1968).

[74]For critiques of the community power literature, see, for example, Polsby, *Community Power and Political Theory*, and "The Sociology of . . ."; Spinrad, "Power in Local Communities"; David

250   CORPORATE POLITICAL POWER: A THREAT?

Rogers, "Community Political Systems: A Framework and Hypothesis for Comparative Studies," in Bert E. Swanson (ed.), *Current Trends in Comparative Community Studies* (Kansas City: Community Studies, Inc., 1962), pp. 31–48; Raymond E. Wolfinger, "Reputation and Reality in the Study of 'Community Power,'" *American Sociological Review*, XXV, No. 5 (October 1960), 636–44; and Dahl, *Modern Political Analysis*, pp. 39–54.

[75]Hunter, *Community Power Structure*; Robert S. Lynd and Helen Merrell Lynd, *Middletown* (New York: Harcourt, Brace & World, Inc., 1956), and *Middletown in Transition* (New York: Harcourt, Brace & World, Inc., 1937); W. Lloyd Warner (ed.), *Yankee City*, abridged ed. (New Haven, Conn.: Yale University Press, 1963), and *Democracy in Jonesville* (New York: Harper & Row, Publishers, 1949); August B. Hollingshead, *Elmtown's Youth* (New York: John Wiley & Sons, Inc., 1949); Roland J. Pellegrin and Charles H. Coates, "Absentee-Owned Corporations and Community Power Structure," *American Journal of Sociology*, LXI, No. 5 (March 1956), 413–19; Mills, *The Power Elite*; and Domhoff, *Who Rules America?*. See also Arthur J. Vidich and Joseph Bensman, *Small Town in Mass Society* (Garden City, N.Y.: Anchor Books, Doubleday & Company, Inc., 1960); Riesman, *The Lonely Crowd*; Rose, *The Power Structure*; E. Digby Baltzell, *An American Business Aristocracy* (New York: Collier Books, a division of Crowell-Collier Publishing Co., 1962); Peter H. Rossi, "The Organizational Structure of an American Community," in Amitai Etzioni (ed.), *Complex Organizations* (New York: Holt, Rinehart & Winston, Inc., 1961), pp. 301–12; and Robert O. Schulze, "The Role of Economic Dominants in Community Power Structure," *American Sociological Review*, XXIII, No. 1 (February 1958), 3–9.

[76]Hunter, *Community Power Structure*, p. 78.

[77]Hunter, *Community Power Structure*, p. 98.

[78]Reprinted from C. Wright Mills, *The Power Elite* (New York: Oxford University Press, Inc., 1959), p. 292.

[79]Dwight D. Eisenhower,"Farewell Radio and Television Address to the American People," January 17, 1961, reprinted in Mason (ed.), *Free Government . . .* , p. 851.

[80]Domhoff, *Who Rules America?*, p. 156.

[81]Jack L. Walker, "A Critique of the Elitist Theory of Democracy," *American Political Science Review*, LX, No. 2 (June 1966), 286.

[82]See, for example, Dahl, *Who Governs?*; Banfield, *Political Influence*; Presthus, *Men at the Top*; Wallace S. Sayre and Herbert

Kaufman, *Governing New York City* (New York: W. W. Norton & Company, Inc., Publishers, 1965); Aaron Wildavsky, *Leadership in a Small Town* (Totowa, N.J.: Bedminster Press, 1964); Edward C. Banfield and James Q. Wilson, *City Politics* (Cambridge, Mass.: Harvard University Press, 1963); Scott Greer, *Governing the Metropolis* (New York: John Wiley & Sons, Inc., 1962); and Roscoe C. Martin, *et al., Decisions in Syracuse* (Bloomington, Ind.: Indiana University Press, 1961).

[83]Robert A. Dahl, *Pluralist Democracy in the United States: Conflict and Consent* (Chicago: Rand McNally & Company, 1967), p. 24.

[84]Dahl, *Who Governs?*, pp. 85–86.

[85]Banfield, *Political Influence*, pp. 287–88.

[86]Sayre and Kaufman, *Governing New York City*, pp. 709–38.

[87]Polsby, *Community Power and . . .*, pp. 123–24.

[88]Polsby, *Community Power and . . .*, p. 138.

[89]For discussions of the theoretical and methodological differences between political scientists and sociologists, see, for example, Presthus, *Men at the Top*, Chaps. 1 and 2; Polsby, "The Sociology of . . . ," and *Community Power and . . .* ; Kaufman and Jones, "The Mystery of Power"; Rose, *The Power Structure*, pp. 253–97; Walker, "A Critique of . . ."; Robert A. Dahl, "Business and Politics: A Critical Appraisal of Political Science," in Robert A. Dahl, Mason Haire, and Paul F. Lazarsfeld, *Social Science Research on Business: Product and Potential* (New York: Columbia University Press, 1959), pp. 31–34; and Bachrach and Baratz, "Two Faces of Power."

[90]See, for example, Hunter, *Community Power Structure*, pp. 61–111.

[91]Reprinted from Arnold M. Rose, *The Power Structure* (London: Oxford University Press, 1967), p. 277.

[92]Reprinted from David Riesman, Nathan Glazer, and Reuel Denney, *The Lonely Crowd* (New Haven and London: Yale University Press, 1961), p. 213.

[93]Reprinted from David Riesman, Nathan Glazer, and Reuel Denney, *The Lonely Crowd* (New Haven and London: Yale University Press, 1961), p. 213.

[94]Schulze, "The Role of . . . ," p. 7.

[95]Schulze, "The Role of . . . ," p. 6.

[96]Reprinted from Arnold M. Rose, *The Power Structure* (London: Oxford University Press, 1967), p. 354.

[97]William V. D'Antonio and William H. Form, *Influentials in Two Border Cities* (Notre Dame, Ind.: University of Notre Dame Press, 1965), p. 222.

[98]Henry S. Kariel, *The Decline of American Pluralism* (Stanford, Calif.: Stanford University Press, 1961).

[99]Kariel, *The Decline* . . . , pp. 47–48.

[100]Mason, "Business Organized as . . ."; and Michael D. Reagan, *The Managed Economy* (Fair Lawn, N.J.: Oxford University Press, Inc., 1963).

[101]For an interesting tabular presentation of the variables affecting corporate involvement and community-power structure, see David Rogers and Melvin Zimet, "The Corporation and the Community: Perspectives and Recent Developments," in Ivar Berg (ed.), *The Business of America* (New York: Harcourt, Brace & World, Inc., 1968), p. 56.

[102]A discussion of recent power models is found in Rose, *The Power Structure*, pp. 286–88.

[103]Rose, *The Power Structure*, pp. 296–97.

[104]For a discussion of United States Steel's role in Birmingham, Alabama, see Clarence C. Walton, *Corporate Social Responsibilities* (Belmont, Calif.: Wadsworth Publishing Company, Inc., 1967), pp. 156–73.

[105]Marshall N. Goldstein, "Absentee Ownership and Monolithic Power Structures: Two Questions for Community Studies," in Swanson (ed.), *Current Trends* . . . , pp. 49–59.

[106]Schulze, "The Role of . . . ," p. 8.

[107]See respectively Dahl, *Who Governs?*, pp. 89–165; and Banfield, *Political Influence*, Chap. 7.

[108]Dahl, *Who Governs?*, p. 79.

[109]Banfield, *Political Influence*, pp. 287–88.

[110]Spinrad, "Power in Local Communities," p. 356.

[111]McConnell, *Private Power and* . . . , p. 337.

[112]McConnell, *Private Power and* . . . , p. 339.

[113]Floyd Hunter, *Top Leadership, U.S.A.* (Chapel Hill, N.C.: The University of North Carolina Press, 1959), p. 246.

[114]Compare Robert Engler, *The Politics of Oil* (Chicago: Phoenix Books, The University of Chicago Press, 1967), especially pp. 267–427, 483–98, with Bauer, Pool, and Dexter, *American Business and* . . . , especially pp. 105–319, 465–90.

[115]Dahl, *Modern Political Analysis*, pp. 15–16.

[116]Kaufman and Jones, "The Mystery of Power," p. 205.

Chapter Nine

Legitimacy:
a Critical Issue

The final argument raised by critics of corporate political activity is that corporations lack legitimacy as political participants. This issue of legitimacy—together with the closely related matter of corporate power discussed in the preceding chapter—goes to the heart of corporate involvement in politics. It raises the normative question of whether corporations *ought* to be political participants—that is, whether there is justification for their historic *de facto* political role. The answer to this query determines whether corporate political activity is consistent with the values of a democratic society or is aberrant behavior that has no place in such a society.

Legitimacy may be defined as a belief in and acceptance of the "rightness, propriety, moral goodness" or "appropriate[ness]" of particular persons, institutions, or modes of behavior.[1] Legitimacy is a vital ingredient for political participation in a democracy since it differentiates political activity that is based purely upon power —effectiveness—from activity predicated on authority—conceded to be rightful or appropriate by members of the society.

A few years ago, Edward S. Mason posed the overriding question concerning the legitimacy of corporate action when he asked whether "Look, Ma, no hands" is an appropriate motto for a corporate society that appears to be running without discernible controls. In describing the relationship of the large corporations to contemporary society, Mason stated:

> What all this seems to add up to is the existence of important centers of private power in the hands of men whose authority is real but whose responsibilities are vague. . . . We are all aware that we live not only in a corporate society but a society of large corporations. The management—that is, the control— of these corporations is in the hands of, at most, a few thousand men. Who selected these men, if not to rule over us, at least to exercise vast authority, and to whom are they responsible? The answer to the first question is quite clearly: they selected themselves. The answer to the second is, at best, nebulous. This, in a nutshell, constitutes the problem of legitimacy.[2]

The question of corporate political legitimacy is, accordingly, twofold in nature. First, there is the *internal* issue of the mode of governance of the corporation—that is, the basis of the authority of managers to make decisions for the firm and the identification of the constituency to which they are responsible. The second or *external* issue concerns the relationship between the corporation and other participants in the American social order. It raises the question of whether the nature of corporate political participation differs fundamentally from that of other actors in the American political process and whether this difference, if discernible, thereby renders the participation improper. The remainder of this chapter is devoted to an examination of these tandem, yet analytically discrete, aspects of corporate political legitimacy.

THE QUESTION OF INTERNAL LEGITIMACY

Generally, the modern corporation does not comport with traditional conceptions of political organizations, and no theory has been developed reconciling it with such conceptions. This divergence from political theory is particularly true with regard to the nature of organizational governance. Unlike the usual forms of private associations found in American society—labor unions, civil-rights groups, agricultural organizations, professional societies and the like—corporations do not have a constituency of definable members, but rather are entities within which the precise relationship between individuals and the organization is amorphous. Thus, the question posed by corporate political involvement is: For whom is the corporation acting and through what source of authority? This issue is relevant; for, although the exercise of power by private groups has been termed the feature "perhaps . . . most characteristic of American democracy,"[3] the obligation to justify this exercise of private political power is of prime importance in a democratic society.

WHO CONSTITUTES THE CONSTITUENCY?

In traditional legal and economic theory, the question of the internal legitimacy of the corporation posed little difficulty. As a result of their property interest, the stockholders were *the* constituency of the firm. Authority within the corporation was analogous to authority within the political state. "The shareholders were the electorate, the directors the legislature, enacting general policies and committing them to the officers for execution. A judiciary was unnecessary, since the state had kindly permitted the use of its own."[4] Corporate managers were considered essentially functionaries or agents to whom the elected board of directors had delegated certain authority to conduct the affairs of the enterprise on behalf of the actual owners—the shareholders. Indicative of the relatively low position given to managers under the legal model, even today in many corporation codes the only officers specifically mentioned are the president, the vice-president, the treasurer, and the secretary. Other categories of corporate managers are not even explicitly recognized, but are lumped together in such catch-all phrases as "such other officers and assistant officers" as the corporation "shall authorize from time to time."[5] According to legal theory, the powers of corporate officers

> are derived from [corporate] bylaws, from resolutions by a board of directors, or by implication through acquiescence in a course of dealing. Authority to bind the corporation is usually not conferred on the officers, with the possible exception of the president, simply by virtue of the offices they hold. In other words, the vice-president has no particular authority simply because the door to his office is labeled "vice-president."[6]

Were this legal model of corporate authority still accurate, the thorny problem of constituency would be resolved. The shareholder would be sovereign and the legitimacy of the action of corporate managers could be judged by the sole criterion of responsiveness to shareholder desires. However, the classic model of the corporation no longer suffices as a description of reality. The myth of shareholder sovereignty has been debunked on innumerable occasions since the appearance in 1933 of Adolf A. Berle, Jr., and Gardiner C. Means' seminal work, *The Modern Corporation and Private Property*, which documented the separation of ownership and control among most of the largest American corporations. The authors described the situation in the following terms:

> It is therefore evident that we are dealing not only with distinct but often with opposing groups, ownership on the one side, control on the other—a control which tends to move further and further away from ownership and ultimately to lie in the hands of the management itself, a management capable of perpetuating its own position.[7]

A study that examined the validity of the Berle and Means thesis as of 1963 concluded that "management control has substantially increased among the 200 largest nonfinancial corporations since 1929," from 44 per cent to 84.5 per cent.[8]   Research by Robert A. Gordon suggests an even greater degree of management control, for not only are corporate managers free of shareholder control, but also they are largely independent of any troublesome constraints by their boards of directors.[9]   In fact, the directors are often selected and dominated by corporate executives.   In the modern, large, publicly held corporation, a very small number of men, the top management, determine the fundamental policies that bind the many.

Accordingly, even those persons who are most sympathetic to the corporation—termed this nation's "representative social institution" since it "sets the standards for the way of life and the mode of living of our citizens . . . and . . . determines our perspectives on our own society"[10]—concede that it does not operate in accordance with democratic norms.   It is surely not a shareholder democracy of individuals who have come together to aggregate their funds for a common purpose.   American shareholders are not the owner-participants of the classic legal literature.   "They are investors, who, for the most part, do not wish to be bothered—except by dividends."[11]   Their relationship with the corporation is distant and fleeting.   It is unrealistic to view the more than 3 million persons and institutions owning nearly 540 million shares of American Telephone and Telegraph stock at mid-1966 as corporate democrats, who elected their representatives (the board of directors) to handle "their" interests.[12]   Moreover, legal redress available to shareholders against the corporation is generally ineffective.   Although dissatisfied shareholders can institute either individual or derivative actions challenging the propriety of the expenditure of company funds for political purposes—depletion of assets, *ultra vires*, and tortious injury to individual stockholders are possible bases for such suits—shareholder success in this litigation is quite unlikely.

This general state of shareholder impotency is further compounded by the fact that at the end of 1966, institutions (insurance and investment companies, noninsured pension funds, nonprofit institutions, common trust funds, bank administered personal trust funds, and mutual savings banks) held more than $157 billion worth, or 33 per cent of the market value, of all stocks listed on the New York Stock Exchange.[13] Despite the fact that these institutions have tended to concentrate their investments in the very largest corporations (in 1964, for example, 14.5 per cent of institutional holdings of listed securities were in the 5 largest companies listed on the New York Stock Exchange; 41 per cent were in the 51 largest issues; and 70.6 per cent in the 171 largest issues)[14] and, accordingly, have the competence and the power to influence corporate management in policy areas, the leaderships of the giant firms have, by and large, been left to their own devices in policy formation. While it is true that on a few occasions mutual funds have actively intervened in struggles for corporate control—usually in the cases of smaller companies or where take-over bids were involved—in the main, institutions have acted as investors, not controllers, and have sought to escape controversy by selling their stock in a firm.

Accordingly, to emphasize that management lacks legitimacy to involve the corporation in politics without the consent of the shareholders is to ignore the facts of modern corporate life. While the ideal might be different, in reality all corporate decisions, from plant expansions to donations to eleemosynary institutions, are made without the approval of stockholders. These decisions are made by corporate managers, assisted by John Kenneth Galbraith's "technostructure," which consists of highly trained specialists who bring expertise to bear in resolving the organization's problems and decide many subpolicy matters.[15]

There is little reason that stockholders should be entitled to a greater voice in the decisions made by business firms in the political area than they are given in other spheres of company activity. The corporation is inherently no more undemocratic in pursuing its political interests than it is in determining and implementing other company objectives. Furthermore, the shareholder is no more—or less—equipped to decide the wisdom of corporate political policy in terms of organizational welfare than he is to evaluate the propriety of other managerial actions. While we may lament the shareholder's basic ineffectiveness, this condition has nothing to do with the political problem under

discussion.   Rather, this ineffectiveness is inherent in the change
of status of the stockholder from an active part owner of the
enterprise to a passive investor whose only connections with the
firm are through the annual report, proxy solicitation, and—hopefully—quarterly dividend checks.   Thus, the truth of the matter
is that

> there is no well-developed *model* for describing stockholder
> status in the larger organizations; and it is perhaps significant
> that in many companies the stockholders are regarded—for or-
> ganizational purposes—as outsiders, though for hortatory rea-
> sons they are always greeted as the "ultimate owners" of the
> business.[16]

The above discussion does not suggest that managers act
capriciously, arbitrarily, or intentionally contrary to the perceived
welfare of the shareholders.   Constraints against such behavior
include the substantial ownership interests that top executives
usually have in their firms as a result of their managerial positions, which give them a general sense of identity with the shareholders; the necessity to cultivate stockholder support to avoid
successful takeover—tender-offer—bids by other firms; the desire
to avoid the unfavorable publicity that results from stockholder
suits; and lastly, the sense of professional responsibility that managers feel towards their shareholders.   To the extent that these
factors increase the responsiveness of management to the stockholders, the internal legitimacy of corporate governance is com-
mensurately enhanced.   However, a model of corporate legitimacy emphasizing the role—or lack of same—of the stockholder
is of limited relevance today.

A NEW CONSTITUENCY?

With the decline of the influence of the shareholder have
come attempts to redefine the corporate constituency.   "A more
spacious conception of 'membership,' and one closer to the facts
of corporate life, would include all those having a relation of
sufficient intimacy with the corporation or subject to its power in

a sufficiently specialized way."[17] In addition to shareholders, groups frequently included as members in the revised model of the corporate constituency are rank-and-file workers, both blue- and white-collar (the former group, frequently represented by labor unions); executive-level officers and directors; suppliers of the corporation; dealers with the company; creditors of the enterprise; and consumers of the company's products. Also mentioned as corporate members are the community in which the enterprise is located and the public-at-large (frequently operating through government).

This expanded model of corporate membership or constituency does not solve the problem of legitimacy, although it is of value in attempting to determine which social interests have claims upon the corporation and, therefore, have reason to expect that the responsible firm will take their welfare into account in making its decisions. In certain situations, the groups mentioned above have formal mechanisms for making claims upon the corporation; but in only very few instances do they participate in the selection of the corporate leadership or have opportunities to limit the authority of top management.

Let us look first at membership participation in the selection of corporate leaders. In Massachusetts, employees may be permitted to elect representatives to the board of directors,[18] but this practice has proved very limited and generally unsuccessful in securing effective worker representation. Creditors occasionally demand and receive representation on the corporate board; however, creditor influence upon corporations has declined greatly since in recent years the bulk (between 60 and 65 per cent)[19] of corporate funds are generated internally. Important customers or suppliers sometimes sit on corporate boards; however, as with virtually all external directors, they tend to be passive, largely rubber-stamping the decisions of management. With the exception of employees, these other interests generally view themselves as outsiders; their basic identifications are with other organizations, with which they spend most of their time and to which they have greatest commitment.

The "new constituency" has but limited institutional mechanisms for curtailing the authority of corporate management.

Labor unions have given employees certain status prerequisites within the enterprise, particularly seniority and job security against arbitrary dismissal, as a result of the establishment of collective bargaining and grievance procedures. The utter dependency of the automobile distributor on the large automobile producers for his franchise resulted in the passage of federal legislation forbidding the cancellation of the dealer's franchise without cause and creating a legal cause of action with prescribed penalties in case of an improper cancellation.[20] General Motors has, moreover, supplemented this legislative requirement with a system of dealer councils—composed of representatives selected by the dealers—to present the views of the dealers to management. As the above illustrations indicate—the dealer councils notwithstanding—the institutionalization of the influence of constituent groups vis-à-vis the corporation has primarily been the result of intervention by the state to require the business firm to consider the claims of a constituent. Most segments of the new constituency lack real representation within the corporation.

Accordingly, the problem of internal legitimacy cannot be resolved simply by expanding the concept of corporate constituency. Corporate governance is basically oligarchical despite expanded labor relations, corporate decentralization and federalism, the advent of philosophies such as participative management, and a new attentiveness to other social interests affected by the corporation. At very best, the business firm constitutes an "absolute democracy" with management adhering to democratic procedures that are determined largely by existing legal requirements. An expert on Soviet politics has noted numerous parallels between the government of the U.S.S.R. and our large industrial enterprises:

> The place of the Communist Party of the Soviet Union within the total political system may be understood more easily if we compare the structure of the USSR to that of a giant Western business corporation. The similarities between these two structures are striking, as scholars are beginning to observe with increased frequency. They go beyond the organizational forms, the absence of truly representative institutions or effectively en-

forced responsibility to a broad constituency in decision-making; they include the thorough bureaucratization of management on all levels. . . . Similarities even include the broad aims of the organizations, which in the cases of both the Soviet Union and the giant corporation are best described as the accumulation of wealth and power and the preservation of the enterprise.[21]

While the analogy is a trifle overdrawn, it does contain much truth, which has prompted Richard Eells to refer to the "constitutional crisis" confronting the corporation and Adolf A. Berle, Jr., while lauding the development of the "conscience of the corporation," to call for the imposition of formal constitutional limitations on corporate actions vis-à-vis individuals.[22] The analogy points up the problem posed by corporate governance—the existence of self-perpetuating oligarchies in the midst of a society espousing democratic principles.

CORPORATE GOVERNANCE AND ORGANIZATIONAL OLIGARCHY

It may be of some small comfort—or perhaps a source of even greater unhappiness—to students of American society to note that, while nondemocratic organizational governance is quite pronounced in business corporations, it is hardly unique to them. Indeed, a number of years ago Max Weber noted the existence of a basic tension between bureaucratic organization, based as it is on a hierarchical ordering of status, and democracy, which seeks to hold a close rein on the wielders of power. In Weber's view:

> Democracy inevitably comes into conflict with the bureaucratic tendencies which, by its fight against notable [status elite] rule, democracy has produced. . . . The most decisive thing here— indeed it is rather exclusively so—is the *leveling of the governed* in opposition to the ruling and bureaucratically articulated group, which in its turn may occupy a quite autocratic position, both in fact and in form.[23] (Emphasis in original.)

Robert Michels provided further insights into the relationship between bureaucratic organizations and democratic governance when he propounded his "iron law of oligarchy" in his classic work, *Political Parties*, first published over a half century ago.[24] Michels argued that hierarchical bureaucratic structure is the inevitable product of formal organization, since organizations that have attained a considerable degree of complexity require a staff of individuals who devote their full activities to the running of the enterprise. The result is the concentration of power at the top and the lessening of membership influence, since the leadership elite possesses many resources that give it an almost insurmountable advantage over the rank and file. The latter, moreover, have little interest in directing the activities of the organization. The interests of the leaders and of the followers frequently conflict, since, as a result of its position at the head of the organization, the elite develops concerns (primary among which is the maintenance of leadership positions) and perspectives not shared by the membership. In making policy, therefore, the will and the interests of the leadership will be reflected rather than those of the masses. In a word—organization results in oligarchy. "Democracy," whether in government, trade unions, political parties, or religious groups, results in domination by an elected few.

Notwithstanding criticisms of Michels' thesis on the grounds that his view of organizational governance is both overly generalized and overly deterministic with regard to elite rule, contemporary social scientists largely agree that the evidence overwhelmingly supports Michels' law of oligarchy as applied to private associations. Significantly, in *Union Democracy*, their study of the internal political system of the International Typographical Union—a deviant example (from Michels' point of view) of democratic organizational governance—Lipset, Trow, and Coleman reaffirm the "iron law." They state:

> The experience of most people as well as the studies of social scientists concerned with the problem of organization would tend to confirm Michels' generalization. In their trade unions, professional societies, business associations, and co-operatives—

in the myriad nominally democratic voluntary organizations—
men have learned, and learn again every day, that the clauses
in the constitutions which set forth the machinery for translating
membership interests and sentiments into organizational purposes and action bear little relationship to the actual political
processes which determine what their organizations do. At the
head of most private organizations stands a small group of men
most of whom have held high office in the organization's government for a long time, and whose tenure and control is rarely
threatened by a serious organized internal opposition. In such
organizations, regardless of whether the membership has a
nominal right to control through regular elections or conventions,
the real and often permanent power rests with the men who
hold the highest positions.[25]

More typical of control in membership organizations than the
unseating of long-time United Steel Workers president, David
McDonald, by Walter Abel or the replacement of veteran SNCC
(Student Nonviolent Coordinating Committee) leader, John J.
Lewis, by Stokely Carmichael is the tenure and organizational
control of George Meany, president of the AFL-CIO, or of Roy
Wilkins, NAACP executive director.

Given the prevalence of oligarchical patterns of governance
in nonbusiness organizations, the presence of the corporation on
the political scene, with effective decision-making control resting with corporate managers rather than in the hands of the
shareholder or an extended constituency, does not significantly
alter the nature of collective political participation. Indeed, in
terms of internal governance, the similarities between corporations and other types of organizations are more striking than
their differences. Probably the outstanding distinction is that
business firms generally do not even pretend to operate in accordance with democratic norms, whereas membership associations do. In practice, however, their governance patterns are
quite similar. As Charles Frankel has noted:

> The contemporary labor union, political party, veterans' asso-
> ciation, or corporation is typically composed of a large inert

membership controlled by a small active minority governing through a one-party or a no-party system. Such organizations may serve their members or stockholders well. But they are service organizations, not participant organizations. Their members are not citizens of the organization but clients, not makers of policy but its customers.[26]

It is hardly coincidental that in their study of formal organizations, Peter M. Blau and W. Richard Scott designated "maintaining membership control, that is, internal democracy" as the "crucial issue" confronting membership, or "mutual benefit," organizations.[27] Blau and Scott divide this central issue into two subthemes, "membership apathy and oligarchical control."[28] Significantly, these same two factors are most frequently mentioned as bases for challenging the legitimacy of corporate internal governance. These fundamental similarities in leadership domination of both business and nonbusiness organizations undercut the argument that corporations inherently lack legitimacy because of the independence of managers from the membership of the firm.

INTERNAL LEGITIMACY RECONSIDERED

The basic commonality between corporate and noncorporate governance is, at best, merely a negative ground upon which to predicate a theory of internal legitimacy. There are also positive arguments supporting such a theory.

In his classic discussion of the nature of authority, Max Weber provided a profound insight into the sources of legitimacy:

There are three pure types of legitimate authority. The validity of their claims to legitimacy may be based on:

1) Rational grounds—resting on a belief in the "legality" of patterns of normative rules and the right of those elevated to authority under such rules to issue commands (legal authority).

2) Traditional grounds—resting on an established belief in the sanctity of immemorial traditions and the legitimacy of the status of those exercising authority under them (traditional authority); or finally,

3) Charismatic grounds—resting on devotion to the specific and exceptional sanctity, heroism or exemplary character of an individual person, and of the normative patterns or order revealed or ordained by him (charismatic authority).[29]

While tradition legitimated the authority of the king during the Middle Ages, and charisma—that "unique force of command"[30] —legitimated the leadership of a Moses, Jesus, Caesar, or Napoleon, the modern bureaucratic organization, under Weber's taxonomy, is characterized by a legal-rational authority structure. Weber noted:

Obedience is owed to the legally established impersonal order. It extends to the persons exercising the authority of office under it only by virtue of the formal legality of their commands and only within the scope of authority of the office . . . the members of the corporate group, in so far as they obey a person in authority, do not owe this obedience to him as an individual, but to the impersonal order."[31]

It is true that aspects of authority based upon tradition can be detected in modern corporations—the family leadership of the Du Ponts, the Firestones, the Fords, and the Kaisers in corporations bearing their names or of the Sarnoffs in RCA—and, perhaps, in rare instances, even upon charisma. However, even in such cases, the real basis of authority is a legal-rational one. The managers have the right to their positions only because they have been elected to office according to the regulations and procedures set forth in corporation codes, articles of incorporation, and the by-laws governing their companies. They have attained their positions and are viewed by the public as having a right to them because they have adhered to the rules of the game relating to the selection of corporate leadership.

In the giant public corporation in which stock ownership

is atomistic, the selection procedure is largely ritualistic, since the incumbent management controls the proxy machinery and the shareholders are largely impotent; nevertheless, the prescribed steps must be followed. The leadership is recognized by shareholders, employees, those dealing with the corporation, and the general public alike as having rightfully come to their offices. While "the ritual process of selection has only historical connection with the real function and concurrent power entrusted to the individuals . . . [and might be replaced] . . . if we were building the American economic system anew,"[32] the real basis of internal corporate legitimacy is public acceptance. The selection process comports with what Adolf A. Berle, Jr., has termed the "public consensus"—"the body of these general, unstated premises which has come to be accepted" within the society by those persons informed about and concerned with corporate operations.[33] This relevant public considers the corporate governance process to be rightful. Therefore, unless public acceptance is withdrawn or the system of leadership selection is altered in the future, the present mode of corporate governance is legitimate.

Internal legitimacy is enhanced by the fact that, increasingly, corporate managers recognize responsibilities beyond minimal legal requirements both to their constituents—vague and amorphous as this constituency may be—and to the general public. The consequence of this recognition "is the rise of *self-restraint* as a hallmark of enterprise management."[34] In the final analysis, therefore, the internal legitimacy of the corporation derives from (1) the selection of corporate leadership in a manner viewed as proper by the public; and (2) "managerial . . . commitment to the enterprise and . . . acceptance of rational, public criteria by which its actions may be judged" resulting in an "innerdynamic" tendency within modern management "toward a progressive reduction in the arbitrariness of decision-making."[35]

THE QUESTION OF EXTERNAL LEGITIMACY

Let us turn now to an examination of the external legitimacy of corporate political activity. As was pointed out in the introduction to this chapter, the basic question concerns the propriety of political involvement by business firms when viewed from the perspective of other political participants and of the total political order. Does corporate political activity fundamentally differ from that of other actors in the American political arena, and if so, is it therefore improper? To resolve the issue of external legitimacy, we must consider a number of factors.

INDIVIDUAL VERSUS GROUP POLITICAL ACTIVITY

An initial challenge to corporate political involvement is one also leveled against political activity by other types of organizations. Challengers argue that *individual* participation is fundamental to the democratic process and that *associational* political activities emasculate the individual, in terms of political powers, and, accordingly, are intrinsically antidemocratic.

Such a call for individual political participation unsullied by the interposition of associational groupings harks back to idyllic, if inaccurate, notions of the political life of Periclean Greece or Emersonian New England. Ernest Barker points out, for example, that Aristotle, in his *Nicomachean Ethics*, recognized that the Greek polis, that fused system of state and society, was an "association of associations."[36] Alexis de Tocqueville noted a half century after the founding of the American Republic that "Americans of all ages, all conditions, and dispositions constantly form associations"[37] for their individual and mutual good.

Political goals have always given significant impetus to collective action. Group theorists such as Arthur F. Bentley, Earl Latham, and David B. Truman have considered the interaction of associational groupings as constituting the warp and woof of American pluralism.[38] This view is not, of course, accepted with unanimity by political scientists. As was discussed earlier, some students of government consider the rationale of the political process to be what has been termed "the quest of the public interest."[39] According to R. M. MacIver, the public may seem to be nothing but the "amorphous residuum that lies outside the contending pressure groups" and the public interest might appear to be nothing but "the diagonal of the forces that constantly struggle for advantage"; however,

> the whole logic of democracy is based on the conception that there is still a national unity and a common welfare. The fact that the interest in the common welfare cannot be organized after the fashion of specific interests should not conceal from us either its existence or the need to sustain it. Democracy itself is the final organization of the common interest. . . . Democracy affirms the community.[40]

The concept of the public interest is plagued by several inherent difficulties. First, the concept is ambiguous in that there exists no totally inclusive public interest within a nation. Differing segments of our society have varying conceptions regarding the nature of this interest. Frank J. Sorauf posed the critical question concerning the public interest when he observed, "But just *whose* standard it is to be remains the problem."[41] To a generation familiar with the conflict over United States involvement in Vietnam during the 1960's, this point is abundantly clear. "Even in war, when a totally inclusive interest should be apparent if it is ever going to be, we always find pacifists, conscientious objectors, spies, and subversives, who reflect interests opposed to those of 'the nation as a whole.' "[42] Similarly, the dilemma over the appropriate public policy regarding minority groups within this country points up conflicts about the nature of the public interest. Significantly, Herbert McClosky has found that "a large proportion of the electorate has failed to grasp certain of the underlying ideas and principles on which the American political system rests."[43] This poorly developed ideological consensus further increases the difficulty of ascertaining the public interests.

A second problem inheres in the intrinsically normative nature of the concept of the public interest, which makes it impossible to formulate universally acceptable standards of measurement to determine what is *the* public interest. Indeed, the many overlapping and conflicting conceptions of the public interest are not susceptible to empirical verification. As Grant McConnell has pointed out, "as a universal principle of moral guidance, it appears to be above tests of mere fact."[44]

I am not proposing that we utterly abandon the search for the public interest. Like such concepts as due process, justice, liberty and equality, it does serve as a polestar—though a vague and flickering one at best—for society. It posits the existence, underlying the political order, of certain basic values that distinguish the interests of American society from the interests of its constituent elements. When viewed in this limited perspective, the public interest is a useful concept.

Returning now specifically to our analysis of the role of group participation in American politics, one further point warrants mention. Neither corporations nor other associations have replaced or should replace individuals as the basic political constituency. One of David B. Truman's outstanding contributions to group theory is his insight that there exists an underlying compatibility between the individual and the group, since these terms are "at most merely convenient ways of classifying behavior, two ways of approaching the same phenomena, not different things."[45] Indeed, he takes pains to point out:

> It is not intended, however, that we should reject the general human values asserted in the militant doctrines of individualism. Since we have assumed the task of developing a conception of the political process in the United States that will enable us to determine the bearing of group organization upon the survival of representative democracy, we have in fact assumed the importance of those values. Far from leaving them out of account, we are primarily concerned with their place in the process of group politics.[46]

Moreover, it must be recalled that despite the emphasis placed in this chapter upon collective activity, our formal political institutions are structured for individual participation. For example, only human persons can exercise the basic political mechanism of a democracy—the vote.

What has been argued here is simply that, while it is quite correct to suggest that individual political participation is basic to a democratic form of government, "the chief social values cherished by individuals in modern society are realized through groups."[47] This is a fact of life within a society in which even the very concept of "individual" is taking on the meaning "social participant," rather than "autonomous person."

Not all public policy results from a conflict between organized social interest groups. Indeed, "the slightest inquiry into empirical evidence would convince the student that many laws are passed not only without the support of organized groups but frequently in opposition to the demands of such organizations."[48] Once again, the example of traffic safety legislation comes to mind. This fact notwithstanding, the existence of social interest groups serves to strengthen citizen political efficacy and is "natural and healthy for a democracy."[49]

COMPARISON OF CORPORATIONS AND OTHER INTEREST GROUPS

Having examined in general terms the role of organizations in American politics, it is now appropriate to look specifically at the political role of business organizations. In contemporary society, corporations are among the most important groups pursuing economic, and increasingly broader social, objectives. While originally intended to shield the corporation from unreasonable intervention by political authority, the assertion in the *Dartmouth College* case that corporations possess neither "political power, [n]or a political character"[50] is totally inappropriate to the realities of twentieth-century America. At this point in our discussion, the existence of corporate political power requires no verification. Corporations also possess a political character analogous to that of other social interests. While corporations do differ in certain respects from such nonprofit organizations as the Ancient Order of Hibernians in America, the United Auto Workers, the National Education Association, the Veterans of

Foreign Wars, the National Grange, and the National Association for the Advancement of Colored People, there are striking similarities between business firms and these organizations.

The objectives pursued by many private associations are often primarily economic in character and are narrowly focused upon fulfilling specific needs of the organization. Consider, for example, the activities of the American Medical Association in attempting to defeat Medicare, the efforts of the American Legion to secure veterans' benefits, or the advocacy by the American Farm Bureau Federation of federal programs for flexible price supports which are particularly favorable to large farmers. As we saw, moreover, in our discussion of corporate internal legitimacy, nondemocratic patterns of organizational governance are not limited to corporations, but are found in many organizations—public and private alike. Conversely, while the social role of the corporation has historically been considered purely economic (producing goods and resources for society and making profits for investors), in recent years corporations have been charged by government and by the general public alike with the responsibility of performing much broader social functions, ranging from the training of minority workers to the development of new methods of increasing the world's food supply.

However, certain differences do exist between corporate and noncorporate organizations. First, for many noncorporate "private governments," political involvement is viewed as an important, albeit not the exclusive, organizational *raison d'être*. The political activity is intended to accomplish the social or economic objectives of the membership, which is the "prime beneficiary" of this type of "mutual benefit" organization.[51] On the other hand, the business corporation exists for the fundamental social purpose of satisfying the economic requirements of American society through the production and distribution of goods and services. In return for fulfilling this function, the corporation is permitted—if possible—to make a profit for the owners of the enterprise. As a result of this difference in basic purpose, the nature of and the reasons underlying organizational affiliation differ for membership organizations and business enterprises.

Second, as a result of social, economic, and political pressures, both the degree of voluntariness in and the intensity of commitment to membership associations vary greatly in the individual case. Affiliation with the Sierra Club, the American Association of University Professors, the Pennsylvania Bar Association, or the American Legion is, to a large degree, voluntary, and results basically from an interest in and identification with the policies and programs of the organization. When joining membership or mutual benefit organizations, individuals are generally aware of the political proclivities of the organization and either consciously or unconsciously weigh this factor when deciding whether to affiliate. Accordingly, membership in such groups constitutes, at least in small measure, a political decision. This is also true for union affiliation; however, in states which permit union shop provisions, the aspect of voluntariness is largely vitiated, although, arguably, this elimination of voluntariness may be essential to the long-run interests of the worker.

On the other hand, affiliation with business corporations is predicated largely on economic grounds with little, if any, consideration given to the political implications of the act. Employees "join" corporations to receive paychecks and security, stockholders become "members" to receive dividends and capital gains. If suppliers, distributors, and creditors are considered to be constituents, the economic basis of their association is all the more apparent. Those who affiliate with the corporation are very often unaware of the political personality of the organization and assume that their relationship is purely economic. Moreover, as indicated earlier, there are few effective means by which, even in theory, the corporate member—with the possible exception of the high-level employee or the large shareholder— can affect the political policies of the organization.

However, despite these distinctions regarding organizational purpose and the reasons for individual affiliation, most membership associations have nonpolitical objectives that are the primary reasons why individuals join them, and their political activities are designed only to effectuate the essentially social and economic goals of the organization. Conversely, modern large corporations are increasingly emphasizing their broad-gauged, noneconomic activities—such as technological advancement, regional development, the support of education and the arts, and equal-employment opportunities—as important functions of the enterprise and are attempting to elicit the support of their membership in effecting them.

While this coalescence in function between corporate and noncorporate organizations must not, of course, be exaggerated, it does point up a basic weakness in distinguishing between the external legitimacy of business and that of membership organizations. In his analysis of the political role of organizations, Alexander Heard arrives at the unavoidable conclusion that

> membership in any organized group [be it a corporation, a trade association, a professional society, or a union] possessed of political interests commits an individual to indirect involvement in the political process. The character of this involvement will be determined by those who dominate the group. There is no escape from politics for the individual.[52]

If the political participation of membership associations is legitimate, so also should be that of corporations. It does not constitute a return to the era of the "personification of corporation"[53] to suggest that the political activities of corporations should be viewed in the same light as those of other associations, full well recognizing that certain differences exist between corporate and noncorporate organizations. As long as the political efforts of business firms conform to practices which are commonly recognized in a democracy as legitimate, their presence in political life is legitimate.

PLURALISM AND INTERDEPENDENCE: BASES OF CORPORATE POLITICAL LEGITIMACY

Two other bases of the legitimacy of political participation by corporations—the pluralistic character of American society and the growth of an interdependent economy—inhere in the nature of our current social environment. Talcott Parsons and Neil J. Smelser have suggested that the goal of the polity is to maximize "the capacity of the society to attain its system goals, i.e., collective goals."[54] Corporations are and must be political participants; in performing their basic social function—the production and distribution of goods and services—they are, in this general process of goal attainment, inextricably bound up with the multitude of institutions and interests present in American society. They are, accordingly, subject to continuous claims by these coexisting interests and institutions and, in return, must seek to effect their own claims. Since the institutions of government are the most important arenas within which these social claims are resolved, corporations must seek access to formal and informal governmental structures in the same manner as do competing social interests. The search for access to and impact upon the foci of governmental decision making is the essence of all politics. This search is particularly widespread in this country. In fact,

> perhaps the outstanding characteristic of American politics . . . is that it involves a multiplicity of co-ordinate or nearly co-ordinate points of access to governmental decisions. The significance of these many points of access and of the complicated texture of relationships among them is great. This diversity assures a variety of modes for the participation of interest groups in the formation of policy, a variety that is a flexible, stabilizing element.[55]

We have already pointed out how important this access is in a mixed, or interdependent, political economy where the interests of the corporation are critically dependent upon government decisions. The very essence of this mix is the joint responsibility of government and business for economic stability and growth. While the future dimensions of this interdependence are, of course, uncertain, it is highly probable that business firms engaged in activities of great public importance increasingly will be subjected to demands by other social interests for governmental supervision of these activities. This development will not be a result of corporate political involvement, but, rather, a consequence of the fact that by performing broad social tasks corporations have become utterly critical to the well-being of American society.

John Kenneth Galbraith predicts that "the industrial system will not long be regarded as something apart from government . . . [but] will increasingly be seen as part of a much larger complex which embraces both the industrial system and the state";[56] more probably, we shall witness in the foreseeable future an uneasy balance between large and powerful industrial units and a large and powerful governmental structure with neither partner being absorbed by the other. Such a relationship would be in keeping with the intrinsically pragmatic character of the American social order and particularly with its character as a business-oriented civilization.

In this uneasy balance, corporate political activity will continue to be an abiding necessity—as it is today—to mitigate constraints. Failure to assume a political posture would result in a diminution of corporate freedom of action and reduce thereby the quality of social pluralism.

The dependence of corporations upon the resources and privileges conferred by government has been mentioned throughout this book. This dependence is basic to an interdependent economy. The net result is to sharpen the political competition between corporations and other social interests—which are also dependent upon governmental favor—as well as among corporations *inter se.* This competition is fundamental to a pluralistic society.

Significantly, it has been argued that, rather than endangering democracy, corporate political participation enhances the quality of pluralism by providing a buffer against the undemocratic tendencies of a mass society. William Kornhauser states the case as follows:

Since big business in highly developed capitalist systems tends to possess a network of organizations for the defense of its interests, as well as a high involvement in voluntary associations of all kinds, its willingness to risk the destruction of an existing democratic order should, in the ordinary course of events, be relatively low. For its multiple stakes in that order require, among other things, that big business protect its position by maintaining continuous access to policy-making institutions, and this access would be jeopardized by support of extremist movements unless they gave strong promise of success.[57]

Today constituting not monolithic but multiple foci of power, interests and affiliation in our society, corporations, together with other social interest groups, contribute to the social pluralism that has characterized American society. It is not coincidental that social pluralism and liberal democracy have had their fullest flowering in the highly urbanized and industrialized societies in which diverse social interests are present and participate in the political order.[58]

Recalling momentarily the internal legitimacy analysis, it is apparent that because leaders of business firms—as well as of other organizations—are not selected on the basis of widespread participation in governance does not mean that they are not representative of the basic interests of those affiliated with the corporation. Survival is the fundamental goal of all organizations, and in its activities, the corporate leadership seeks to insure the longevity of the firm—an objective essential to the entire membership. In representing and having to balance the claims of the diverse interests associated with the corporation—however we define this constituency—professional leadership and bureaucratic management help to maintain the texture of a pluralistic society. They thereby contribute to the pattern of carefully ordered conflict that is characteristic of the American political order.

A word of summation is necessary. Throughout this book, the importance of social pluralism and economic interdependence in contemporary American society has been emphasized. These two fundamental characteristics of our social order have required corporations to be active political participants and thereby underlie the external legitimacy of corporate political involvement.

PUBLIC ACCEPTANCE OF CORPORATE EXTERNAL LEGITIMACY

Inherent in the notion of legitimacy is an acknowledgement of the propriety of particular modes of behavior. Public acceptance of corporate political involvement provides, therefore, yet an additional basis of legitimacy.

In the University of Michigan Institute for Social Research study cited in Chapter Seven, control over political activities was mentioned by less than 2 per cent of those polled as constituting one of the "desired areas of government control over big business activities." Significantly, only 3 per cent of the persons surveyed were of the opinion that big business had "too much power over other institutions—government, newspapers, schools, etc." Interestingly, the federal government was picked as the most powerful institution, with labor unions second, big business third, state governments fourth, and "not big" business fifth. Those polled revealed the following desired ordering of power: the national government was selected first, state governments second, big business third, labor unions fourth, and "not big" business fifth. It is noteworthy that more than half of those surveyed desired big business either to move up (16 per cent) in the power ordering or not to shift (40 per cent), while the vast majority desired labor unions to move down (54 per cent) or to remain the same (32 per cent) in the power rankings.[59] The findings of the Michigan survey indeed indicate that "big business was not a scare word to the public at large."[60] This conclusion is confirmed by a Gallup Poll conducted in 1968 among over 1500 people across the nation. In response to the question ". . . which of the following do you think will be the biggest threat to democracy in the future—big business, big labor, or big government?", 46 per cent of those surveyed designated big government; 26 per cent, big labor; 12 per cent, big business; and 16 per cent, no opinion.[61] Thus, only a small percentage of respondents feel threatened by the role which big business—large corporations—plays in American society.

Significantly, even union members—supposedly the most rabid enemies of business political involvement—acknowledge the legitimacy of such involvement. In their study of the voting behavior of members of the United Auto Workers during the 1952 Presidential election, Kornhauser, Sheppard, and Mayer found that 78 per cent of those polled (351 persons) felt that it was "all right for businessmen and business groups to work for Eisenhower" while only 12 per cent viewed such action as improper.[62] The remaining 10 per cent expressed no opinion. As to whether it was "all right for the unions to work for Stevenson," 78 per cent replied that it was, while 14 per cent indicated that it was not; 8 per cent had no opinion. The authors of the study concluded that the results indicate a "significant expression of overwhelming sentiment in favor of organized political participation in the presidential campaign *both* by unions and by business."[63] Significantly, even though 35 per cent of the workers polled indicated that they did not trust the recommendation of business groups (12 per cent did not trust those of labor groups), 42 per cent felt that business should either have more influence on government (19 per cent) or have neither more nor less influence (23 per cent).[64] Forty-one per cent expressed the view that business should have less influence, while 17 per cent registered no opinion. Accordingly less than half of the union respondents thought that corporate influence on government should be reduced. When one recalls the nature of the constituency—Detroit auto-workers—this response is, surprisingly, supportive of corporate political action.

What factors have contributed to this public acceptance of the legitimacy of corporate political activity during the post-World War II era, whereas such activity encountered deep-seated hostility during the early days of this century? Three factors are important. First, America has completed the transition from a rural-agrarian to an urban-industrial nation. The unfavorable experiences that farmers had with the banks, railroads, and mills during the Populist Era have faded into the historical past. Moreover, as we have seen, agrarian values have been largely replaced by values compatible with a business society.

Second, no longer is the corporation divided into two distinct socioeconomic classes—the owners and the workers—that are fundamentally hostile toward each other. Rather, the work force of the corporation spans the entire spectrum of class identifications. The "we-they" mentality, which was prevalent in the past, has largely been dissipated because of the existence of many, almost imperceptible, class graduations among corporate employees. Thus, the class-based hostility toward and fear of corporate political activity has been weakened. Finally, the very growth in the size and power of government and other social interests—for example, labor unions—during the past several decades has lessened public fear of political domination by business interests. Other formidable protagonists are now on the political scene. There exists a greater awareness and acceptance of the presence and the necessity, in our society, of multiple centers of power, which serve to restrict the exercise of excessive power by any single social interest. As a consequence of these developments and of others discussed in this book, "the position of business within society was never more solidly entrenched. . . . Its legitimacy is now virtually complete, its acceptance without exception. For perhaps the first time in American history there is no longer any substantial intellectual opposition to the system of business nor any serious questioning of its economic privileges and benefits."[65]

GOVERNMENTAL RECOGNITION OF CORPORATE POLITICAL LEGITIMACY

A final indication of the acceptance of the legitimacy of corporate political activities is the acknowledgement of corporate politics by government. Business firms are formally co-opted into the administrative process by requiring regulatory bodies to consult with them apropos matters affecting their interests. Furthermore, corporations are permitted—as are other interest groups—to make expenditures to influence legislation, without violating the Federal Regulation of Lobbying Act.[66] We have also seen that businessmen are frequently called upon to consult with and to advise governmental officials.

There has been legal recognition of the legitimacy of corporate political participation. We have already pointed out that corporations have been accorded the status of persons. Business firms have been granted the protection of the First and Fourteenth Amendments in cases involving communications, collective bargaining, and libel.[67] It will be recalled, moreover, that in *Eastern R.R. Presidents Conference v. Noerr Motor Freight, Inc.*, a case specifically focusing upon the question of the propriety of business political involvement, the Supreme Court refused to prohibit such involvement.[68] In recognizing the right of a group of railroads to engage in an extensive publicity campaign concerning legislation regulating the long-distance trucking business, the Court expressed concern over the constitutionality of any ban on the activities of the Railroad Conference.

Section 610 of the Federal Criminal Code prohibiting corporations—and labor unions—from making campaign contributions and expenditures on behalf of candidates or parties constitutes the *sole* federal limitation generally applicable to corporations.[69] As such, the section raises questions concerning the legitimacy of this aspect of corporate political behavior. It is illuminating, therefore, to see the reaction of the Supreme Court to the statutory prohibition.

Although the Court has never been called upon to apply Section 610 to a corporation—both of the cases reaching the Supreme Court have involved labor organizations—in *United States v. Congress of Industrial Organizations* the majority (by way of a strong dictum) commented:

> If [Section 610] were construed to prohibit the publication, by corporations and unions in the regular course of conducting their affairs, of periodicals advising their members, stockholders or customers of danger or advantage to their interests from the adoption of measures, or the election to office of men espousing such measures, *the gravest doubt would arise in our minds as to its constitutionality.* . . . It would require explicit words in an act to convince us that Congress intended to bar a trade journal, a house organ or a newspaper, published by a corporation, from

expressing views on candidates or political proposals in the regular course of its publication. It is unduly stretching language to say that the members or stockholders are unwilling participants in such normal organizational activities, including the advocacy thereby of governmental policies affecting their interests, and the support thereby of candidates thought to be favorable to their interests.[70] (Emphasis added.)

Although this pronouncement relates primarily to the issue of the internal legitimacy of corporate political activity since it concerns political communications between a corporation and its members, it recognized, by implication, the necessity and propriety of such involvement in the American political environment and questions the constitutionality of the legislative limitation. While, in a subsequent case, *United States v. International Union United Automobile, Aircraft and Agricultural Implement Workers of America (UAW-CIO)*,[71] the Court refused to extend the notion of internal communications to include union-sponsored programs on commercial television stations, it did not retract or comment upon the dictum expressed in the CIO case. The Court has yet to decide the constitutionality of Section 610.

Significantly, in the more than sixty years during which the statutory prohibition has been in effect, there have been only two recorded lower-court cases involving corporations, one in 1916 and the other in 1966.[72] In *United States v. United States Brewers' Ass'n.*, the defendant corporations pleaded guilty to contributing money in connection with an election for members of the House of Representatives. The latter case, *United States v. Lewis Food Company, Inc.*, involved a small closely held family firm which had published a newspaper "scorecard" rating candidates in congressional primaries. The matter was eventually resolved when the defendant entered a plea of *nolo contendere*— not admitting, but not contesting the charges—and received a nominal fine.[73] Once again, however, there was no resolution of the constitutionality of the statutory provision.

SUMMATION

While in terms of the traditional perspective of democratic theory, corporate political participation poses a troublesome question, it does not follow that a verdict of "no legitimacy" inevitably follows. The factors examined in this chapter provide, if not a comprehensive model for corporate political legitimacy, then at least the foundation blocks.

With regard to the issue of internal political legitimacy, definition of the corporate constituency and the nondemocratic pattern of corporate governance present problems, but a number of elements support a finding that business political activities are, indeed, appropriate. While managers are no longer accountable to shareholders in the manner suggested by the traditional legal-economic model of the firm and instead constitute a self-perpetuating oligarchy, this condition inheres in the present relationship of the stockholder to the large corporation and is not confined to political activities of the organization. The patterns of accountability and governance are not altered, moreover, if the "membership" of the firm is widened to include other interests intimately associated with or affected by the corporation. These facts notwithstanding, managers generally do not act capriciously with regard to the interests of either shareholders or these other constituents.

The pattern of organizational oligarchy and independence of membership control described above is not, however, unique to corporations. As Michels pointed out a number of years ago, hierarchical nondemocratic governance is an inevitable product of formal organization and can be found in a wide variety of social groups. If corporate governance is considered illegitimate because of the lack of effective democratic procedures, so too must the leadership of other organizations.

More importantly, because corporate managers come to their positions of authority according to the procedures specified by law and by proper corporate practice, they enjoy public acceptance. Under Weber's schema of authority, they exercise legal-rational authority. This public acceptance of business leaders, which provides the underlying positive rationale of the internal legitimacy of corporate politics, is enhanced by two other factors: (1) the acknowledgement by corporate leaders of greater responsibility to a broader constituency and (2) a progressive decline in the arbitrariness of managerial decision making.

Similarly, the external legitimacy of corporate politics is

grounded on a number of factors. Notwithstanding the search by some social scientists for the elusive "public interest," American politics has been basically group politics, characterized by the competition of diverse social interests. Individuals maximize their political interests through membership and participation in interested groups. While corporations differ in certain respects from other organizations in terms of both basic purpose and constituency, these distinctions lose much of their significance when one considers the similarities between business and nonbusiness organizations in terms of actual social involvement and reasons for membership affiliation.

Equally important with regard to external legitimacy are the presence of social pluralism and economic interdependence in the United States. Corporations constitute one of the diverse social interests that compete for access and influence within government. In an economy characterized by interdependence, the importance of governmental decisions for the corporation has become all the more acute. Political involvement is, therefore, essential to protect corporate interests both in their competition with other social groups, equally as important, and *inter se.* Corporate political involvement enhances the quality of pluralism and provides an additional safeguard against the authoritarian potential of a mass society.

Another source of external legitimacy is derived from the general public acceptance, over the years, of corporate political involvement. Indeed, even union members have acknowledged the propriety of business political activities. Finally, various branches of government have formally co-opted corporations and their leaders into the public decision-making process. The Supreme Court has reaffirmed the right of business firms to participate in specified political activities and has expressed its reservations regarding the constitutionality of attempts to prohibit this involvement, although it has not specifically decided this issue.

Consequently, although political theory has not kept pace with political fact, there are cogent reasons for recognizing both the internal and the external legitimacy of corporate political participation. To acknowledge this legitimacy does not mean, however, that the political activities of corporations—just like those of other political participants—should not be subject to public scrutiny and review. Political involvement is not an either-or proposition; it is a matter of kind and degree. The fundamental question persists and requires continual reevaluation: What manner and what scope of corporate political activity are acceptable in a pluralistic democracy? This question focuses attention on the appropriateness of existing restrictions upon corporate political activity and the desirability of totally removing these constraints or, in the alternative, of substituting a different set of limitations. Even more importantly, the question calls for the formulation of a relevant theoretical guideline for evaluating the political participation of business firms. This guideline should reflect the fact that, although in certain ways corporations are unique, in most respects relevant to the political process they share common characteristics with other social interest groups. The concluding chapter of this book will be addressed to these thorny matters.

NOTES

[1]Robert A. Dahl, *Modern Political Analysis* (Englewood Cliffs, N.J.: Prentice-Hall, Inc., 1963), p. 19; and Seymour Martin Lipset, *Political Man* (Garden City, N.Y.: Anchor Books, Doubleday & Company, Inc., 1963), p. 64. See also Max Weber, *The Theory of Social and Economic Organization*, trans. A. M. Henderson and Talcott Parsons, ed. by Parsons (New York: The Free Press, 1964), pp. 124–32, 324–407; Herbert A. Simon, *Administrative Behavior*, 2d ed. (New York: The Free Press, 1957), pp. 123–53; and Chester I. Barnard, *The Functions of the Executive* (Cambridge, Mass.: Harvard University Press, 1964), pp. 161–84.

[2]Edward S. Mason, "Introduction" in Edward S. Mason (ed.), *The Corporation in Modern Society* (Cambridge, Mass.: Harvard University Press, 1959), pp. 4–5. See also Robert A. Dahl and Charles E. Lindblom, *Politics, Economics, and Welfare: Planning and Politico-*

Economic Systems Resolved into Basic Social Processes (New York: Torchbooks, Harper & Row, Publishers, 1963), pp. 480–83.

[3]Grant McConnell, *Private Power & American Democracy* (New York: Alfred A. Knopf, Inc., 1966), p. 3.

[4]Abram Chayes, "The Modern Corporation and the Rule of Law," in Mason (ed.), *The Corporation in . . .* , p. 39.

[5]Pennsylvania Business Corporation Law, Purdon's Pennsylvania *Statutes Annotated*, Title 15, Ch. 11, § 1406 (Philadelphia: George T. Bisel Company, 1967).

[6]Dow Votaw, *Modern Corporations* (Englewood Cliffs, N.J.: Prentice-Hall, Inc., 1965), p. 63. On this subject, see also Norman D. Lattin, *Lattin on Corporations* (Brooklyn, N.Y.: Foundation Press, 1959), pp. 227–36; Henry Winthrop Ballantine, *Ballantine on Corporations*, rev. ed. (Chicago: Callaghan and Company, 1946), pp. 137–55; and Ralph J. Baker and William L. Cary, *Cases and Materials on Corporations*, 3d ed., unabridged (Brooklyn, N.Y.: Foundation Press, Inc., 1959), pp. 127–41.

[7]Adolf A. Berle, Jr., and Gardiner C. Means, *The Modern Corporation and Private Property* (New York: The Macmillan Company, Publishers, 1933), p. 124.

[8]Robert J. Larner, "Ownership and Control in the 200 Largest Nonfinancial Corporations, 1929 and 1963," *American Economic Review*, LVI, No. 4 (Sept. 1966), 780. Compare Robert Sheehan, "Proprietors in the World of Big Business," *Fortune*, LXXV, No. 7 (June 15, 1967), 178–83, 242.

[9]Robert Aaron Gordon, *Business Leadership in the Large Corporation* (Berkeley, Calif.: University of California Press, 1961), esp. Chaps. 3, 6.

[10]Peter F. Drucker, *Concept of the Corporation* (Boston: Beacon Press, Inc., 1960), pp. 5–6.

[11]J. A. Livingston, *The American Stockholder*, rev. ed. (New York: Collier Books, a division of Crowell-Collier Publishing Co., 1963), p. 33.

[12]*1967 Fact Book* (New York: New York Stock Exchange, May 1967), pp. 24–25.

[13]*1967 Fact Book*, p. 37.

[14]Daniel Jay Baum and Ned B. Stiles, *The Silent Partners* (Syracuse, N.Y.: Syracuse University Press, 1965), pp. 53–54.

[15]John Kenneth Galbraith, *The New Industrial State* (Boston:

Houghton Mifflin Company, 1967), pp. 60–71. See also Mason Haire, "The Concept of Power and the Concept of Man," in George B. Strother (ed.), *Social Science Approaches to Business Behavior* (Homewood, Ill.: Dorsey Press, Inc. and Richard D. Irwin, Inc., 1962), pp. 163–83.

[16]Richard Eells, *The Government of Corporations* (New York: The Free Press, 1962), p. 87.

[17]Chayes, "The Modern Corporation . . . ," in Mason (ed.), *The Corporation in . . . ,* p. 41.

[18]*Massachusetts General Laws Annotated* (Boston: Boston Law Book Co., 1958), ch. 156, § 23 (1919).

[19]President of the United States, *Economic Report of the President, Together with the Annual Report of the Council of Economic Advisors* (Washington, D.C.: U.S. Government Printing Office, 1968), p. 294 (Table B-72).

[20]15 U.S.C.A. § 1222 (1956).

[21]Alfred G. Meyer, *The Soviet Political System* (New York: Random House, Inc., 1965), p. 112. For additional insight into parallels between the corporation and Soviet economic organization, see David Granick, *The Red Executive* (Garden City, N.Y.: Anchor Books, Doubleday and Company, Inc., 1961). See also, Dahl and Lindblom, *Politics, Economics, and Welfare,* p. 278.

[22]See, respectively, Eells, *The Government . . . ,* pp. 16–28; and Adolf A. Berle, Jr., "Constitutional Limitations on Corporate Activity —Protection of Personal Rights from Invasion through Economic Power," *University of Pennsylvania Law Review,* 100, No. 7 (May 1952), 933–55. See also his *The 20th Century Capitalist Revolution* (New York: Harvest Books, Harcourt, Brace & World, Inc., 1954), pp. 61–115.

[23]H. H. Gerth and C. Wright Mills, *From Max Weber: Essays in Sociology* (Fair Lawn, N.J.: Oxford University Press, Inc., 1958), p. 226.

[24]Robert Michels, *Political Parties: A Sociological Study of the Oligarchical Tendencies of Modern Democracy* (New York: Collier Books, a division of Crowell-Collier Publishing Co., 1962).

[25]Seymour Martin Lipset, Martin A. Trow, and James S. Coleman, *Union Democracy* (Garden City, N.Y.: Anchor Books, Doubleday & Company, Inc., 1962), pp. 2–3. See also Robert Presthus, *The Organizational Society* (New York: Vintage Books, Random House,

Inc., 1965), pp. 27–58; and Charles Frankel, *The Democratic Prospect* (New York: Harper Colophon Books, Harper & Row, Publishers, 1962), pp. 30–48. Compare Seymour Martin Lipset, "Introduction" in Michels, *Political Parties*, pp. 15–39; David B. Truman, *The Governmental Process* (New York: Alfred A. Knopf, Inc., 1951), pp. 129–55; Robert A. Dahl and Charles E. Lindblom, *Politics, Economics, and Welfare* (New York: Harper Torchbooks, Harper & Row, Publishers, 1963)., pp. 227–86; and John D. May, "Democracy, Organizations, Michels," *American Political Science Review*, LIX, No. 2 (June 1965), 417–29.

[26]Frankel, *The Democratic Prospect*, pp. 57–58.

[27]Peter M. Blau and W. Richard Scott, *Formal Organizations* (San Francisco: Chandler Publishing Company, 1962), pp. 27–58.

[28]Blau and Scott, *Formal Organizations*, pp. 27–58.

[29]Weber, *The Theory of* . . . , p. 328.

[30]Robert A. Nisbet, *The Sociological Tradition* (New York: Basic Books, Inc., Publishers, 1966), p. 143.

[31]Weber, *The Theory of* . . . , pp. 328, 330.

[32]Adolf A. Berle, Jr., *Power Without Property* (New York: Harvest Books, Harcourt, Brace & World, Inc., 1959), p. 107.

[33]Berle, *Power Without Property*, p. 111.

[34]Philip Selznick, "Private Government and the Corporate Conscience" (unpublished manuscript prepared for Symposium on Business Policy, April 8–11, 1963, Graduate School of Business Administration, Harvard University), p. 23.

[35]Selznick, "Private Government . . . ," p. 25.

[36]Ernest Barker, *Principles of Social and Political Theory* (London: Oxford University Press, 1951), p. 5.

[37]Alexis de Tocqueville, *Democracy in America* (New York: Vintage Books, Random House Inc., 1954), Vol. II, p. 114.

[38]Arthur F. Bentley, *The Process of Government* (Cambridge, Mass.: The Belknap Press, Harvard University Press, 1967); Earl Latham, *The Group Basis of Politics; A Study in Basing-Point Legislation* (Ithaca, N.Y.: Cornell University Press, 1952); and Truman, *The Governmental Process*.

[39]McConnell, *Private Power* . . . , pp. 336–68. See also Peter H. Odegard, "A Group Basis of Politics: A New Name for an Ancient Myth," *Western Political Science Quarterly*, XI, No. 3 (Sept. 1958), 689–702; E. E. Schattschneider, *The Semi-Sovereign People* (New

York: Holt, Rinehart & Winston, Inc., 1960), Chap. 2; and Sheldon S. Wolin, *Politics and Vision* (Boston: Little, Brown and Company, 1960), Chap. 10.

[40]Robert M. MacIver, *The Web of Government*, rev. ed. (New York: The Free Press, 1965), p. 165. Copyright R. M. MacIver 1965.

[41]Frank J. Sorauf, "The Conceptual Muddle," in Carl J. Friedrich (ed.), *Nomos V—The Public Interest* (New York: Atherton Press, 1967), p. 184.

[42]Truman, *The Governmental Process*, p. 50.

[43]Herbert McClosky, "Consensus and Ideology in American Politics," *American Political Science Review*, LVIII, No. 2 (June 1964), 365.

[44]McConnell, *Private Power* . . . , p. 364. For comprehensive criticisms of the "public interest" concept, see Sorauf, "The Conceptual Muddle," in Friedrich (ed.), *Nomos V* . . . , pp. 183–90; and Glendon Schubert, "Is There a Public Interest Theory?" in Friedrich (ed.), *Nomos V* . . . , pp. 162–76.

[45]Truman, *The Governmental Process*, p. 48.

[46]Truman, *The Governmental Process*, p. 49.

[47]Earl Latham, "The Group Basis of Politics: Notes for a Theory," *American Political Science Review*, XLVI, No. 2 (June 1952), 376. For a perceptive and relevant analysis of the changing role of the individual in contemporary society, see John William Ward, "The Ideal of Individualism and the Reality of Organization," in Earl F. Cheit (ed.), *The Business Establishment* (New York: John Wiley & Sons, Inc., 1964), pp. 37–76.

[48]Harmon Zeigler, *Interest Groups in American Society* (Englewood Cliffs, N.J.: Prentice-Hall, Inc., 1964), p. 24.

[49]Zeigler, *Interest Groups* . . . , p. 39.

[50]*Dartmouth College* v. *Woodward*, 4 Wheaton 518, 636 (1819).

[51]This terminology is drawn from Blau and Scott, *Formal Organizations*, pp. 27–58.

[52]Alexander Heard, *The Costs of Democracy* (Chapel Hill, N.C.: The University of North Carolina Press, 1960), p. 210.

[53]Thurman W. Arnold, *The Folklore of Capitalism* (New Haven, Conn.: Yale University Press, 1937), pp. 185–206.

[54]Talcott Parsons and Neil J. Smelser, *Economy and Society* (New York: The Free Press, 1956), p. 48.

⁵⁵Truman, *The Governmental Process*, p. 519.

⁵⁶John Kenneth Galbraith, *The New Industrial State* (Houghton Mifflin Company), p. 392.

⁵⁷William Kornhauser, *The Politics of Mass Society* (New York: The Free Press, 1959), p. 197. See also Joseph A. Schumpeter, *Capitalism, Socialism, and Democracy* (New York: Harper & Row, Publishers, 1947), p. 55.

⁵⁸For further discussion of this point, see Kornhauser, *The Politics of Mass Society*, pp. 227–38; Gerard DeGré, "Freedom and Social Structure," *American Sociological Review*, II, No. 5 (Oct. 1946), 529–36; and Seymour Martin Lipset, "Some Social Requisites of Democracy: Economic Development and Political Legitimacy," *American Political Science Review*, LIII, No. 1 (March 1959), 69–105.

⁵⁹Burton R. Fisher and Stephen B. Withey, *Big Business as the People See It* (Ann Arbor, Mich.: The Survey Research Center Institute for Social Research, University of Michigan, 1951), pp. 22, 51, 128.

⁶⁰Richard Hofstadter, "What Happened to the Antitrust Movement?" in Cheit (ed.), *The Business Establishment*, p. 132.

⁶¹" 'Big Government' is Feared in Poll," *The New York Times*, August 18, 1968, p. 51, col. 1.

⁶²Arthur Kornhauser, Harold L. Sheppard, and Albert J. Mayer, *When Labor Votes* (New York: University Books, Inc., 1956), p. 100.

⁶³Kornhauser, Sheppard, and Mayer, *When Labor Votes*, p. 101.

⁶⁴Kornhauser, Sheppard, and Mayer, *When Labor Votes*, pp. 106, 112.

⁶⁵Robert L. Heilbroner, *The Limits of American Capitalism* (New York: Harper & Row, Publishers, 1965), p. 55.

⁶⁶2 U.S.C. §§ 261–270 (1946).

⁶⁷These cases are collected in Edwin M. Epstein, *Corporations, Contributions, and Political Campaigns: Federal Regulation in Perspective* (Berkeley: Institute of Governmental Studies, University of California, May 1968), p. 194, fns. 279–81.

⁶⁸365 U.S. 127 (1961).

⁶⁹18 U.S.C. § 610 (1951). For an analysis of this provision, see Epstein, *Corporations, Contributions, and. . . .*

⁷⁰335 U.S. 106 (1948) at 121–23.

[71]352 U.S. 567 (1957).

[72]*United States* v. *United States Brewers' Ass'n,* 239 F. 163 (W.D. Pa. 1916) and *United States* v. *Lewis Food Company, Inc.,* 366 F.2d 710 (9th Cir. 1966), *reversing,* 236 F. Supp. 849 (S.D. Cal. 1964).

[73]For an analysis of the *Lewis Food Company* case, see Epstein, *Corporations, Contributions, and* . . . , pp. 35–42.

Chapter Ten

Conclusion: Corporate Political Activity In Perspective

The role of economic interest groups in American political and social life has been a subject of abiding concern from the very earliest days of our national existence. Reference was made in Chapter Eight to the tenth of the Federalist Papers, in which James Madison warned of the dangers of economic "faction" and suggested that the principal task of government was the "regulation of these various and interfering interests."[1] Although the precise issues that concerned Madison have been replaced in the ensuing two centuries by new problems, reflecting a vastly different economy and society, his basic point is still well taken. These new and considerably more complex problems have resulted, in large measure, from the appearance of an economic organization of which he was but remotely aware and whose impact he could not anticipate—the business corporation. As we have seen, by the end of the nineteenth century the nation had become highly industrialized, and the large corporation had emerged as the single most important institution in American society. The hegemony of agriculture had been broken, and the balance of political power was dispersed among diverse business interests.

TWO CONSEQUENCES OF THE RISE OF CORPORATIONS

Closely associated with the emergence of the national and international corporation as the dominant means of conducting economic activity are two other trends that have influenced American political life. These developments are (1) the organizational commitment of the new middle class to the corporation and (2) the growth of the interdependent economy, with the resultant blurring of the distinction between public and private activities.

THE NEW MIDDLE CLASS AND POLITICS

Just as the atomization of economic life that characterized the initial three-quarters of a century of our national existence gave way to the more concentrated industrial scene of the post-Civil War period, so too the multiplicity of individual identifications and affiliations has diminished in a predominantly organizational society. Particularly for the white-collar group[2] (the upper stratum of the segment of the population that C. Wright Mills has designated the "New Middle Class"), the primary focus of personal commitment and identification has been the economic organization to which the individual belongs, rather than the community, the polity, or often even the profession of which he is a member.

The critical importance of the corporation to the life of the individual enhances its political significance in the following way. Since for many upper-level white-collar employees, the fulfillment of personal objectives is inextricably tied up with the accomplishment of corporate objectives, they tend naturally to identify with the policies and goals of the firm, including its political policies and goals. This identification broadens the political base of the corporation.

It is not my intention to overdramatize either the prevalence or the significance of these associated phenomena. There is evidence that managerial identification with the corporation is declining somewhat as executives (particularly younger ones) become (a) more mobile—shifting from one company to another —and (b) better educated and increasingly professionally oriented.[3] Without question, moreover, substantial numbers of white-collar managerial and professional employees still retain extra-corporate affiliations of a meaningful sort and feel no political commitment—and, perhaps, even political hostility—to the firm. The important point, however, is that the development discussed above is still very much apparent and has had the effect of enhancing the political significance of the corporation.

THE BLURRING OF PUBLIC AND PRIVATE IN THE INTERDEPENDENT ECONOMY

The second—and unquestionably the more important—trend is the continued blurring of the distinction between public and private activities that has resulted from the emergence of an interdependent economy. We have seen that many business firms, particularly our largest enterprises, increasingly devote a substantial proportion of their activities to matters of defense, space exploration, the management of governmental installations, and the conduct of scientific research for governmental agencies. Other companies participate in governmental social programs, such as running Job Corps centers and assisting in regional planning and development programs. Still other corporations, as their primary business activities, direct our nation's communications and transportation facilities, operate our utilities, and provide the raw materials and finished products necessary to our national well-being.

Thus the notion of the corporation as a "creature of the state" has now come full circle from the early nineteenth century, although in a profoundly different way. In fulfilling the diverse tasks specified above, the business corporation is, in a real sense, doing the public's work. In this manner, the public interest, as it is manifested in specific governmental policies and programs, becomes the private interest when the corporation serves as the vehicle for the accomplishment of public tasks.

Looking now at the other side of the coin—the projection of governmental authority into areas that previously had been considered sacrosanctly private—we have examined various manifestations of this "intrusion." These include wage and price guidelines, licensing activities, investment restrictions, strategic material and natural resources priorities and a wide range of regulatory provisions, not to mention the commitments undertaken by the federal government to maintain full employment and to assure equal employment opportunities for all Americans.

As a consequence of this two-pronged development, corporate activity is fraught with public policy implications more explicitly than ever before in our nation's history. Indeed, the notion of degrees of publicness and privateness is replacing the traditional public-private dichotomy. The service by corporations as instrumentalities of public policy is, therefore, of great concern to our governmental order. It raises a question of propriety: Should those who carry out public policy also have, through political activities, a significant role in its formulation? In a very imperfect way, this question is reminiscent of the classic issue in public administration concerning the feasibility and desirability of separating politics from administration in the operations of governmental bureaucracy. Analogies from that dispute may be relevant and helpful in analyzing the appropriate role of the corporation as an instrument of governmental policy.

CORPORATIONS AND PUBLIC
BUREAUCRACIES COMPARED

It would, of course, be inaccurate to suggest that the corporation is the exact counterpart of the governmental bureaucracy. The basic theoretical assumptions underlying the two differ fundamentally. We assume that governmental bodies are public and are specifically intended to fulfill the public's business. On the other hand, by tradition, we have assumed that the corporation is a private organization intended to accomplish private purposes and to serve the public only as an indirect consequence of its activities.[4]

Just as the corporation, however, now has "publicness" as one of the aspects of its organizational role as it fulfills the manifold social functions delegated to it, so too does the public bureaucracy have a dimension of "privateness," as it seeks to further organizational policies and objectives in which it has a vested interest. For example, in his study of the Tennessee Valley Authority, Philip Selznick noted the hostility which the TVA encountered during its early days from the Department of Agriculture because the new agency was viewed by the older body as encroaching upon its interests.[5] Similarly, existing agencies that regulated transportation were generally opposed to the establishment of the Department of Transportation in 1966, since the new department would inevitably usurp part of their spheres of influence. Thus, both public agencies and business corporations have their private oxen to gore through the political process. Moreover, political scientists now generally agree that while the public bureaucracy should be primarily instrumental in its operations—fulfilling delegated objectives—it is not a political cipher in the governmental process and has an important political role to play in the formulation of public policy. Similarly, even though it may serve as a vehicle for fulfilling public functions, a corporation retains a private side, which gives it distinct organizational goals and necessities which must be realized through the political process.

As a consequence of these factors, a complete separation between politics and the administration of public tasks is no more possible in the private (corporate) context than it is in the public sphere. Indeed, the history of publicly owned corporations in the United States, Great Britain and Italy—as well as that of the state-controlled enterprises in the Soviet Union—indicates that even direct public ownership does not remove industrial organizations or their managers from the political arena. A comment by Dwight Waldo regarding the politics-administration controversy is particularly apropos to this general point. He observed:

> Like so many grand and simple truths politics-administration tells us nothing so far as particular actions are concerned. *It tells us nothing at all about the organs to which these functions should be assigned, or the desirable relationships among these organs.*[6]

Similarly, the question of the appropriateness of political activity by corporations that serve as public instrumentalities goes to the heart of the relationship between corporations and other social interests and, accordingly, does not lend itself to facile *Yes* or *No* answers. Such corporations have proper and important political roles to play as long as their participation does not impair the openness of our political order and the participation of competing social interests. The same conclusion holds true for the political activities of all other political participants.

Unavoidably, such a position raises anew the issue of the political implications of corporate power. Because this issue is so central to the conclusion that I have reached regarding the appropriateness of business political involvement, I shall at this point recapitulate and place in perspective some previously discussed aspects of power.

CORPORATE POWER REVISITED

We saw that corporations do indeed have political power resulting from their possession of requisite resources and their willingness to utilize those resources available to them, but that no standards exist to measure the quantum of this power. As was emphasized earlier, the critical point is rather that particular corporations, acting either individually or in concert, seek to exercise political power in particular situations, at particular times, over particular persons, groups or institutions, and to varying degrees. As is the case with all other social actors, corporate power is contextual or relational and does not lend itself to definitive categorization in simplistic terms. Accordingly, we are warranted in making only the most general statements concerning the over-all impact of corporate political activities.

Looking first at the relationship between corporations and the various organs of government, we have seen that business firms, like other client groups, have had influence on the policies of agencies and departments charged with their regulation. Indeed, business regulation has been described as a system of intergroup mediation in which the political system has been called upon to "mediate among social groups to maintain both the peace and a rough equity in the relations of men."[7] During periods of our history, this equity may indeed have been quite rough and particular governmental institutions especially supine in the face of private interests. On balance, however, no single group has been able to dominate the multiple points of access to governmental decisions. Business firms have experienced political success, but so too have other social interests including labor, farmers, and, recently, various minority groups. Moreover, it is frequently the case that the success of one corporation constitutes the failure of another in their competition for political favor.

While the above comments have been made primarily in the context of corporate political involvement in the administrative and executive spheres—the primary areas of business political influence—the same observations are appropriate with regard to legislative activities. Notwithstanding hoary stories from bygone days about bought legislatures and kept representatives, the reasoned view is that today "the influence of interest groups in the legislative process depends more on the harmony of values between the group and the legislators than it does on the ability of a group to wield its 'power' either through skillful techniques or presumed electoral influence."[8] Access to and influence with a given legislator are often more a function of accentuating and exploiting the local preoccupations of the legislator than of applying pressure. Interestingly enough, certain legislative enactments are generally—and often erroneously—considered to represent business victories. Taxation expert Stanley S. Surrey reports, for example, that percentage depletion allowances for oil and gas production and the deduction permitted for intangible drilling expenses emerged from legislative compromises and administrative interpretations which "for the most part do not appear to have been planned as special-interest relief."[9] The active (and successful) legislative efforts by the petroleum companies have been applied to retaining these advantages.

There is no direct correlation between the economic power of the corporation and its political power. For example, any suggestion that General Motors is more powerful politically than any other firm because of its position at the head of the *"Fortune* Directory" would stem from an oversimplified view of political dynamics. Similarly, the economic position of GM does not make it paramount over all other social groups and institutions. Were this the case, the National Traffic and Motor Vehicle Safety Act of 1966 would never have become law, given the united opposition of the automobile manufacturers, which in 1966 included three of the nation's five largest companies as ranked by sales.[10]

Although on the level of the individual firm, the line between the political and economic aspects of organizational activity is quite blurred, economic power constitutes merely one of the ingredients important for political effectiveness. On a systemic level, R. M. MacIver has pointed out the intrinsic fallacy in equating economic power with political power, noting:

> Economic power is always prominent. But we cannot simplify the issue and claim with the Marxists that economic power is always primary in capitalistic society and that political power is both its offspring and its servant. For in the first place economic power is multi-centered and is the scene of internecine warfare. . . . Every economic position is relative, every economic gain to one group is a cost from the viewpoint of some other group, and the greater the gain the greater the cost. . . . The second reason why we cannot, even under the reign of capitalism, assign to economic power the simple dominance postulated by Marxian socialism is that economic power cannot be segregated from other forms of social power as though

it operated by itself and sought objectives inherent in its own nature.[11]

The above considerations are not advanced to belittle the importance of economic power, but rather to place it in perspective. In a pluralistic society, the bases and means of power—including economic power—are widely distributed among many social interests. While corporations do indeed possess political power, neither they nor any other class of political participant has achieved hegemony over our political order.

A GUIDELINE FOR CORPORATE POLITICAL ACTIVITIES

Given the pluralistic character of American political life, what guidelines should determine public policy regarding participation by corporations and their managers in the political process? It is my contention that in a democratic society all limitations upon political activities should be judged by the following criterion:

Does the nature and the quality of political participation by any given social interest (whether individual or collective) or combination of interests threaten unduly to deny on a continuing basis to other interests in the society effective access to and potential influence upon foci of governmental decision-making?

Among the questions that readily come to mind when applying this criterion are: What "interests"? Which "foci of governmental decision making"? What amount and quality of "effective" access and influence? When does particular behavior "threaten unduly . . . on a continuing basis"? How and by whom is a violation to be determined?

There can be no completely satisfactory answers to the above inquiries. For years, political scientists have been evaluating the impact of the behavior of political actors, and only now are they beginning to develop techniques of measurement. The question of whether the activities of a particular social interest group violate the above standard must accordingly be determined on a pragmatic case-by-case basis. Limitations should be imposed upon political actors only to the extent necessary to maintain access and potential influence for other social interests that desire to participate in the political decision-making process.

It is unrealistic to expect that the proposed guideline would achieve precise political parity among the many interests present in American society. Political resources and the desire and ability to utilize those resources are never uniformly distributed among political participants. Accordingly, to obtain parity is, as a practical matter, an impossibility. Moreover, the effort to prescribe equal effectiveness for all interests (if such were possible) would be, by the very nature of the undertaking, inherently undemocratic. A basic premise of a democratic society is that competing social interests attempt to achieve a *modus vivendi* through their participation in the political process. This position of equipoise is not to be determined in accordance with any preconceived notion of the proper balance, but by means of the efficacious utilization of available resources by competing social interests.

The point is not that access and influence should be distributed evenly in our society. Rather, the crucial factor is that sufficient political access should exist to permit any given social interest the opportunity to pursue its objectives through a resort to politics. There can be no guarantee that a particular actor will be successful in achieving its political objectives, nor should public policy be pointed toward this end. "The only authentic public concern is to keep the ends of life open and uncongealed, to provide the conditions for, but not the substance of, our various private lives."[12] The continuing possibility, rather than the present ability, of being an effective political actor is the essential characteristic of what Robert A. Dahl terms the "'normal' American political process . . . one in which there is a high probability that an active and legitimate group in the population can make itself heard effectively at some crucial stage in the process of decision."[13]

Virtually all interests in our society possess political access and influence, although the quantity and quality of such access and influence varies substantially. For example, the black American possessed only minimal political access and influence as we entered the post-World War II era; however, there has been a continuous increase in the political efficacy of this group, although the rate of increase has hardly fulfilled the expectations of most blacks and some whites. Another, less obvious, example is the dramatic increase in the scope of political access and the general influence of the professional scientist as a consequence of the all-pervasive impact of science and technology upon American society.

Turning now specifically to the application of the proffered standard to political activities of the business corporation, several observations are in order. Although the political power of business firms and their managers is very real and pervasive, it does not presently constitute a danger to the American pluralistic democracy, which continues to produce legislation, rulings, decisions, and programs that are contrary to the desires of significant corporate interests. For example, in the past few years, Congress has acted to benefit the consumer and to prevent air and water pollution, despite the vigorous opposition of some of the nation's largest companies. Similarly, the National Labor Relations Board continues to incur the ire of business firms by rulings unfavorable to them, while the Federal Trade Commission and the antitrust division of the Department of Justice have achieved victories in proceedings instituted under the various antitrust statutes. Further, much to the consternation of some business managers, the federal courts have not been averse to deciding against the interests of large companies in matters of rate-making and of merger policy.

Even within those governmental areas where corporations have traditionally carved out spheres of influence through "client-control" of executive or administrative agencies, the public interest has not gone unrepresented. Of late, the Food and Drug Administration, the Interstate Commerce Commission and the Securities and Exchange Commission have followed the lead of the Federal Trade Commission in scrutinizing corporate activities far more carefully than in the past.

The critical point is that political effectiveness is not an all-or-nothing proposition, as some critics of corporate political activity would have us believe. While business firms do indeed experience frequent success in the political sphere on given issues, so also they meet with defeat on particular matters. As a class of political participant, corporations possess no monopoly over political access or influence. Even among themselves, they vary dramatically in their political effectiveness as a result of such factors as size, strategic economic position, available resources, ability to utilize these resources, and a host of other variables which were discussed in earlier chapters (particularly Chapters Seven and Eight). Accordingly, there is an inherent difficulty in attempting to formulate accurate generalizations concerning corporate political participation, since the nature and the quality of this participation vary so substantially among business firms.

This same difficulty attaches to efforts to develop a comprehensive public policy governing corporate political involvement. The question is raised, therefore, whether the political activities of corporations and their executives should be subject to statutory restrictions that are not generally applicable to other political participants. In this author's opinion, the answer is clearly No. Since the most important legislative limitation upon corporate politics is in the sphere of electoral politics, it is appropriate to look there first.

FEDERAL STATUTORY LIMITATIONS ON CORPORATE ELECTORAL POLITICS[14]

Current federal legislation dating from the Progressive Era (Section 610 of the United States Criminal Code, popularly known by the former name of the act, of which it is a part, the Federal Corrupt Practices Act) prohibits corporations (and, since 1947, labor organizations) from making a "contribution or expenditure in connection with any [federal] election."[15] Although the enactment of the statute was motivated in part by a desire to protect shareholders from the use of corporate funds by officers and directors for political purposes to which the shareholders had not assented, its primary purpose was to destroy the influence over elections that corporations had exercised through their financial contributions during the late nineteenth and early twentieth centuries. However appropriate the legislation may have been at the time of its enactment in 1907, several reasons compel the conclusion that it should be repealed completely, leaving corporations (and labor organizations) subject only to those provisions regarding the public reporting of contributions and expenditures that apply to other social interests.[16]

THE CONSTITUTIONAL ISSUE

In the first place, as we saw in Chapter Nine, the restrictions of Section 610 against corporations are of questionable constitutional validity. Although the United States Supreme Court has been presented with the constitutional issue in two cases involving labor organizations, it has carefully avoided rendering an opinion on the subject. In both cases, however, a substantial number of justices expressed either grave doubts as to the legality of the legislation or the outright belief that it is in violation of the First Amendment.[17] The net effect of this constitutional uncertainty is that the statute has been suspect in the eyes of both government officials, who have been exceedingly reluctant to institute actions under it—seven reported decisions (two involving corporations) in 61 years—and lower federal courts, which have been quick to discover or create loopholes in the statutory language. Consequently, the likelihood that effective criminal sanctions will be brought to bear against an errant corporation and its officials is so small as to deter practically no one.

INEFFECTIVENESS OF THE RESTRICTIONS

A second ground for eliminating the present restriction is its ineffectiveness in actually preventing corporate campaign contributions and expenditures. As we saw during our discussion of corporate electoral activities, corporate moneys find their way into campaign chests through a variety of direct and indirect means. This ineffectiveness is not unique to the United States. Recently, the specially appointed Canadian Committee on Election Expenses commented that "it is a striking feature of laws concerning election expenses generally that they are widely disobeyed. . . . It may be that direct prohibition of corporate donations is almost unenforceable."[18]

Two factors inherent in the American political process underlie the ineffectiveness of Section 610. The first is that campaign costs have been rising inexorably as a result of the expenses associated with the saturation style of electioneering (including the use of mass media, public opinion polls, and rapid transportation) that now characterizes American campaigning. In 1964, the presidential race alone cost more than $29 million, and the cost of campaigns at all levels that year is estimated at more than $200 million.[19] Consequently, parties and candidates need increased funds and are obliged to seek assistance from sources that have helped in the past. Thus corporations and business executives are constantly called upon to extend largess. This call will continue in the future, until such time as a comprehensive system of financing election campaigns with public moneys is developed that renders obsolete the necessity for private funds. Although an abortive—and not notably well-conceived—beginning was made with the passage of the now-repealed Presidential Election Campaign Fund Act of 1966,[20] public financing of elections still appears to be years off.

The second underlying factor—the need for political access in an interdependent economy—has already been discussed at great length. The critical point is that the political necessities of business encourage corporate financial involvement in electoral campaigns. The selection of governmental officials who are sympathetic to the company's concerns is of considerable importance to every corporation. As we have seen, political donations enhance the access that a firm enjoys. On the other hand, corporations are occasionally subject to dunning by politicians. Even where open and blatant pressure is not present, companies recognize the wisdom of ingratiating themselves with officials who make decisions of great consequence to business.

Accordingly, corporations will continue to make contributions until candidates and parties neither want nor need contributions from private sources. This eventuality is not likely to occur in the foreseeable future.

CHANGE IN CORPORATE ELECTORAL BEHAVIOR IS UNLIKELY

Third, although the danger of a flood from corporate financial sluices is always present if current prohibitions are removed, in light of the fact that corporate moneys already find their way into the political financial stream in substantial amounts, the advent of "wide-open" activity would not, in all likelihood, basically alter the existing level of electoral involvement. Most companies would not substitute overt political activity for existing *sub rosa* methods for fear of offending customers, employees, shareholders, organized labor, and others who deal with them. Also, government officials might be prompted to respond to overt corporate involvement with undesired rulings, regulations, legislation, or litigation. Moreover, political fund-raising groups are likely to eschew contributions from corporate sources, which would have to be reported publicly, for fear of appearing to be subject to business domination. There is virtually no evidence of excessive corporate financial involvement in those states where corporate electoral contributions and expenditures are not prohibited by law in state and local elections.

A related factor suggesting the unlikelihood of a change in corporate electoral behavior is that the "public-be-damned" attitude, which characterized some business leaders of the past, has been replaced, in large measure, by a desire to affect and even to effect social responsibility. Basically, this change in approach reflects a desire by business managers to preserve their autonomy by accommodating to public expectations. Excessive or heavy-handed political activity could incur public ire and, in the extreme instance, pervasive governmental restrictions, an effect diametrically opposite to corporate intentions.

Despite historical and cultural variations, experience of

other countries with corporate political contributions is illuminating. Spending by big business (and big labor) in Great Britain has been termed "quite tolerable."[21] Following the repeal of prohibitory legislation in 1930, politics in Canada did not come under the domination of corporate interests. Indeed the 1907 Canadian statute, which was modeled after the American act, was recently called by the Committee on Election Expenses "the most ridiculous chapter in an uninspiring story of ineffective legislation."[22] Regulatory efforts appear to be virtually confined to the United States. Great Britain, Australia, Israel, Norway, Italy, the Philippines, Sweden, the Netherlands, and Japan all permit corporations to make political contributions. Yet, in a number of these countries, despite the lack of prohibitions, companies still prefer to contribute secretly in order to avoid possible unfavorable public reaction.[23] Accordingly, although one can never predict the future with certainty, it is quite unlikely that most American firms would appreciably alter their present behavior if Section 610 were repealed. As a practical matter, the primary effect of the repeal of Section 610 would likely be that requests (or demands) by candidates for assistance would be directed to the firm itself, rather than to the individual managers.

POLICY INCONGRUITIES

A fourth reason that the retention of Section 610 is undesirable is the section's basic incongruity with other aspects of federal regulatory policy. For example, a corporation (or any other interest group) can make expenditures to influence legislation without violating the Federal Regulation of Lobbying Act of 1946.[24] The same corporation may not, however, actively support the campaign of a candidate who favors such legislation. Yet, as we have seen, it is basic to the effectiveness of any social-interest group to be able to promote the election of representatives who are sympathetic to the group's legislative goals. There is little reason for upholding an exclusionary policy in the case of electoral politics while recognizing the propriety of corporate involvement in the governmental sphere.

ANACHRONISTIC POLICY BASES

Finally, the present statutory prohibition should be eliminated because it rests upon two anachronistic policy bases: (1) the protection of the interests of the shareholders and (2) the maintenance of the purity of elections, free from corporate financial dominance. These policies were pertinent to the situation at the turn of the twentieth century, when corporate electoral activity was characterized by certain excesses. Since the appropriate role of the shareholder was extensively discussed in the examination of the internal legitimacy of corporate political activities in Chapter Nine, this issue need not be reexamined. Suffice it to say that protection of the shareholder is not an appropriate ground for retention of Section 610.

Concerning the second policy basis underlying the section —elimination of corporate moneys from elections—the necessary refutations have already been made in this chapter. Historically, Section 610 has been virtually ineffective in preventing corporate campaign contributions and expenditures, and it is highly improbable that business firms would change their present electoral practices if the prohibition were eliminated.

In summation, Section 610 makes inappropriate distinctions, in terms of both the political legitimacy of the corporation and its impact upon democratic pluralism in this country, between the political activities of corporations (and labor organizations) and those of other social-interest groups that are not covered by the statute. There is, accordingly, little justification for retaining the provision.

A PROPOSAL FOR REMOVAL OF CURRENT CORPORATE ELECTORAL RESTRICTIONS

The elimination of Section 610, which was proposed in the preceding section, should be accompanied by new legislation requiring corporate contributions and expenditures—and those of all other individuals and groups—to be reported to a designated national governmental agency (such as the recently proposed Federal Elections Commission)[25] and to a designated local agency (such as the Clerk of the United States District Court or the office of the Secretary of Commonwealth or State) in the area where the funds were received or used in connection with an election. Such legislation would have the advantage of subjecting corporate political support—along with all other contributions—"to the white light of public scrutiny."[26] Though corporations should be entitled to participate fully in electoral politics, the public has the right to be informed about such participation.

The legislation would offer several additional benefits both to the corporation and to the political process. First, it would eliminate the constitutional ambiguities surrounding the current restrictions. Second, it would comport with political reality by recognizing that corporations function in a political environment and, accordingly, have needs and objectives that require them to be political actors irrespective of existing restrictions. The taint of illegality surrounding corporate electoral activities would be eliminated and corporations would be placed legally where they belong—on a par with other social interests. A third and related benefit would result from the fact that corporate managers would no longer be thrust into the position of knowingly violating legislation that they consider inconsistent with the realities of both business and political life. Such knowing violations of legal restrictions foster in many executives cynicism regarding the political process, as well as a general disrespect for the law.

In the event that most corporations did alter their political behavior by publicly reporting their campaign contributions and expenditures, a fourth advantage would result. The electorate would be informed of the extent to which parties, candidates, and issues are backed by particular business interests—just as they would be similarly informed of the activities of labor, agricultural, and other social groups which provide electoral support to candidates and parties. To the extent that this information would be available, voters would be in a better position to make their electoral decisions. Even if corporations continue to conduct their electoral activities covertly, the proposed elimination of existing restrictions would not aggravate the existing political climate or adversely affect the interests of other political participants. Political fund-raisers now obtain corporate moneys in substantial sums, while the electorate remains largely unaware of both the sources and the amounts. In short, whether corporations report or not, the situation would not be worse than it is with Section 610 in effect. If, indeed, business firms do report their contributions, this is a substantial improvement over the present situation. Accordingly, there is little to lose and much to gain by a repeal of this anachronistic provision.

SOME ALTERNATIVE PROPOSALS

However much the outright repeal of Section 610 might logically commend itself, several factors render such repeal an impossibility at the present time. In the first place, many members of Congress consider the section such an article of faith with the electorate that, notwithstanding their personal misgivings concerning both the wisdom and the efficacy of the provision, they dare not take the political risk of publicly supporting its repeal. Second, pure expediency on the part of those benefiting from the legislation contributes to congressional inactivity. The existence of the statute permits certain elected officials and corporate contributors to conduct their activities under the pretext that effective legislation has eliminated corporate moneys from election financing. A public sense of security is thereby generated by the mere existence of the section. At the same time, since the restriction poses little practical difficulty for either contributor or recipient, those benefiting from the arrangement have little incentive to rock the boat. Finally, there is the psychological unwillingness, for largely historical reasons, on the part of some members of the public to equate the political activities of General Motors (or the United Auto Workers) with the activities of the American Medical Association or the Veterans of Foreign Wars.

Unfortunately, therefore, the best that can be hoped for at this time by way of reform of Section 610 is the passage of legislation modifying the coverage of the provision. Several alternatives are available, each of which would be a distinct improvement over the present statutory arrangement. It should be noted that the first two suggestions are equally applicable to the electoral activities of labor organizations and other group interests.

1. Direct corporate contributions to candidates or political committees could be legalized, but limited to an aggregate sum (for example, $100,000) or, alternatively, as in India, to a maximum based on a designated percentage of company assets.[27] Likewise, Congress could impose limits on company contributions to individual candidates or groups. As suggested in the preceding section, the corporation would be required to report such contributions both nationally and locally. Although there are obvious drawbacks to any limitations or ceilings on contributions, it is still preferable to designate a certain amount as legal, rather than to prohibit all contributions.

Contributions in kind—such as the assignment or donation of advertising space or media time to parties and the loan of company premises or personnel for partisan purposes—would also be permitted, subject to the dollar limitations and reporting requirements suggested above. The monetary value of such contributions would be based on the fair market value of the goods or services provided.

2. Corporations could be permitted to make direct expenditures for the purpose of publicizing the firm's position on candidates for federal office by means of the mass media and distribution of literature to the general public. All such expenditures would be subject to national and local reporting requirements, as well as to the dollar limitations discussed under Proposal 1. Moreover, any advertising sponsored or materials distributed by the corporation would have to be prominently designated as a "Paid Political Advertisement," with the name of the company clearly indicated. While this proposal could result in the further proliferation of already voluminous political advertising, such a consequence is preferable to maintaining the current obfuscation of the sources of significant amounts of campaign literature. Moreover, this proposal would eliminate a number of constitutional problems that surround the present ban.

3. As a third alternative, a distinction could be made in

the present Section 610 between the political activities of large, publicly owned firms possessing tens of thousands of shareholders and assets running into the billions of dollars and those of small closely held firms with but a few stockholders and limited financial resources. The latter are in essence merely the legal shells within which owner-managers conduct their operations. This distinction is not novel in the law, since corporations have been differentiated by size for certain purposes, including taxation and securities regulation. Increasingly, "in America today there is developing some recognition that a closely held concern may in fact function upon an entirely different basis than a public corporation."[28] Corporations could be distinguished by such criteria as total assets, number of shareholders, and the distribution of equity interest among the stockholders. If it is corporate size and wealth that are so greatly to be feared, there is little reason to subject an incorporated neighborhood food market to the same restrictions as General Electric or Standard Oil of New Jersey. This proposal might, however, be subject to constitutional challenge on the ground that it provides for an arbitrary—and hence, illegal—pattern of classification among corporations.

None of these suggestions offers a panacea for the problem of secrecy surrounding corporate moneys in election campaigns. Indeed, as has been suggested, either outright repeal or modification of Section 610 might effect no alteration in current corporate practices. However, in comparison with the current situation, such repeal or modification would encourage open contributions and expenditures, so that, to some degree at least, the electorate might be informed of the origins, extensiveness, and beneficiaries of corporate campaign moneys. Equally important, alteration of the statutory status quo would effect recognition of the fact that corporations have a legitimate interest in the electoral process which they should legally be permitted to pursue.

If the object of public policy regarding campaign financing is to maintain the integrity of elections, either public financing or the attainment of a broad base of electoral financial support is a more important goal than outlawing contributions and expenditures by corporations, labor unions, or other large contributors. These financing alternatives would reduce the overall dependence of parties and candidates on any particular private source of funds and would lessen the likelihood of large donors exercising a disproportionate degree of political influence.

PUBLIC POLICY TOWARD CORPORATE GOVERNMENTAL POLITICS

Turning now to an examination of an appropriate public policy toward corporate political involvement of a general governmental character, little modification of current public policy is necessary, since restrictions on the day-to-day activities of corporations are virtually nonexistent. The Federal Regulation of Lobbying Act of 1946[29] does not require corporations either to register or to report expenditures that they make for the purpose of directly influencing legislation. A Senate committee investigating political activities, lobbying and campaign contributions reported that

> a corporation or other group can spend several million dollars to obtain passage of legislation, designed solely to line its own pockets, and yet does not have to furnish Congress with any information concerning its activities, providing it spends its own money.[30]

Moreover, the Lobbying Act is applicable only to efforts to influence legislation through direct communication with members of Congress, in instances where the lobbying group has obtained money for the "principal purpose" of influencing such legislation. Corporations, accordingly, are not required to register under the provisions of the act, nor are their employees, except those who devote substantially all their time to attempting to influence legislation by direct communication. Consequently, only a handful of firms register representatives.

Similarly, few corporations report making expenditures for

lobbying purposes. For example, despite extensive legislative involvement by corporations during 1967, individual firms constitute less than 5 per cent of the 146 business groups that reported expenditures for lobbying activities.[31] In 1964, less than 10 per cent of business groups reporting lobbying expenditures were corporations.[32] Of even greater interest, although the debate over automobile safety raged during 1966 and involved strenuous efforts by the automobile industry to block legislation, none of the Big Three automobile makers reported expenditures for lobbying activities during the year.[33]

Despite the many shortcomings in the reporting requirements of the present Lobbying Act, since its passage the public has had available more comprehensive data concerning the political activities of corporations and other interest groups attempting to influence Congress than during any other period in our national history.

Efforts to strengthen the Lobbying Act have consistently failed. One such measure, the Legislative Activities Disclosure Act of 1957,[34] provided that an officer or employee of a business firm who devoted the major portion of his time to the regular business of the firm must nevertheless report even occasional direct contacts with Congress if he received $300 or more as compensation or expenses (exclusive of personal travel expenses) for the purpose of influencing legislation by means of such direct communication. Presumably such a provision would have applied to corporate Washington representatives maintained by a number of companies. The bill went beyond congressional lobbying to encompass under its provisions direct communications with any agency or department of the executive branch. This measure was intended to correct the fact that the Lobbying Act does not apply to efforts to influence Congress by having administrative agencies come to Congress asking legislative action on behalf of a "client." The modification would not, however, have brought within the coverage of the Lobbying Act those lobbying activities that are intended solely to obtain a favorable administrative decision from an executive agency. In this context, it should be pointed out that while selected classes of corporations (for example, public utilities) and their representatives who are engaged in lobbying activities are required to register with a number of administrative agencies (such as the Securities and Exchange Commission, the Federal Power Commission, and the Department of Commerce), there is no comprehensive legislation requiring firms to register with or to report their lobbying expenditures to regulatory bodies or executive departments.

In 1967, another serious effort was made to amend the Lobbying Act. Key sections of the measure—Title V of the Legislative Reorganization Act of 1967—(1) required registration of persons who solicit or receive money "a substantial part of which is to be used to aid, or a substantial purpose of which person is to aid" in obtaining the passage or defeat of legislation; (2) provided that where contributions were received or expenditures made in part for lobbying purposes and in part for other purposes, persons or organizations filing financial statements were to indicate the portion of funds devoted to lobbying purposes and "if the relative proportions cannot be ascertained with reasonable certainty," such statements were to indicate total receipts and expenditures together with an estimate of the percentage allocable to lobbying; and (3) specified that the office of the Comptroller General was to administrate the provisions of the Lobbying Act, and to refer to the Justice Department for appropriate action all violations of the Act.[35] The "substantial purpose" provision was designed to broaden the scope of applicability of the Lobbying Act, while the estimating provision was intended to close the loophole which permitted persons to avoid reporting by claiming that they could not calculate precisely the amount received for lobbying. Although the measure handily passed the Senate, it was never reported out of the House Rules Committee.[36]

Accordingly, corporations are virtually unrestricted in their government activities. Indeed, in the omnibus tax bill of 1962, Congress permitted businesses to deduct from their federal income tax expenditures incurred in connection with appearances before or communications to committees and members of Congress or other legislative bodies with respect to legislation or proposed legislation of "direct interest" to the taxpayer.[37] Expenses intended to influence the general public regarding legislation are not deductible however.

REGISTRATION AND REPORTING DESIRABLE

In keeping with the suggestions made in the preceding section dealing with statutory restrictions of corporate electoral activities, one further modification of current lobbying policy seems appropriate. Although firms should not be subjected to special prohibitions, it is advisable that they—and other social-interest groups—be required to register under the Lobbying Act if they seek to influence the passage or defeat of any legislation before Congress, even though they utilize their own funds and are represented solely by corporate employees. While such registration requirements would apply to company employees and representatives whose regular sphere of activities includes contacts with governmental units, they would not encompass an official who merely appears infrequently as a witness before or has an occasional meeting with a public agency. For example, a corporate executive would not be required to register unless, over the course of a year, the value of his time allocable to governmental appearances exceeds a specified amount, say $1,000. Similarly, all expenditures made by corporations (and other social interests) to influence the passage or defeat of legislation —even expenditures for so-called informational or educational purposes—should be reported if the amount within a year exceeds a sum specified by Congress, say $500. To remedy the current virtual nonenforcment of the Lobbying Act, an independent governmental agency, such as the office of the Comptroller General, should be given the responsibility of insuring compliance with the legislation.

COVERAGE OF ADMINISTRATIVE AND EXECUTIVE LOBBYING

Lobbying activities before administrative agencies and executive departments to secure the passage or defeat of rulings or the award of contracts, franchises, or licenses should be subject to these proposed regulations under an amended Lobbying Act. This proposal is reinforced by the conclusion of a number of students of American politics that the political impact of corporations and other social interests is maximal in the executive and administrative spheres. As in the case of lobbying activities before Congress, the registration of company representatives and the reporting of corporate expenditures connected with administrative and executive lobbying would constitute a sound approach to the problem.

Although the effectiveness of current registration and publicity statutes has been the subject of much justifiable criticism, V. O. Key, Jr., has observed that "so mild a requirement [for lobbyists to file financial reports that are available for public inspection] may be of more significance than might be supposed, if one judges from the dodges employed to evade it."[38] If nothing else, the above proposals would have the effect of better informing the public of the interests of corporations and other social groups in legislative, administrative, and executive decisions, and contributing, thereby, to the maintenance of our pluralistic system. Once again, there is little to lose and much to gain from their adoption.

It is interesting to note that there is generally little difficulty identifying corporate "judicial lobbyists" because of the requirement that parties to a litigation or those seeking to appear before the court in an *amicus* capacity file their appearance with the relevant court, so that their activity then becomes a matter of record. Occasionally, however, corporations involved in judicial proceedings may be concealed from public view by their use of a straw party or surrogate whose connection with the firm is not publicly known. The occasional use of this subterfuge by corporations and other social interests has not posed a serious problem because of the public and adversary nature of the legal process.

PROPOSALS TO GOVERN ALL
SOCIAL-INTEREST GROUPS

The above proposals, which would require corporations to register their political representatives and to report publicly their expenditures and contributions for both governmental and electoral political activities, should not be viewed as a derogation from the author's basic thesis that, at the present time, corporations should not be subject to special restrictions limiting the nature or extent of their political involvement. Indeed, the crucial point is that the requirements should be applicable to *all* associational political participants (including labor unions, agricultural associations, professional societies, consumer organizations, and other interest groups), except for those activities which are of an incidental character. This proposal permits social interests complete freedom as political participants, while at the same time guaranteeing, to the greatest extent possible, that the public is aware of their activities. Moreover, it would seem that the suggested registration and reporting requirements do not violate the freedoms guaranteed by the First Amendment —freedom to speak, publish, and petition the government, and freedom of association.

The requirements would not have the effect of inhibiting or harassing social interests that desire to influence public policy. For example, they do not require that shareholder, employee, or membership lists be disclosed, thereby possibly exposing persons on such lists to economic, social, or political pressure.[39] Rather, the requirements are designed to apprise other groups and individuals within our society of any efforts to affect important governmental decisions, thus giving to these other social interests an opportunity to assert their positions before public bodies. The net result of the proposal would be to increase the openness of our political system and to enhance the quality of American pluralism.

Except for the registration of company representatives and the reporting of corporate political expenditures, no further restrictions should be imposed on corporate governmental activities. Although frequent comment has been made in this book concerning the high degree of political effectiveness of business firms within certain governmental bodies, no restrictions should be placed on such activities. Rather than by limiting the involvement of corporations, the protection of other social groups can better be insured by (1) requiring the appointment of their representatives to the myriad of governmental advisory boards and committees that are now heavily populated by business executives; and (2) requiring public officials to consult with them prior to making any decision that affects their interests. Where no particular group or groups appear to be the obvious representatives of opposing social interests, the governmental body should be obligated to consult with individuals from a broad spectrum of private life in order to assure a wide range of opinion on important questions of public policy. The "closed politics" which has characterized much of the administrative decision-making in the past would thereby be reduced and the influence of any particular social interest minimized.

The above policy recommendations pertaining to corporate governmental activities are made—just as were the proposals relating to electoral politics—in light of existing political conditions. They do not constitute guidelines that are invariable in time and circumstance. While it is not likely to be the case, if these policies should threaten to interfere with the political access and potential influence of other social interests in a manner inconsistent with the formula suggested earlier in this chapter, then additional restrictions upon corporate activities, consistent with constitutional safeguards, could be developed to safeguard these interests. At the present time, however, such restrictions are unnecessary.

CORPORATE MANAGERS AND POLITICS

There is little danger that the public will be overwhelmed by the businessman-politician. The *Harvard Business Review* studies mentioned in Chapters Five and Eight clearly demonstrate that the absolute level of personal political involvement by businessmen is low.[40] Only a small percentage of managers were what might be called political activists and even these came primarily from smaller companies rather than from large national firms. As already mentioned, moreover, political apathy generally characterizes the corporate middle class, political education programs notwithstanding. Accordingly, it is likely that, rather than becoming a widespread undertaking among businessmen, business political activity will remain the province of a few high-level specialists and top leaders within the corporation who are concerned with organizational objectives.

NO LIMITATIONS ON MANAGERS ARE NECESSARY

On occasion, the question has been raised whether corporate leaders, particularly those of large enterprises intimately involved with areas of public concern—primarily defense contractors and transportation and communication carriers—should be restricted from any political activities, with the exception of the minimal rights of voting, partisan affiliation, and personal free speech. Underlying this inquiry is the contention that, as Adolf A. Berle, Jr., has maintained in another context, corporate managers "are in the same boat with public office-holders."[41] Because of this characterization, it has been suggested that executives should be subject to limitations similar to those found in the federal Hatch Act and in comparable state laws that preclude civil servants from certain forms of partisan political involvement.[42]

Needless to say, any singling out of corporate managers for political prohibitions is fraught with constitutional dangers, although the history of the Hatch Act might possibly provide the necessary precedents. As a matter of policy, however, such limitations would be justified only if political activity by corporate officials threatened to impair the political access and potential influence of other interests and thereby to render political institutions supine to corporate desires. Such domination has not occurred and is only remotely possible in contemporary American politics. Accordingly, any special limitations on the electoral activities of corporate managers are unjustifiable. Similarly, no restrictions on the governmental involvement of individual business leaders is appropriate, except for the registration requirements already discussed. Such involvement is proper and indeed quite necessary in our interdependent economy.

A final point warrants mention. Despite this interdependence, corporate managers have, in the past, often assumed a negative posture toward the activities of government and the operation of the political process. A basic lack of understanding and a distrust of democratic pluralism has led some businessmen to view politics as the province of fools and knaves. Combined with a dislike for governmental involvement in areas considered to be private, this distrust has occasionally been coupled with a peculiar myopia which has prevented managers from identifying their own activities as political in nature or from admitting that their firms had needs and goals that could be realized only through political participation. As a consequence, businessmen were sometimes in the anomalous position of arguing that political activity was either (1) to be avoided at all costs or (2) to be undertaken in order to save the American System. Neither posture is tenable or desirable.

Regarding the first position, business firms are and must continue to be active political participants because their daily activities bring them into contact with all levels of government and with the competing claims of other social interests. In the words of Hans F. Morgenthau, "We are in the presence of a revival of a truly political economy, whose major economic problems are political in nature."[43] Pursuit of the firm's interests through the political process should, therefore, be viewed by managers as a necessary organizational activity, which they are willing to acknowledge and for which they are willing to assume public responsibility. For example, while one may question from a policy viewpoint the wisdom of General Motors' stance on auto-safety legislation, GM needs no excuse to use regular political processes to defeat measures that it views as inimical to its organizational interests. Company officials must recognize, however, that their efforts to prevent such legislation involve them in politics and unavoidably may engender criticism of the firm.

A CALL FOR A POSITIVE VIEW OF POLITICS

Concerning the second position, a factor that will be of importance in determining the propriety of future political involvement by corporations and their managers is the frame of reference within which companies conduct their political activities. If political participation by business firms is undertaken solely with a narrow conception of company interest which fails to recognize that there are many legitimate viewpoints concerning the nature of the public interest in American society, then corporate political activity will of necessity have a negative quality. Similarly, if business managers undertake political involvement to bring the governmental process—together with other political participants—to heel, then corporate political activity will constitute a distinct danger to a democratic society.

If, however, corporate executives regard political participation in a positive way as (1) a necessary, appropriate, but limited organizational activity intended merely to enhance the ability of the corporation to accomplish its primary functions of fulfilling the economic and social needs and expectations of American society and (2) an activity that must always be carried out in accordance with the norms of a pluralistic democracy, then corporate political involvement offers little to be feared and should be viewed in the same light as the political participation of any other legitimate interest.

Fortunately, as mentioned earlier, there is reason to believe that this positive and, in the author's view, much more realistic perspective on political activity is prevailing among corporate leaders of our largest and most politically significant enterprises. This change in perspective has resulted both from personal experience with the governmental process and from a heightened sensitivity to the expectations of other social interests. This sensitivity arises from the very character of our socioeconomic order, which is requiring business managers to view the activities of their firms within a broad social context.

CORPORATE POLITICAL PARTICIPATION: A NECESSARY ASPECT OF AMERICAN PLURALISM

By its very nature, the maintenance of an open political system is an exceedingly delicate process. As Pendleton Herring has stated:

The faith of democracy, for all its shibboleths and hypocrisies, is still based on the fundamental tenet that society can continue peacefully even though men agree to disagree. Out of this one attitude we may be able to make the continuing adjustments to each other and to our environment that are inevitable in any social process but which have seldom been accomplished in the past through methods short of violence.[44]

As a part of these "continuing adjustments" to our environment must come a modification of the traditional concepts of political participation, including a reappraisal of the political role of the corporation. Such a reappraisal should result in the explicit recognition that the corporation is a necessary and legitimate participant in the political process—a participant that, together with other social interests, contributes to the maintenance of pluralistic democracy in America rather than endangers it.

NOTES

[1]James Madison, "The Federalist, No. 10" in Alexander Hamilton, James Madison, and John Jay, *The Federalist Papers* (New York: New American Library of World Literature, Inc., 1961), p. 79.

[2]See C. Wright Mills, *White Collar* (Fair Lawn, N.J.: Oxford University Press, Inc., 1956), pp. 63–76.

[3]See, for example, Eugene E. Jennings, *The Mobile Manager: A Study of the New Generation of Top Executives* (Ann Arbor, Michigan: University of Michigan, 1967), and Robert C. Albrook, "Why It's Harder to Keep Good Executives," *Fortune*, LXXVIII, No. 6 (November 1968), 136.

[4]For an analysis of the blurring distinction between "public" and "private," see Robert A. Dahl and Charles E. Lindblom, *Politics, Economics, and Welfare: Planning and Politico-Economic Systems Resolved into Basic Social Processes* (New York: Torchbooks, Harper & Row, Publishers, 1963), pp. 3–54.

[5]Philip Selznick, *TVA and the Grass Roots* (New York: Torchbooks, Harper & Row, Publishers, 1966), pp. 47–82.

⁶Dwight Waldo, *The Administrative State* (New York: The Ronald Press Co., 1948), p. 115.

⁷V. O. Key, Jr., *Politics, Parties, and Pressure Groups*, 5th ed. New York: Thomas Y. Crowell Co., 1964), p. 76.

⁸Harmon Zeigler, *Interest Groups in American Society* (Englewood Cliffs, N.J.: Prentice-Hall, Inc., 1964), p. 274.

⁹Stanley S. Surrey, "The Congress and the Tax Lobbyist—How Special Provisions Get Enacted," *Harvard Law Review*, LXX, No. 7 (May 1957), 1152.

¹⁰"The *Fortune* Directory—The 500 Largest U.S. Industrial Corporations," *Fortune*, LXXV, No. 7 (June 15, 1967), 196–97.

¹¹R. M. MacIver, *The Web of Government*, rev. ed. (New York: The Free Press, 1965), pp. 68–69. Copyright R. M. MacIver 1965.

¹²Henry S. Kariel, "The Corporation and the Public Interest," *Annals of the American Academy of Political and Social Science*, CCCXLIII (September 1962), 44.

¹³Robert A. Dahl, *A Preface to Democratic Theory* (Chicago: Phoenix Books, The University of Chicago Press, 1956), p. 145.

¹⁴This section is drawn from Edwin M. Epstein, *Corporations, Contributions and Political Campaigns: Federal Regulation in Perspective* (Berkeley: Institute of Governmental Studies, University of California, 1968). For additional discussion of many of the points raised here, see the above-cited publication.

¹⁵18 U.S.C. § 610 (1951). The Public Utility Holding Company Act of 1935, 15 U.S.C. § 79 (*1*) (h) (1935), similarly prohibits holding companies or their subsidiaries from making contributions.

¹⁶See 2 U.S.C. § 244 (1925); 18 U.S.C. § 608 (1948); and 18 U.S.C. § 612 (1950).

¹⁷See concurring opinion in *United States* v. *Congress of Industrial Organizations*, 335 U.S. 106, 129 (1948), *affirming*, 77 F.Supp. 355 (D.D.C. 1948); and dissenting opinion in *United States* v. *International Union United Automobile, Aircraft and Agricultural Implement Workers of America (UAW-CIO)*, 352 U.S. 567, 593 (1957), *reversing*, 138 F.Supp. 53 (E.D. Mich. 1956). In a recent Court of Appeals decision the court refused to determine the constitutionality of the section as it applies to corporations. See *United States* v. *Lewis Food Company*, 366 F.2d 710 (9th Cir. 1966). For discussions of the constitutional aspects of the problem, see, for example, Donald B. King, "Corporate Political Spending and the First Amendment,"

University of Pittsburgh Law Review, XXIII, No. 4 (June 1962), 847–79; Jeremiah D. Lambert, "Corporate Political Spending and Campaign Finance," *New York University Law Review*, XL (December 1965), 1033–78; Vincent P. Haley, "Limitations on Political Activities of Corporations," *Villanova Law Review*, IX, No. 4 (Summer 1964), 593–618; Comment, "Constitutionality of Section 610 of the Federal Corrupt Practices Act," *California Law Review*, XLVI, No. 3 (August 1958), 439–46; Comment, "Corporate Political Affairs Programs," *Yale Law Journal*, LXX, No. 5 (April 1961), 821–62; and Note, "Statutory Regulation of Political Campaign Funds," *Harvard Law Review*, LXVI, No. 7 (May 1953), 1259–73.

[18]*Report of the Committee on Election Expenses* (Ottawa, Canada: Queen's Printer and Controller of Stationery, 1966), pp. 28, 93.

[19]Herbert E. Alexander, *Financing the 1964 Election* (Princeton, N.J.: Citizen's Research Foundation, 1966), pp. 8, 13.

[20]Int. Rev. Code of 1954, § 6096.

[21]Frank C. Newman, "Money and Elections Law in Britain—Guide for America?" *Western Political Quarterly*, X, No. 3 (September 1957), 602.

[22]*Report of the Committee* . . . , p. 18.

[23]Foreign experience is discussed in a series of articles in Richard Rose and Arnold J. Heidenheimer (eds.), "Comparative Studies in Political Finance," *Journal of Politics*, XXV, No. 4 (November 1963), 643–811.

[24]2 U.S.C. §§ 261–270 (1946).

[25]See H.R. 18162, 89th Cong., 2d Sess. (1966); H.R. 11233, 90th Cong., 1st Sess. (1967); and S. 596, 90th Cong., 1st Sess. (1967).

[26]Louise Overacker, *Presidential Campaign Funds* (Boston: Boston University Press, 1946), p. 70.

[27]For a discussion of the Indian approach, see A. H. Somjee and G. Somjee, "India," in Rose and Heidenheimer (eds.), "Comparative Studies . . . ," pp. 686–702, esp. pp. 686, 694–95.

[28]Ralph J. Baker and William L. Cary, *Cases and Materials on Corporations*, 3d ed., unabridged (Brooklyn: Foundation Press, Inc., 1959), p. 250.

[29]2 U.S.C. §§ 261–270 (1946).

[30]*Report No. 395: Final Report . . . Pursuant to S. Res. 219 of*

the 84th Congress, as extended by S. Res. 47 and S. Res. 128 of the
85th Congress, U.S. Congress, Senate, Special Committee to Investigate Political Activities, Lobbying, and Campaign Contributions, 85th
Cong., 1st Sess. (Washington, D.C.: U.S. Government Printing Office,
1957), p. 69.

[31]*Legislators and the Lobbyists*, 2d ed. (Washington, D.C.:
Congressional Quarterly Inc., 1968), pp. 41–42.

[32]*Legislators and the Lobbyists* (Washington, D.C.: Congressional Quarterly Inc., 1965), pp. 44–46.

[33]See Congressional Quarterly Incorporated, *Weekly Report*,
XXV, No. 27 (July 7, 1967), pp. 1161–68.

[34]S. 2191, 85th Cong., 1st Sess. (1957). For a discussion of
the proposed act, see Belle Zeller, "Regulation of Pressure Groups and
Lobbyists," *Annals*, CCCXIX (September 1958), 101–3; and *Report
No. 395* . . . (Senate, Special Committee . . .), pp. 96–105.

[35]S.335, 90th Cong., 1st Sess. (1967). See also, U.S. Congress,
Senate, Special Committee on the organization of the Congress, 90th
Cong., 1st Sess. (Washington, D.C.: U.S. Government Printing Office,
1967), pp. 53–55.

[36]For a detailed legislative history of the measure, see *Legislators and Lobbyists*, 2d ed., pp. 18–19.

[37]Int. Rev. Code of 1954, § 162(e).

[38]Key, *Politics, Parties, and* . . . , p. 151.

[39]Such pressure was applied, for example, against the National
Association for the Advancement of Colored People (NAACP) by a
number of southern states during the late 1950's. The United States
Supreme Court ruled, however, that private membership lists were
protected by the First Amendment from public disclosure. See, for
example, *NAACP* v. *Alabama ex rel. Patterson*, 357 U.S. 449 (1958).

[40]Stephen A. Greyser, "Business and Politics (Problems in Review), 1964," *Harvard Business Review*, XLII, No. 5 (September-
October 1964), 22–32a, 177–86; and "Business and Politics, 1968
(Special Report)," *Harvard Business Review*, XLVI, No. 6 (November-December, 1968), 4–12, 184–88.

[41]Adolf A. Berle, Jr., *The 20th Century Capitalist Revolution*
(New York: Harcourt, Brace & World, Inc., 1954), p. 60.

[42]The Hatch Act provisions are found at 18 U.S.C. 594–605
(1958) and 5 U.S.C. 118i–118n (1958).

[43]Hans F. Morgenthau, quoted in Robert F. Lenhart and Karl

Schriftgiesser, "Management in Politics," *Annals,* CCCXIX (September 1958), 33.

[44]Pendleton Herring, *The Politics of Democracy* (New York: W. W. Norton & Company, Inc., Publishers, 1965), pp. 432–33.

Appendix

Since there is a conspicuous lack of empirical studies pertaining to the business corporation and the political process, there are many opportunities for original research in this field. I have set forth below a number of questions that currently interest me in hopes of attracting fellow toilers to the vineyards. This listing is merely illustrative and thus hardly inclusive of all the available subjects. Topics are not listed in any order of research priority but are classified in two main categories for purposes of convenience. For additional suggestions, see Robert A. Dahl's essay in *Social Science Research on Business: Product and Potential*.[1]

INTRACORPORATE POLITICAL ORGANIZATION

1. What is the role of corporate public affairs and governmental relations departments? Who are

the personnel and what are the responsibilities, objectives, organizational prestige, and perceived effectiveness of such departments?

2. What role, if any, do business corporations play in the political socialization of corporate employees? Is there a discernible shift in employee political attitudes as a consequence of corporate affiliation?

3. What impact, if any, do corporate political education programs have in stimulating political participation by corporate employees?

4. How and by whom are the nature, extent, and direction of corporate political activities determined? What are the relevant factors in arriving at such decisions?

5. What variables are critical in determining the nature and amount of corporate resources that are devoted to political activities?

6. What are the attitudes of nonmanagerial employees regarding the political participation of their firms? Are such employees subject to political "coercion" by corporate superiors?

7. What are the views of shareholders concerning corporate political activities? What distinctions, if any, do shareholders make between corporate electoral and governmental activities?

POLITICAL ATTITUDES AND BEHAVIOR OF CORPORATE MANAGERS AND THEIR FIRMS

8. What do top corporate managers consider to be the political role of the corporation (if any), and how does this managerial perspective affect the political behavior of the organization?

9. What are the political attitudes of high corporate executives and middle managers regarding specified issues of public policy? Are there discernible attitude patterns among these businessmen based on age, length of affiliation with the organization, professional training, function within the company, and socioeconomic background?

10. What corporate officers and employees engage in polit-

ical activities on behalf of the organization and what is the nature of these activities?

11. What, in the opinion of corporate managers, are the political constraints upon managerial decision making and to what political pressures, if any, do they see themselves as subject?

12. What has been the political role of the Business Council? How do corporate leaders who serve as members perceive their function as Presidential advisors?

13. Regarding what types of social issues do corporate managers view their firms as having organizational interests? How does the effectiveness of the corporation (measured in terms of achieving its political objectives) vary with the issue?

14. What differences, if any, are discernible in the political attitudes and behavior of corporate managers whose firms have extensive involvement with government—local, state, or federal— as opposed to firms with minimal governmental contacts? What differences, if any, are discernible in the attitude of managers of these two categories of corporations regarding the role of government?

15. Are there discernible differences in the political attitudes and behavior of managers of subdivisions and subsidiaries of the same corporation?

16. What are the partisan affiliations and voting behavior of corporate leaders? Are there discernible differences in managerial political preferences and behavior regarding local, state, and federal politics? What are the salient differences, if any, in partisan affiliation and voting behavior between top and middle management?

17. What differences, if any, are discernible between the political attitudes and behavior of business managers in the United States and their counterparts in other nations regarding the political role of the firm and its relationship with government?

18. In what critical ways, if any, do corporations and their managers differ in their patterns of political behavior from other specified social interest groups and their leaders?

19. What are the views of corporate managers regarding

the probable character of corporate electoral behavior if current restrictions on corporate contributions and expenditures were removed?

20. What relationship, if any, do corporations engaged in international business have to the formulation and implementation of American foreign policy in geographical areas where they do business or have interests?

21. How do various categories of public officials regard the legitimacy and effectiveness of political participation by business corporations? Are there discernible differences in attitude toward corporate electoral as compared with governmental activities?

22. What are the attitudes of the public regarding the legitimacy of corporate political participation and what variables determine differences in public opinion concerning this issue? How do public views regarding corporate participation differ, if at all, from views concerning the political activities of labor or other social interest groups? Does public opinion differ regarding the propriety of corporate electoral as compared with governmental activities?

23. From the public's point of view, what impact, if any, do business firms and their managers have as molders of public opinion?

24. What impact, if any, does corporate political participation have on the political involvement of other specified social-interest groups?

25. What impact, if any, do selected corporations have within particular arenas on specified issues? (A call for case studies of particular instances of corporate political involvement.)

NOTE

[1]Robert A. Dahl, "Business and Politics: A Critical Appraisal of Political Science," in Robert A. Dahl, Mason Haire, and Paul F. Lazarsfeld, *Social Science Research on Business: Product and Potential* (New York: Columbia University Press, 1959), pp. 3–44.

Selected Reading List

BOOKS AND MONOGRAPHS

ADAMS, CHARLES FRANCIS, JR., and HENRY ADAMS, *Chapters of Erie.* Ithaca, N.Y.: Great Seal Books, Cornell University Press, 1956. 193 pp.

ALEXANDER, HERBERT E., *Financing the 1964 Election.* Princeton, N.J.: Citizens' Research Foundation, 1966. 137 pp.

BAILEY, STEPHEN KEMP, *Congress Makes a Law.* New York: Columbia University Press, 1950. 282 pp.

BALTZELL, E. DIGBY, *An American Business Aristocracy.* New York: Collier Books, Crowell Collier Publishing Co., 1962. 511 pp.

———, *The Protestant Establishment.* New York: Vintage Books, 1966. 429 pp.

BANFIELD, EDWARD C., *Political Influence.* New York: The Free Press, 1961. 354 pp.

BAUER, RAYMOND A., ITHIEL DE SOLA POOL, and LEWIS ANTHONY

DEXTER, *American Business and Public Policy*. New York: Atherton Press, 1964. 499 pp.

BAUMER, WILLIAM H., and DONALD G. HERZBERG, *Politics Is Your Business*. New York: The Dial Press, Inc., 1960. 187 pp.

BENTLEY, ARTHUR F., *The Process of Government*. Cambridge, Mass.: The Belknap Press, Harvard University Press, 1967. 501 pp.

BERLE, ADOLF A., JR., *Power Without Property*. New York: Harcourt, Brace & World, Inc., 1959. 184 pp.

———, *The 20th Century Capitalist Revolution*. New York: Harcourt, Brace & World, Inc., 1954. 192 pp.

BERNSTEIN, MARVER H., *Regulating Business by Independent Commission*. Princeton, N.J.: Princeton University Press, 1955. 306 pp.

BLAISDELL, DONALD C., *American Democracy Under Pressure*. New York: The Ronald Press Company, 1957. 324 pp.

BRADY, ROBERT A., *Business as a System of Power*. New York: Columbia University Press, 1947. 340 pp.

BRAYMAN, HAROLD, *Corporate Management in a World of Politics*. New York: McGraw-Hill Book Company, 1967. 272 pp.

CARY, WILLIAM L., *Politics and the Regulatory Agencies*. New York: McGraw-Hill Book Company, 1967. 149 pp.

CHERINGTON, PAUL W., and RALPH L. GILLEN, *The Business Representative in Washington*. Washington, D.C.: The Brookings Institution, 1962. 134 pp.

COCHRAN, THOMAS C., *The American Business System*. New York: Harper & Row, Publishers, 1957. 297 pp.

———, and WILLIAM MILLER, *The Age of Enterprise*. New York: Harper & Row, Publishers, 1961. 396 pp.

DAHL, ROBERT A., *Modern Political Analysis*. Englewood Cliffs, N.J.: Prentice-Hall, Inc., 1963. 118 pp.

———, *Pluralist Democracy in the United States: Conflict and Consent*. Chicago: Rand McNally & Company, 1967. 471 pp.

———, *A Preface to Democratic Theory*. Chicago: Phoenix Books, The University of Chicago Press, 1956. 154 pp.

———, *Who Governs?* New Haven, Conn.: Yale University Press, 1962. 355 pp.

———, MASON HAIRE, and PAUL F. LAZARSFELD, *Social Science Research on Business: Product and Potential*. New York: Columbia University Press, 1959. 185 pp.

———, and CHARLES E. LINDBLOM, *Politics, Economics, and Wel-*

fare: Planning and Politico-Economic Systems Resolved into Basic Social Processes. New York: Torchbooks, Harper & Row, Publishers, 1963. 557 pp.

DOMHOFF, G. WILLIAM, *Who Rules America?* Englewood Cliffs, N.J.: Prentice-Hall, Inc., 1967. 184 pp.

DOWNS, ANTHONY, *An Economic Theory of Democracy.* New York: Harper & Row, Publishers, 1957. 310 pp.

EDELMAN, MURRAY, *The Symbolic Uses of Politics.* Urbana, Ill.: The University of Illinois Press, 1967. 201 pp.

ENGLER, ROBERT, *The Politics of Oil.* Chicago: Phoenix Books, The University of Chicago Press, 1967. 565 pp.

EPSTEIN, EDWIN M., *Corporations, Contributions, and Political Campaigns: Federal Regulation in Perspective.* Berkeley: Institute of Governmental Studies, 1968. 222 pp.

FRIEDRICH, CARL J. (ed.), *Nomos V—The Public Interest.* New York: Atherton Press, 1962. 256 pp.

GALBRAITH, JOHN KENNETH, *American Capitalism.* Boston: Houghton Mifflin Company, 1956. 208 pp.

———, *The New Industrial State.* Boston: Houghton Mifflin Company, 1967. 427 pp.

GALLIGAN, DAVID J., *Politics and the Businessman.* New York: Pitman Publishing Corporation, 1964. 126 pp.

GILB, CORINNE LATHROP, *Hidden Hierarchies.* New York: Harper & Row, Publishers, 1966. 307 pp.

HAMILTON, WALTON, *The Politics of Industry.* New York: Vintage Books, Random House, Inc., 1957. 169 pp.

HEARD, ALEXANDER, *The Costs of Democracy.* Chapel Hill, N.C.: The University of North Carolina Press, 1960. 493 pp.

HERRING, PENDLETON, *The Politics of Democracy.* New York: W. W. Norton & Company, Inc., 1940. 468 pp.

HOFSTADTER, RICHARD, *The Age of Reform.* New York: Vintage Books, Random House, Inc., 1955. 330 pp.

HUNTER, FLOYD, *Community Power Structure.* Garden City, N.Y.: Anchor Books, Doubleday & Company, Inc., 1963. 294 pp.

JOSEPHSON, MATTHEW, *The Politicos.* New York: Harvest Books, Harcourt, Brace & World, Inc., 1938. 760 pp.

———, *The Robber Barons.* New York: Harvest Books, Harcourt, Brace & World, Inc., 1934. 474 pp.

KARIEL, HENRY S., *The Decline of American Pluralism.* Stanford, Calif.: Stanford University Press, 1961. 339 pp.

KEY, V. O., JR., *Politics, Parties, and Pressure Groups* (5th ed.). New York: Thomas Y. Crowell Co., 1964. 738 pp.

KOLKO, GABRIEL, *The Triumph of Conservatism.* New York: The Free Press, 1963. 344 pp.

KORNHAUSER, ARTHUR, HAROLD L. SHEPPARD, and ALBERT J. MAYER, *When Labor Votes.* New York: University Books, Inc., 1956. 352 pp.

LANE, EDGAR, *Lobbying and the Law.* Berkeley, Calif.: University of California Press, 1964. 224 pp.

LANE, ROBERT E., *The Regulation of Businessmen: Social Conditions of Government Economic Control.* New Haven, Conn.: Yale University Press, 1954. 144 pp.

LATHAM, EARL, *The Group Basis of Politics, A Study in Basing-Point Legislation.* Ithaca, N.Y.: Cornell University Press, 1952. 244 pp.

Legislators and the Lobbyists. Washington, D.C.: Congressional Quarterly Inc., 1965. 78 pp.

Legislators and the Lobbyists, 2d ed. Washington, D.C.: Congressional Quarterly Inc., 1968. 92 pp.

LIPSON, LESLIE, *The Democratic Civilization.* Fair Lawn, N.J.: Oxford University Press, Inc., 1964. 614 p.

LYND, ROBERT S., and HELEN MERRELL LYND, *Middletown.* New York: Harvest Books, Harcourt, Brace & World, Inc., 1929. 550 pp.

——, *Middletown in Transition.* New York: Harvest Books, Harcourt, Brace & World, Inc., 1937. 604 pp.

MACIVER, ROBERT M., *The Web of Government* (revised ed.). New York: The Free Press, 1965. 373 pp.

MASON, EDWARD S. (ed.), *The Corporation in Modern Society.* Cambridge, Mass.: Harvard University Press, 1961. 335 pp.

MCCONNELL, GRANT, *Private Power & American Democracy.* New York: Alfred A. Knopf, Inc., 1966. 397 pp.

——, *Steel and the Presidency—1962.* New York: W. W. Norton & Company, Inc., 1963. 119 pp.

MICHELS, ROBERT, *Political Parties: A Sociological Study of the Oligarchical Tendencies of Modern Democracy.* New York: Collier Books, Division of Crowell-Collier Publishing Co., 1962. 379 pp.

MILBRATH, LESTER W., *The Washington Lobbyists.* Chicago: Rand McNally & Company, 1963. 431 pp.

MILLER, ARTHUR SELWYN, *The Supreme Court and American Capitalism.* New York: The Free Press, 1968. 259 pp.

MILLS, C. WRIGHT, *The Power Elite.* Fair Lawn, N.J.: Oxford University Press, Inc., 1959. 423 pp.

———, *White Collar.* Fair Lawn, N.J.: Oxford University Press, Inc., 1956. 378 pp.

NOSSITER, BERNARD D., *The Mythmakers.* Boston: Beacon Press, 1964. 244 pp.

PALAMOUNTAIN, JOSEPH CORNWALL, JR., *The Politics of Distribution.* Cambridge, Mass.: Harvard University Press, 1955. 270 pp.

POLSBY, NELSON W., *Community Power and Political Theory.* New Haven, Conn.: Yale University Press, 1963. 144 pp.

PRESTHUS, ROBERT, *Men at the Top.* Fair Lawn, N.J.: Oxford University Press, Inc., 1964. 485 pp.

PROTHRO, JAMES W., *The Dollar Decade, Business Ideas in the 1920's.* Baton Rouge, La.: Louisiana State University Press, 1954. 256 pp.

Public Affairs in National Focus (Public Affairs Conference Report No. 5). New York: National Industrial Conference Board, Inc., 1966. 147 pp.

REAGAN, MICHAEL D., *The Managed Economy.* Fair Lawn, N.J.: Oxford University Press, Inc., 1963. 288 pp.

RIESMAN, DAVID, NATHAN GLAZER, and REUEL DENNEY, *The Lonely Crowd.* New Haven, Conn.: Yale University Press, 1961. 315 pp.

The Role of Business in Public Affairs (Studies in Public Affairs, No. 2). New York: National Industrial Conference Board, Inc., 1968. 40 pp.

ROSE, ARNOLD M., *The Power Structure.* Fairlawn, N.J.: Oxford University Press, Inc., 1967. 506 pp.

SCHATTSCHNEIDER, E. E., *Politics, Pressures and the Tariff.* Hamden, Conn.: Archon Books, 1963. 301 pp.

———, *The Semisovereign People.* New York: Holt, Rinehart & Winston, Inc., 1960. 147 pp.

SCHRIFTGIESSER, KARL, *Business Comes of Age.* New York: Harper & Row, Publishers, 1960. 248 pp.

———, *Business and Public Policy.* Englewood Cliffs, N.J.: Prentice-Hall, Inc., 1967. 254 pp.

———, *The Lobbyists: The Art and Business of Influencing Lawmakers.* Boston: Little, Brown and Company, 1951. 297 pp.

SHONFIELD, ANDREW, *Modern Capitalism: The Changing Balance of Public and Private Power.* Fair Lawn, N.J.: Oxford University Press, Inc., 1965. 456 pp.

SUTTON, FRANCIS X., SEYMOUR E. HARRIS, CARL KAYSEN, and JAMES TOBIN, *The American Business Creed.* New York: Schocken Books, 1962. 414 pp.

TRUMAN, DAVID B., *The Governmental Process.* New York: Alfred A. Knopf, Inc., 1951. 544 pp.

VOTAW, DOW, *Modern Corporations.* Englewood Cliffs, N.J.: Prentice-Hall, Inc., 1965. 120 pp.

WALTON, CLARENCE C., *Corporate Social Responsibilities.* Belmont, Calif.: Wadsworth Publishing Company, Inc., 1967. 177 pp.

WARNER, W. LLOYD (ed.), *Yankee City* (abridged ed.). New Haven, Conn.: Yale University Press, 1963. 432 pp.

WESTIN, ALAN F. (ed.), *The Uses of Power.* New York: Harcourt, Brace & World, Inc., 1962. 376 pp.

WIEBE, ROBERT H., *Businessmen and Reform.* Cambridge, Mass.: Harvard University Press, 1962. 283 pp.

WILDAVSKY, AARON, *Dixon-Yates, A Study in Power Politics.* New Haven, Conn.: Yale University Press, 1962. 351 pp.

WOLIN, SHELDON S., *Politics and Vision.* Boston: Little, Brown and Company, 1960. 529 pp.

ZEIGLER, HARMON, *Interest Groups in American Society.* Englewood Cliffs, N.J.: Prentice-Hall, Inc., 1964. 343 pp.

———, *The Politics of Small Business.* Washington, D.C.: Public Affairs Press, 1961. 150 pp.

ARTICLES

ALEXANDER, HERBERT E., and HAROLD B. MEYERS, "The Switch in Campaign Giving," *Fortune*, LXXII, No. 5 (November 1965), 170.

BACHRACH, PETER, and MORTON S. BARATZ, "Two Faces of Power," *American Political Science Review*, LVI (December 1962), 947–52.

BARATZ, MORTON S., "Corporate Giants and the Power Structure," *Western Political Quarterly*, IX (June 1956), 406–15.

BAZELTON, DAVID T., "Big Business and the Democrats," *Commentary*, XXXIX, No. 5 (May 1965), 39–46.

BERLE, ADOLPH A., JR., "Constitutional Limitations on Corporate Activity—Protection of Personal Rights from Invasion through Economic Power," *University of Pennsylvania Law Review*, 100 (May 1952), 933–55.

BERNSTEIN, MARVER H., "Political Ideas of Selected Business Journals," *Public Opinion Quarterly*, XVII (September 1953), 258–67.

BUNZEL, JOHN H., "The General Ideology of American Small Business," *Political Science Quarterly*, LXX (March 1955), 87–102.

CHEIT, EARL F., "Why Managers Cultivate Social Responsibility," *California Management Review*, VII (Fall 1964), 3–22.

CLELLAND, DONALD A., and WILLIAM H. FORM, "Economic Dominants and Community Power: A Comparative Analysis," *American Journal of Sociology*, LXIX (March 1964), 511–21.

"Corporate Political Affairs Programs," Comment, *Yale Law Journal*, LXX (1961), 821–62.

"Corporations Make Politics Their Business," *Fortune*, LX (December 1959), 100.

DAHL, ROBERT A., "The Concept of Power," *Behavioral Science*, II (July 1957), 201–15.

DEXTER, LEWIS ANTHONY, "Where the Elephant Fears to Dance Among the Chickens: Business in Politics? The Case of DuPont," *Human Organization*, XIX (Winter 1960), 188–94.

FALTERMAYER, EDMUND K., "What Business Wants from Lyndon Johnson," *Fortune*, LXXI (February 1965), 122.

FENN, DAN H., JR., "Business and Politics (Problems in Review)," *Harvard Business Review*, XXXVII (March-April 1959), 37–47.

FINER, S. E., "The Political Power of Private Capital," Part I, *Sociological Review*, III (December 1955), 279–94; Part II, *Sociological Review*, IV (July 1956), 5–30.

GABLE, RICHARD W., "NAM: Influential Lobby or Kiss of Death?" *Journal of Politics*, XV (May 1953), 254–73.

GARCEAU, O., and C. SILVERMAN, "A Pressure Group and the Pressured: A Case Report," *American Political Science Review*, XLVIII (September 1954), 672–91.

GLAD, PAUL W., "Progressives and the Business Culture of the 1920s," *Journal of American History*, LIII (June 1966), 75–89.

GOLDSTEIN, MARSHALL N., "Absentee Ownership and Monopolistic Power Structures: Two Questions in Community Studies," in Bert E. Swanson (ed.), *Current Trends in Comparative Community Studies* (Public Affairs Monograph Series, No. 1), Kansas City, Mo.: Community Studies, Inc., 1962, pp. 49–59.

GREENEWALT, CRAWFORD H., "A Political Role for Business," *California Management Review*, II (Fall 1959), 7–11.

GREYSER, STEPHEN A., "Business and Politics, 1964 (Problems in Review)," *Harvard Business Review*, XLII (September-October 1964), 22.

———, "Business and Politics, 1968 (Special Report)," *Harvard Business Review*, XLVI (November-December 1968), 4.

HACKER, ANDREW, "The Elected and the Anointed: Two American Elites," *American Political Science Review*, LV (September 1961), 539–49.

———, "Politics and the Corporation," in Andrew Hacker (ed.), *The Corporation Take-Over*, New York: Harper & Row, Publishers, 1964, pp. 246–69.

———, and JOEL D. ABERBACH, "Businessmen in Politics," *Law and Contemporary Problems*, XXVII (Spring 1962), 266–79.

HARSANYI, JOHN C., "Measurement of Social Power, Opportunity Costs, and the Theory of Two-Person Bargaining Games," *Behavioral Science*, VII (January 1962), 67–80.

HECTOR, LOUIS J., "Problems of the CAB and the Independent Regulatory Commissions," *Yale Law Journal*, LXIX (May 1960), 931–64.

JESSUP, JOHN KNOX, "A Political Role for the Corporation," *Fortune*, XLVI (August 1952), 112.

KARIEL, HENRY S., "The Corporation and the Public Interest," *Annals of the American Academy of Political and Social Science*, CCCXLIII (September 1962), 39–47.

KAUFMAN, HERBERT, and VICTOR JONES, "The Mystery of Power," *Public Administration Review*, XIV (Summer 1954), 205–12.

KING, DONALD B., "Corporate Political Spending and the First Amendment," *University of Pittsburgh Law Review*, XXIII (June 1962), 847–79.

KOISTINEN, PAUL A. C., "The 'Industrial-Military Complex' in Historical Perspective: World War I," *Business History Review*, XLI (Winter 1967), 378–403.

KORNHAUSER, WILLIAM, "'Power Elite' or 'Veto Groups'?" in Reinhart Bendix and Seymour Martin Lipset, *Class, Status, and Power* (2d ed.), New York: The Free Press, 1966, pp. 210–18.

LAMBERT, J. D., "Corporate Political Spending and Campaign Finance," *New York University Law Review*, XL (December 1965), 1033–78.

LATHAM, EARL, "The Group Basis of Politics: Notes for a Theory," *American Political Science Review*, XLVI (1952), 376–97.

LENHART, ROBERT F., and KARL SCHRIFTGIESSER, "Management in Politics," *Annals of the American Academy of Political and Social Science*, CCCXIX (September 1958), 32–40.

LEVITT, THEODORE, "Business Should Stay Out of Politics," *Business Horizons*, III (Summer 1960), 45–51.

LIPSET, SEYMOUR MARTIN, "Some Social Requisites of Democracy: Economic Development and Political Legitimacy," *American Political Science Review*, LIII (March 1959), 69–105.

MCCLOSKY, HERBERT, "Consensus and Ideology in American Politics," *American Political Science Review*, LVIII (June 1964), 361–82.

MADISON, JAMES, "The Federalist, No. 10," in Alexander Hamilton, James Madison, and John Jay, *The Federalist Papers*, New York: New American Library of World Literature, Inc., 1961, pp. 77–84.

MANNING, BAYLESS, "Corporate Power and Individual Freedom: Some General Analysis and Particular Reservations," *Northwestern Law Review*, LV (March-April 1960), 38–53.

MASON, ALPHEUS T., "Business Organized as Power: The New Imperium in Imperio," *American Political Science Review*, XLIV (June 1950), 323–42.

MONSEN, R. JOSEPH, JR., and ANTHONY DOWNS, "A Theory of Large Managerial Firms," *Journal of Political Economy*, LXXIII (June 1965), 221–36.

NORTON-TAYLOR, DUNCAN, "How to Give Money to Politicians," *Fortune*, LIII (May 1956), 112.

ODEGARD, PETER H., "A Group Basis of Politics: A New Name for an Ancient Myth," *Western Political Quarterly*, XI (September 1958), 689–702.

PELLEGRIN, ROLAND J., and CHARLES H. COATES, "Absentee-Owned Corporations and Community Power Structure," *American Journal of Sociology*, LXI (March 1956), 413–19.

POLSBY, NELSON W., "The Sociology of Community Power: A Reassessment," *Social Forces*, XXXVII (March 1959), 232–36.

REAGAN, MICHAEL D., "The Seven Fallacies of Business in Politics," *Harvard Business Review*, XXXVIII (March-April 1960), 60–68.

ROGERS, DAVID, and MELVIN ZIMET, "The Corporation and the Community: Perspectives and Recent Developments," in Ivar Berg (ed.), *The Business of America*, New York: Harcourt, Brace & World, Inc., 1968, pp. 39–80.

ROSE, RICHARD, and ARNOLD J. HEIDENHEIMER (eds.), "Comparative Studies in Political Finance," *Journal of Politics*, XXV (November 1963), 643–811.

RUETTEN, R. T., "Anaconda Journalism: The End of an Era," *Journalism Quarterly*, XXXVII (1960), 3–12.

SCHULZE, ROBERT O., "The Role of Economic Dominants in Community Power Structure," *American Sociological Review*, XXIII (February 1958), 3–9.

SHELDON, HORACE E., "Business Must Get Into Politics," *Harvard Business Review*, XXXVII (March-April 1959), 37–47.

SMITH, RICHARD AUSTIN, "The Company's Man in Washington," *Fortune*, LXXIII (April 1966), 132.

SPINRAD, WILLIAM, "Power in Local Communities," *Social Problems*, XII (Winter 1965), 335–56.

SURREY, STANLEY S., "The Congress and the Tax Lobbyist—How Special Tax Provisions Get Enacted," *Harvard Law Review*, LXX (May 1957), 1145–82.

VOSE, CLEMENT E., "Litigation as a Form of Pressure Group Activity," *Annals of the American Academy of Political and Social Science*, CCCXIX (September 1958), 20–31.

VOTAW, DOW, "The Politics of a Changing Corporate Society," *California Management Review*, III (Spring 1961), 105–118.

WALTON, CLARENCE C., "Big Government, Big Business, and the Public Interest," in Ivar Berg (ed.), *The Business of America*, New York: Harcourt, Brace & World, Inc., 1968, pp. 83–118.

GOVERNMENT PUBLICATIONS

1956 Presidential and Senatorial Campaign Contributions and Practices: Hearings . . ., pt. 2. U.S. Congress, Senate, Committee on Rules and Administration, Subcommittee on Privileges and Elections, 84th Cong., 2d Sess. Washington, D.C.: U.S. Government Printing Office, 1956.

Hearings . . . Pursuant to S. Res. 219 of the 84th Congress. U.S. Congress, Senate, Special Committee to Investigate Activities, Lobbying and Campaign Contributions, 84th Cong., 2d Sess. Washington, D.C.: U.S. Government Printing Office, 1957.

Report, 1956 General Election Campaigns. U.S. Congress, Senate, Committee on Rules and Administration, Subcommittee on Privileges and Elections, 85th Cong., 1st Sess. Washington, D.C.: U.S. Government Printing Office, 1957.

Report No. 395: Final Report . . . Pursuant to S. Res. 219 of the 84th Congress, as extended by S. Res. 47 and S. Res. 128 of the 85th Congress . . . U.S. Congress, Senate, Special Committee to Investigate Activities, Lobbying and Campaign Contributions, 85th Cong., 1st Sess. Washington, D.C.: U.S. Government Printing Office, 1957.

CASES, STATUTES, AND MISCELLANEOUS

Dartmouth College v. *Woodward,* 4 Wheaton 518 (1819).

Eastern Railroad Presidents Conference v. *Noerr Motor Freight, Inc.,* 365 U.S. 127 (1961).

Santa Clara Co. v. *Southern Pacific Railway Co.,* 118 U.S. 394 (1886).

United States v. *Congress of Industrial Organizations,* 335 U.S. 106 (1948).

United States v. *International Union United Automobile, Aircraft and Agricultural Implement Workers of America* (UAW-CIO), 352 U.S. 567 (1957).

United States v. *Lewis Food Company, Inc.,* 366 F.2d 710 (9th Cir. 1966), *reversing* 236 F. Supp. 849 (S.D. Cal. 1964).

2 U.S.C. Sec. 610 (1951) (United States Criminal Code)—popularly known by the former name of the act of which it is a part, the Federal Corrupt Practices Act.

18 U.S.C. Secs. 261–70 (1946) (Federal Regulation of Lobbying Act of 1946).

Congressional Quarterly Weekly Report. *Special Report: 1964 Political Campaign Contributions and Expenditures.* No. 3, Part I of II Parts (January 21, 1966), pp. 57–240.

Index